Personalized Anaesthesia

Personalized Anaesthesia

Targeting Physiological Systems for Optimal Effect

Edited by

Pedro L. Gambús
Hospital Clínic de Barcelona, Spain

Jan F. A. Hendrickx
Aalst General Hospital, Belgium

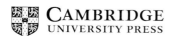

CAMBRIDGE
UNIVERSITY PRESS

CAMBRIDGE
UNIVERSITY PRESS

University Printing House, Cambridge CB2 8BS, United Kingdom

One Liberty Plaza, 20th Floor, New York, NY 10006, USA

477 Williamstown Road, Port Melbourne, VIC 3207, Australia

314–321, 3rd Floor, Plot 3, Splendor Forum, Jasola District Centre, New Delhi – 110025, India

79 Anson Road, #06–04/06, Singapore 079906

Cambridge University Press is part of the University of Cambridge.

It furthers the University's mission by disseminating knowledge in the pursuit of education, learning, and research at the highest international levels of excellence.

www.cambridge.org
Information on this title: www.cambridge.org/9781107579255
DOI: 10.1017/9781316443217

First published 2020

Printed in Singapore by Markono Print Media Pte Ltd

A catalogue record for this publication is available from the British Library.

Library of Congress Cataloging-in-Publication Data
Names: Gambus, Pedro, editor.
Title: Personalized anaesthesia : targeting physiological systems for optimal effect / edited by Pedro Gambus, Hospital CLINIC de Barcelona, Spain, Jan Hendrickx, Aalst General Hospital, Belgium.
Description: Cambridge, United Kingdom ; New York : Cambridge University Press, 2019. | Includes index.
Identifiers: LCCN 2019027233 (print) | LCCN 2019027234 (ebook) | ISBN 9781107579255 (paperback) | ISBN 9781316443217 (epub)
Subjects: LCSH: Anesthesia. | Anesthetics – Physiological effect.
Classification: LCC RD82 .P44 2019 (print) | LCC RD82 (ebook) | DDC 617.9/6–dc23
LC record available at https://lccn.loc.gov/2019027233
LC ebook record available at https://lccn.loc.gov/2019027234

ISBN 978-1-107-57925-5 Paperback

Contents

v

Contributors

Pedro Amorim MD
Center for Clinical Research in Anesthesia, Serviço de Anestesiologia, Centro Hospitalar do Porto, Porto, Portugal

Brian J. Anderson MB ChB, PhD, FANZCA, FCICM
Department of Anaesthesiology, University of Auckland, New Zealand

Michael M. Beck MD, MBA
Mountain West Anesthesia, Utah Society of Anesthesiologists, UT, USA

Xavier Borrat PhD, MD
Department of Anesthesiology, Hospital Clínic de Barcelona, University of Barcelona, Barcelona, Spain

Emmanuel Boselli MD, PhD
Pierre Oudot Hospital Center, Bourgoin-Jallieu, APCSe Unit, VetAgro Sup UPSP 2016.A101, University Lyon I Claude Bernard, University of Lyon, France

Michael K. Cahalan MD
Department of Anesthesiology, University of Utah School of Medicine, Salt Lake City, UT, USA

Luis I. Cortinez MD
Departamento de Anestesiología, Hospital Clínico Pontificia Universidad Católica de Chile, Santiago, Chile

Andre M. De Wolf MD
Department of Anesthesiology, Feinberg School of Medicine, Northwestern University, Chicago, IL, USA

Vincent Degos MD, PhD
Department of Anesthesiology and Intensive Care of Pitié Salpetrière Hospital, Paris, France

Douglas J. Eleveld PhD
Department of Anaesthesiology, University Medical Center Groningen, University of Groningen, Groningen, The Netherlands

Neus Fabregas MD, PhD, DESA
Department of Anaesthesiology, Hospital Clínic de Barcelona, Universitat de Barcelona, Spain

Malin Jonsson Fagerlund MD, PhD, DESA
Perioperative Medicine and Intensive Care, Karolinska University Hospital and Karolinska Institutet, Stockholm, Sweden

Lluís Gallart MD
Department of Anaesthesiology, Hospital del Mar, Universitat Autonoma de Barcelona, Spain

Pedro L. Gambús MD, PhD
Systems Pharmacology Effect Control and Modeling (SPEC-M) Research Group, Department of Anesthesiology, Hospital Clínic de Barcelona, Biomedical Engineering Degree, Universitat de Barcelona, Barcelona, Spain

María J. Garrido PhD
Pharmacometrics and Systems Pharmacology, Department of Pharmaceutical Technology and Chemistry, School of Pharmacy and Nutrition, Universidad de Navarra, Pamplona, Spain

Adrian W. Gelb MBChB, FRCPC
Department of Anesthesia and Perioperative Care, University of California San Francisco, San Francisco, CA, USA

Pauline Glasman MD
Department of Anesthesiology and Intensive Care of Pitié Salpetrière Hospital, Paris, France

Robert G. Hahn MD, PhD
Anesthesia and Intensive Care, Research Unit, Södertälje Hospital, Södertälje, Sweden

Jacqueline A. Hannam PhD
Department of Pharmacology and Clinical Pharmacology, School of Medical and Health Sciences, University of Auckland, Auckland, New Zealand

Jan F. A. Hendrickx MD, PhD
Department of Anesthesiology/CCM, OLV Hospital, Aalst, Belgium

Jeffrey B. Horn MD
Department of Anesthesiology, University of Utah, UT, USA

Alice Jacquens MD
Department of Anesthesiology and Intensive Care of Pitié Salpetrière Hospital, Paris, France

Sebastián Jaramillo MD
Systems Pharmacology Effect Control and Modeling (SPEC-M) Research Group, Department of Anesthesiology, Hospital Clínic de Barcelona, Barcelona, Spain

Mathieu Jeanne MD, PhD
Anesthesia and Intensive Care, University Hospital of Lille, France

Erik W. Jensen PhD
Research and Development Department, Quantium Medical, Systems Pharmacology Effect Control and Modeling (SPEC-M) Research Group, Anesthesiology Department, Hospital Clínic de Barcelona, Centre for Biomedical Research (CREB), Automatic control and Informatics (ESAII) Department, UPC-Barcelonatech, Barcelona, Spain

Ken B. Johnson MD
Center for Patient Simulation, Department of Anesthesiology, University of Utah, UT, USA

R. Ross Kennedy MD, ChB, PhD
Department of Anaesthesia, Christchurch Hospital and University of Otago, Christchurch, New Zealand

Oliver Kimberger MD
Medical University of Vienna, Department of Anesthesiology, General Intensive Care and Pain Medicine, Vienna, Austria

Kai Kuck PhD
Department of Anesthesiology, University of Utah School of Medicine, Salt Lake City, UT, USA

Umberto Melia PhD
Research and Development Department, Quantium Medical, Barcelona, Spain

Jordi Mercadal MD
Department of Anesthesiology, Hospital Clínic de Barcelona, University of Barcelona, Barcelona, Spain

Catarina Nunes MSci, PhD, MIEEE, MIET, FHEA
Center for Clinical Research in Anesthesia, Serviço de Anestesiologia, Centro Hospitalar do Porto, Porto, Portugal

Klaus T. Olkkola MD, PhD
Department of Anaesthesiology, Intensive Care and Pain Medicine, University of Helsinki and Helsinki University Hospital, Helsinki, Finland

Timothy G. Short MD, FANZCA
Department of Anaesthesia and Perioperative Medicine, Auckland City Hospital, Auckland, New Zealand

Natalie Silverton MD
Department of Anesthesiology, University of Utah School of Medicine, Salt Lake City, UT, USA

Iñaki F. Trocóniz PhD
Pharmacometrics and Systems Pharmacology, Department of Pharmaceutical Technology and Chemistry, School of Pharmacy and Nutrition, Universidad de Navarra, Pamplona, Spain

José F. Valencia PhD
Department of Electronic Engineering, Universidad de San Buenaventura, Cali, Colombia

Sergio Vide MD
Center for Clinical Research in Anesthesia, Serviço de Anestesiologia, Centro Hospitalar do Porto, Porto, Portugal; Systems Pharmacology Effect Control and Modeling (SPEC-M) Research Group, Anesthesiology Department, Hospital Clínic de Barcelona, Barcelona, Spain

Foreword

Anaesthesia, the state of oblivion and non-responsiveness that permits surgical invasion of our bodies, is among the most important medical discoveries in history. In Henry Jacob Bigelow's famous report of William Morton's first public demonstration of ether anaesthesia, he not only describes successful surgery under ether anaesthesia, but also his subsequent investigations to determine the nature of the anaesthetizing agent. [1]

Morton, hoping to profit from his discovery, declined to reveal that ether was responsible for the miracle of anaesthesia. In his famous case report, Bigelow conducted his own experiments: 'The first experiment was with sulphuric ether, the odor of which was readily recognized in the preparation employed by Dr. Morton. Ether inhaled in vapor is well known to produce symptoms similar to those produced by nitrous oxide. In my own former experience, the exhilaration has been quite as great, though perhaps less pleasurable, than that of this gas, or of the Egyptian haschish.'

Bigelow then describes the drug delivery system: 'A small two-necked glass globe contains the prepared vapor, together with sponges to enlarge the evaporating surface. One aperture admits the air to the interior of the globe, whence, charged with vapor, it is drawn through the second into the lungs. The inspired air thus passes through the bottle, but the expiration is diverted by a valve in the mouth-piece and escaping into the apartment is thus prevented from vitiating the medicated vapor.'

Bigelow goes on to describe the time course of drug effect in a series of dental cases he observed: onset in 3–5 minutes, requirement for increased drug during dental extraction, and recovery ranging from 10 minutes to an hour. He notes the accumulation of anaesthetic effect with continued administration: 'When the apparatus is withdrawn at the moment of unconsciousness, it continues, upon the average, two or three minutes, and the patient then recovers completely or incompletely, without subsequent ill effects. But if the respiration of the vapor be prolonged much beyond the first period, the symptoms are more permanent in their character. In one of the first cases, that of a young boy, the inhalation was continued during the greater part of ten minutes, and the subsequent narcotism and drowsiness lasted more than an hour.'

Finally Bigelow describes measurement of anaesthetic effect: 'The pulse has been, as far as my observation extends, unaltered in frequency, though somewhat diminished in volume, but the excitement preceding an operation has, in almost every instance, so accelerated the pulse that it has continued rapid for a length of time. The pupils are in a majority of cases dilated; yet they are in certain cases unaltered.'

There it is! The very first published report about anaesthesia linked 1) the pharmacology of anaesthetic drugs, 2) the physiology of the body's response to the drugs, and 3) monitoring drug effect and patient status to the (now daily) miracle of rendering a person insensible to surgical pain.

However, that was only the start of the enduring entwining of anaesthesia, pharmacology, technology and patient safety. The *following year* John Snow published an account of eighty operations with ether anaesthesia. [2] He begins by describing five 'degrees' of ether anaesthesia: a first degree 'whilst he still retains a capacity to direct his volunteer movements', a second degree with 'voluntary actions performed, but in a disorganized manner', a third degree with 'no evidence of mental function', a fourth degree with 'no movements ... except those of respiration' and patients 'incapable of being influenced by external impressions' (sounds like 1 MAC), and a fifth degree, where 'respiratory movements are more or less paralyzed.' He also notes ether uptake, which starts at 'about two drachms of ether per minute.' The ensuing chapter describes each stage in detail. Snow then presents the basic concepts of anaesthetic uptake and distribution. He has already figured out some of the subtle details. For example, recovery is initially rapid, but slows because 'when he is inhaling the vapour he is quickly removed from {the second} into the third degree, but when inhalation is discontinued the vapour is got rid of, in a ratio varying directly with the quantity in the blood, which is a constantly decreasing ratio.' Snow then introduces a novel drug administration technology, a temperature controlled ether vaporizer, because 'a knowledge of the strength of the vapour as being essential to a correct determination of the state of the patient at all times.'

Snow concludes this book, published just a year after Morton's demonstration, with an appendix describing his experiments anaesthetizing frogs! John Snow is widely credited as having founded two scientific disciplines: anaesthesiology and epidemiology. In our minds, John Snow should also be recognized as the founder of clinical pharmacology.

It has been nearly two centuries since Bigelow's report and John Snow's book(!). The fundamentals of anaesthesia practice to which these authors alluded have not changed. What has changed is the precision of our practice. Our drugs target their biological sites of action more precisely than ether. The onset and offset of our anaesthetics is far faster than with ether, enabling more precise control of anaesthetic depth. Our knowledge of physiology is far more precise. We can achieve desired drug effects and mitigate adverse effects by targeting specific ligands in nearly every tissue in the body. Our monitoring is more precise, with the ability to capture neurological and cardiopulmonary status in real time.

Despite these advances, anaesthesia remains a mystery. We understand precisely where the intravenous hypnotics bind, but we have not been able to translate that knowledge into understanding how they induce and maintain the anaesthetic state. Decades of research using the most advanced tools in pharmacology and neuroscience have failed to identify the site of action of inhaled anaesthetics. We have no idea how isoflurane, sevoflurane, nitrous oxide and xenon produce unconsciousness. Understanding the mechanism of inhaled anaesthetic action remains among the oldest and most puzzling mysteries in pharmacology and neuroscience.

Although anaesthesia remains mysterious, mathematics is infinitely more so. Mathematics can describe paradoxes of the quantum world that defy common sense. Mathematics can describe the behaviour of distant galaxies, the expansion of the universe, the relative sizes of infinities and the first moments after the Big Bang. As noted by physicist Eugene Wigner, 'The miracle of the appropriateness of the language of mathematics for the formulation of the laws of physics is a wonderful gift which we neither understand nor deserve. We should be grateful for it and hope that it will remain valid in future research and that it will extend, for better or for worse, to our pleasure, even though perhaps also to our bafflement, to wide branches of learning.' [3]

Personalized anaesthesia, as described in this book, is the marriage of these two mysteries: anaesthesia and mathematics. Personalized anaesthesia applies the power of mathematics to the elements of anaesthesia described in Bigelow's report and Snow's book. This, too, has a long history in our specialty. John Severinghaus built a career from applying mathematics to physiological measurement. [4] E.I. ('Ted') Eger II developed mathematical models of inhaled anaesthetics while stationed at Fort Leavenworth, Kansas. [5] His mathematical models predicted the second gas effect, verified clinically.

We had the good fortune to be among dozens of investigators combining mathematics and computer modelling with precise measurements of drug concentrations following intravenous administration and with precise measurements of drug effect. [6] The authors of this book represent the current generation of leaders in personalized anaesthesia. They are not the intellectual descendants of Morton, who pursued anaesthesia solely to find fame and fortune, but of Bigelow, who presciently described anaesthesia as 'one of the most important discoveries of the age' [1] and Snow, who turned Morton's clinical parlour trick into a science. [2] Seeking to advance scientific understanding and patient care, the authors of this book combine the latest scientific findings and the most sophisticated tools of technology with the nearly infinite power of mathematics.

We are proud to have contributed to this long and distinguished history. We applaud the authors for their continuing efforts advancing the daily miracle and mystery of anaesthesia.

Steven L. Shafer, MD
Professor of Anesthesiology, Perioperative and Pain Medicine, Stanford University School of Medicine
Adjunct Associate Professor of Bioengineering and Therapeutic Sciences, University of California at San Francisco

Donald R. Stanski, MD
Emeritus Professor of Anesthesiology, Perioperative and Pain Medicine, Stanford University School of Medicine

References

1. Bigelow HJ. Insensibility during surgical operations produced by inhalation. Boston Med Surg J 1846;35:309–17.

2. Snow J. *On the Inhalation of the Vapour of Ether in Surgical Operations*. John Churchill publisher, London, 1847.

3. Wigner EP. The unreasonable effectiveness of mathematics in the natural sciences. Communications on Pure and Applied Mathematics 1960;12:1–14.

4. Severinghaus JW. Career perspective: John W. Severinghaus. Extrem Physiol Med 2013;2:29.

5. Eger EI II. *Autobiography of a Persistent Anesthesiologist*. Ed Shafer SL, 2019.

6. Shafer SL, Fisher DM. Pharmacokinetic and pharmacodynamic modeling in anesthesia (Chapter 40) *Wondrous History of Anesthesia*, Eds Eger EI II, Saidman LJ, Westhorpe RN. Springer, New York, 2014.

Introduction

Pedro L. Gambús and Jan F. A. Hendrickx

This book aims to provide the modern anaesthesiologist and interested clinician with the tools to understand how anaesthesia and surgery influence human physiology, how information about the anaesthetic state and the different homeostatic systems of the human body is collected and processed, and how this information can be integrated to optimize and individualize care to the patient by helping us to swiftly respond to changes: personalized anaesthesia.

The book is based upon the concept of general anaesthesia being a constellation of galaxies (see Fig. 1). By providing hypnosis, antinociception/analgesia and immobility, anaesthesia makes surgery possible. But anaesthesia and surgery also generate a number of changes in different systems of the body. Some of these are expected and intended to protect the patient against the harmful effects of the surgical process. Others are a consequence of the relative non-specificity of the drugs used or derive from the procedure *per se*. It is the anaesthesiologist's task to keep this galaxy stable.

Current knowledge about physiology and pharmacology allows the anaesthesiologist to understand to some degree what is going on in the human body. Concurrently, technology has grown exponentially. We are now able to determine the 'depth' of the anaesthetic state. We measure signals from almost any organ system in the body that provide us with an indication of the well-being of the homeostatic systems in the individual patient. All this allows us to titrate drugs, fluids, blood products, heat and other

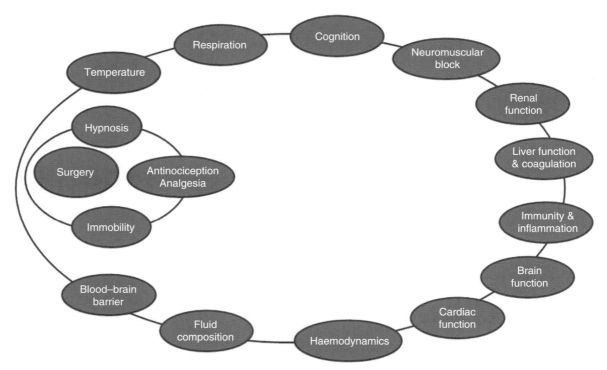

Fig. 1 Cascade of changes triggered by surgery and anaesthesia. The combined effects of surgery and anaesthetic drugs generate direct and indirect physiological changes that should be kept within normal limits.

factors, more and more with the help of automated closed-loop systems to maintain the anaesthetic state 'on target' while also preserving internal homeostasis in the individual patient. This is the basis of 'personalized anaesthesia'.

Being able to titrate anaesthesia to an individual's personal needs is bound to become more and more important because we face an increasingly older population of patients. Some patients are in good physical condition, but others are very sick, not only because of their surgical diagnosis *per se* but also and mainly because of concurrent chronic conditions. The number of patients presenting for ever-more complex surgery keeps increasing at a rate that prompted the World Health Organization (WHO) to warn of a future shortage of anaesthesia providers.

Integration of clinical knowledge, technology that allows us to measure parameters indicative of the anaesthetic state and organ homeostasis, data collection and mathematical modelling allows us to move from the old 'reactive' paradigm, where we take action after changes have taken place, to not only a 'proactive'

paradigm, where we take action before something happens, but ultimately a 'predictive' paradigm where past and present information are processed and analysed into predictions about short- or long-term outcomes.

We challenged ourselves to integrate this vision about 'personalized anaesthesia' in this book (Fig. 2), which has two parts. The first part presents the fundamentals of the quantitative approach: pharmacological concepts, signal and response analysis, modelling principles, covariate analysis, individualization principles and how they are integrated in an updated view of 'anaesthesia'. The second part describes the different effects of surgery and anaesthesia on each galaxy component from a common quantitative perspective, and where applicable the automated closed-loop systems that can help keep these systems stable. For each of these chapters we invited the world's experts.

Without any doubt, time will make the content of a book that seeks to explain personalized anaesthesia outdated – and for the better: new technologies, new information, new data analysis methods, different approaches to information, etc. are bound to be developed in the future. Artificial intelligence, including machine learning and other related approaches, is certainly going to be one of the major forces that will drive this change. New knowledge and technological innovations will continue to contribute more and more to individualized anaesthesia care, ultimately improving patient safety, outcomes and quality of life.

The editors want to thank the Gambús family members, the Hendrickx family members, their own mentors, the many expert authors that contributed to this book, and the patient staff of Cambridge University Press.

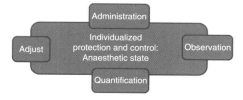

Fig. 2 Scheme of proactive and predictive anaesthesia action. Clockwise: drug administration will induce effects that are quantitated with adequate technology. In the event that prior and present information has been processed and analysed, adjustments will be done according to information-based predictions to avoid undesired outcomes.

Principles of Quantitative Clinical Pharmacology

Pedro L. Gambús and Sebastián Jaramillo

Introduction

Because there is no disease condition that can be treated with the administration of anaesthetic medications, the specialty of anaesthesiology does not possess a curative effect in itself. Nevertheless, achieving the state of anaesthesia or the anaesthetic state relies completely on the use of drugs. Drugs used in anaesthesia are very powerful and able to transiently break the most deeply rooted physiological defence mechanisms. Some of the effects induced include lack of consciousness, absence of response to pain, absence of muscle tone, immobility, lack of breathing and dysfunction of the autonomic nervous system, to name just a few. Some of these effects might be considered target or 'therapeutic effects', such as unconsciousness, analgesia or immobility, but others are 'side effects' that are induced because of the relative low specificity of currently used anaesthetic drugs.

Both the therapeutic and side effects are highly dynamic in their time course and they reach clinically effective ranges in a matter of seconds or minutes. If some of the collateral effects like respiratory depression are not adequately managed with measures such as securing the airway and providing mechanical ventilation, severe morbidity or even mortality might result. Fortunately, the current practice of anaesthesia relies on preoperative evaluation of patients as well as on several technological advances to try to predict and control the physiological changes in the patient. In addition, the effects of modern short-acting anaesthetic drugs fade very fast after discontinuing their administration.

It is of high importance to understand the fundamentals of pharmacology to be able to rationally dose anaesthetic drugs. Dosing has to be adjusted and individualized according to the characteristics of the patient, to the characteristics of the surgical or diagnostic procedure, and to the timing and events occurring during every procedure.

The present chapter will review basic concepts of clinical pharmacology. A quantitative perspective will be used. For instance, we will explain how mathematical models help understand drug effects, and how this will help us to define such concepts as onset of effect, peak effect and its time course, offset of effect after a bolus or continuous administration, context-sensitive decrement times, and the relevance of interindividual variability in anaesthetic drug response. These will serve as the basis for rational individualized drug dosing. Other chapters in this book will introduce topics such as estimating and characterizing inter-individual variability in drug response, incorporating covariate factor effects to decrease variability, signal analysis to measure actual responses to drugs with the goal of understanding, quantitating and individualizing drug responses in individual patients, for specific procedures, and for specific events during surgery.

The study of the principles governing the relation between dose and drug concentrations in the body constitutes pharmacokinetics (PK), and will be treated first. The relationship between drug concentration and effect will be presented in the pharmacodynamic (PD) concepts section.

Pharmacokinetic Concepts

Pharmacokinetics is the branch of pharmacology that studies the time course of the concentration of a drug resulting from initial drug dosing, its distribution to the different organs and tissues, and its disposal by the body through biotransformation and elimination. It also describes how it is absorbed when the drug is not intravenously administered. In real life, these processes occur simultaneously. The fundamental PK concepts are volume of distribution and clearance, the basic building blocks of the compartment models that are used to explain PK and PD of intravenous drugs (Fig. 1.1). For inhaled agents, physiological models are most often (but not exclusively) used.

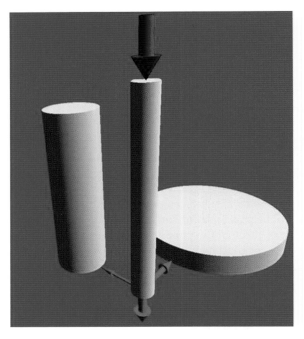 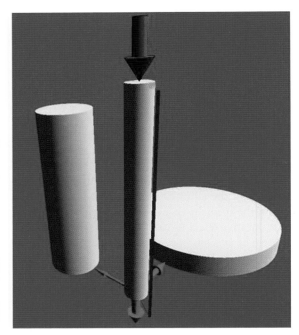

Fig. 1.1 Classical compartment model description. The left panel shows a three-compartment pharmacokinetic model. Drug input is marked by the red arrow and clearance, metabolic and intercompartmental, by the green arrows. The right panel shows a PK model with the addition of an effect site in the form of a long blue rectangle with no volume to meet the assumptions required for the modelling approach (generated with the use of the Cylinders software available at www.pkpdtools.com).

Volume of Distribution

The volume of distribution describes the relationship between the amount of drug in the body and its blood concentration [1]. When a bolus dose of any drug is administered intravenously, the drug gets diluted by and in the blood. It can be seen as analogous to introducing a substance into a bucket of water or fluid where physical laws regulate the speed and degree of dissolution. However, in the case of drugs and tissues, the degree to which a substance is diluted or how it reaches the tissues will also depend on drug properties such as lipophilicity, protein binding, partitioning into tissues and the flow of blood to the different organs and tissues.

Once the drug is in the fluid, which most often is the blood within the context of anesthesia, its presence can be measured as a concentration. If the concentration of a drug and the amount of drug administered are known, the volume of distribution can be estimated:

$$Volume\ of\ distribution = Dose\ of\ drug\ /\ Concentration\ of\ drug \qquad (1)$$

A volume of distribution is an apparent volume, i.e. a calculated value that does not have to bear a resemblance to any anatomical entity; it does not need to be equal to the volume of tissues in the body. For example, if a drug is highly bound to tissues, its concentration in blood will be very low, and therefore the estimation of the distribution volume can be very high, higher than any rational estimate of human body volume.

Volume of Distribution in the Central Compartment versus Peripheral Compartments

The central compartment is defined as the compartment into which a drug is initially injected and from which samples are taken for measurement. In the context of anaesthetic drugs, it is usually the volume of blood contained in the heart and blood vessels. The volume of distribution of the central compartment is the ratio of the administered dose over the first measured drug concentration. The 'maximal' concentration, i.e. at the time of injection, is obtained by back extrapolation of the concentration–time curve to time zero. The 'volume of distribution' concept is calculated with this concentration, which obviously is a theoretical construct because there is not yet a single drug molecule in the circulation at time zero because it takes some time for the drug to be transported from the vein to the central circulation.

There are several factors that affect estimation of the volume of distribution of the central compartment. Some are related to study design, for instance the sampling site and the timing of the samples. The sampling site, venous versus arterial blood, may affect the estimation because the concentration is lower in the venous than in the arterial blood: the estimation of volume of distribution based on venous blood samples thus will be significantly larger than that based on arterial blood. Timing of the first sample also has an effect: the longer it takes to obtain the first sample, the lower the 'initial' concentration will be because distribution and elimination start immediately after the drug enters the body, and thus the larger the calculated volume of distribution will be, leading to an overestimate. Erroneous distribution volume estimates will have consequences when they are going to be used for dosing guidelines because the recommended dose to achieve a given concentration will be much larger if the volume of distribution has been overestimated. This will result in excessively high actual concentrations. It also underscores the need for prospective testing of a model.

While it is known that several anaesthetic drugs undergo some initial distribution and degradation in the lungs, estimates of central volume do not usually take this into account. The study and integration of the changes taking place during the initial phase of mixing and distribution of drugs in the blood, its first-pass through the lung circulation, and possible degradation of drugs by the lungs is what is known as 'front-end kinetics'. Front-end kinetics has been studied and characterized, and more complex models have been proposed that could be implemented in infusion devices [2–4].

Depending on the characteristics of drugs and their ability to reach peripheral tissues, compartments other than the central compartment might be added and estimated. For most anaesthetic drugs it is assumed that the drug permeates rapidly from the central compartment to a group of highly perfused tissues, considered to be a fast peripheral compartment, and more slowly to a group of poorly perfused tissues, a slow peripheral compartment, mainly composed of fat. A drug that has reached fat tissues slowly will also slowly return to the central compartment. However, the possibility of a drug returning from fat to blood in significant quantities is very unlikely with the rapidly acting drugs that we use nowadays, therefore the probability of significant side effects related to significant amounts of drug back from fat to blood is very low.

To determine whether a one, two, or three compartment model best describes the time course of drug concentration, an adequate number of blood samples has to be drawn at predefined times, otherwise the whole PK process may not be accurately described.

At this point it is important to remark that PK not only describes the relation between dose and concentration of drugs, but that it is an important driver for pharmacological effect over time. Volumes of distribution and clearances not only have a combined influence on the PK, but also on the time course of the effect of each drug. This can be seen in Fig. 1.2 where a larger volume of distribution slows the onset of effect and decreases the duration of effect as well.

Clearance

Clearance describes the relation between the concentration of a drug and the rate of elimination of the drug from the body. Clearance reflects a real

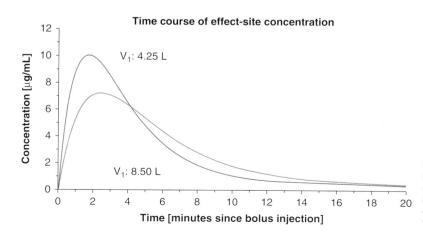

Time course of effect-site concentration

V_1: 4.25 L

V_1: 8.50 L

Concentration [μg/mL]

Time [minutes since bolus injection]

Fig. 1.2 Decay of effect-site concentration at two extreme values of volume of distribution. Doubling volume of distribution alters the dynamics of the effect by delaying onset, decreasing intensity and slowing the fall of effect site concentration.

physiological phenomenon, namely the ability of the body to eliminate an external substance, in this case a drug. It is measured in flux units (volume per time unit, i.e. litres/hour), and it describes how many litres of blood are irreversibly cleared of the drug in one hour.

Intuitively, clearance can be compared to a vacuum cleaner absorbing dust from the air in a room: clearance deals with the ability to clear 'the solvent (air or plasma)' from 'the solute (dust or drug)' per unit of time rather than with the amount of the solute (dust or drug) that is being removed. It can apply to a single organ (hepatic clearance for instance) or to the whole body (sometimes referred to as 'metabolic clearance') [5].

Clearance describes the intrinsic ability of the body to extract drugs from blood or plasma – it is not the rate of elimination or removal of the absolute amount of the drug per time unit. The amount of drug eliminated will depend on the concentration of the drug present in the blood at any moment. If drug clearance is constant at 1 L/h, the drug elimination rate will be zero if there is no drug but would be 1 mg/h if the concentration is 1 mg/L, and 100 mg/h if the concentration is 100 mg/L. Clearance is the proportionality constant that relates the rate of elimination to the measured concentration.

Clearance parameters, expressed in units of flow (L/min or L/kg/min), simply quantify the volume of plasma from which the drug is completely cleared per unit of time. Clearance is constant and independent of drug concentration for drugs that have a so-called linear behaviour meaning that doubling the dose will result in doubling of the drug concentration.

Clearance has been extensively used to calculate drug dosing schemes:

$$Maintenance\ dose\ rate = Clearance \times Target\ Concentration \qquad (2)$$

Age affects clearance: as adults grow older, their capacity to clear a drug is also decreasing. Organ failure can also affect the clearance by that particular organ. Concomitant drugs can also affect the clearance of a subject, for instance by altering cardiac output or simply by interfering with metabolic mechanisms. The two main organs with clearance ability are the liver and the kidneys.

As mentioned before for volume of distribution, clearance is a key component of the PK of any drug, but it also has an important influence on the time course of effect. Figure 1.3 presents the predicted effect-site concentration of propofol with normal and with doubled (metabolic) clearance to illustrate the effect of PK changes on drug effect.

Hepatic Clearance

From a clearance point of view, the liver is the most important organ. The liver clears drugs from the blood or the plasma. Two different drug classes are discerned, those with a high and those with a low extraction ratio. The first class are those drugs for which the only limiting factor for hepatic clearance is the flow of blood to the organ, and these drugs are said to have a high 'extraction ratio', close to one, as is the case for propofol. Drugs in the second class are those where the ability of the liver to clear blood or plasma is limited by the function of the hepatocyte, due to its internal

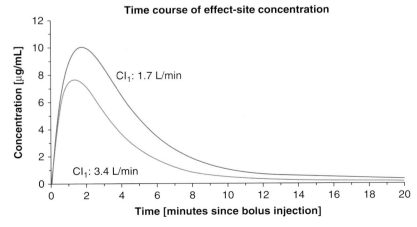

Time course of effect-site concentration

Fig. 1.3 Decay of effect-site concentration at two extreme values of clearance. Doubling clearance hastens the peak of effect but decreases its intensity and hastens the fall of the effect-site concentration.

enzymatic mechanisms or because some drug characteristics make it difficult to enter the cell. Drugs with these characteristics are said to have a low extraction ratio (well below one). Alfentanil is a good example of this class of drugs.

Renal Clearance

Renal clearance is composed of two different mechanisms: glomerular filtration, and secretion at the tubular level. As with any other organ, ageing affects kidney function and consequently drug clearance, causing drug concentrations after the same dose to be higher and thus causing their effects to last longer. Some anaesthetic agents undergo liver biotransformation to generate water soluble compounds that can be excreted through the kidney. A classical, now historical, example is the neuromuscular blocking agent pancuronium, 85% of which is excreted by the kidneys. Many anaesthetic drugs also alter kidney function by altering renal blood flow.

Distributional Clearance

Distributional clearance reflects the transfer of a drug from the central volume of distribution, blood or plasma, to peripheral tissues. It will depend on the blood flow to each tissue or organ and on the permeability of capillary walls to different drugs. For propofol, a highly lipophilic hypnotic drug, the sum of metabolic clearance plus distribution clearance is almost as high as cardiac output, and this is because it is avidly captured by peripheral tissues. When it comes to drugs undergoing plasma enzymatic metabolism, such as remifentanil or Dynorphin A 1–13, the sum of metabolic and distributional clearance is higher than cardiac output. Distributional clearance is responsible for terminating a drug's effect after the initial bolus.

Compartment Models Applied to Pharmacology

When a bolus of a drug is administered and blood samples are collected to quantitate plasma drug concentrations, a certain concentration decay pattern can be observed. This pattern is similar when the same drug dose(s) and blood sampling sequence are repeated in a number of individuals. As can be seen in Fig. 1.4, Panel A, there is a common trend or tendency: there is a fast decay after the initial administration that subsequently slows down. Panel B represents how there is

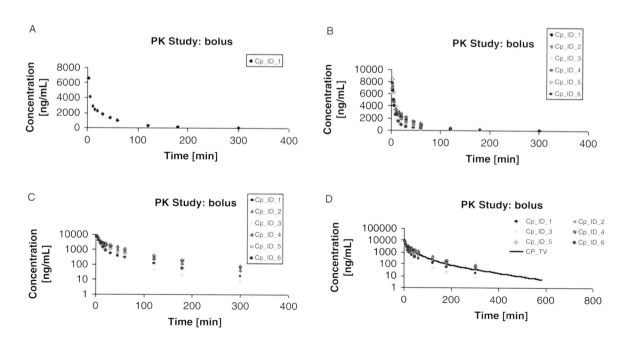

Fig. 1.4 Constructing a PK model. Panel A shows the time course of concentrations for a single subject. Panel B shows the common time course pattern for six individuals. If the results are plotted on a graph with a semi-logarithmic concentration on the Y-axis, three different decay phases can be observed in Panel C. Panel D shows the typical curve describing the time course of drug concentrations for all individuals and for the curve representative of the population or 'typical' individuals.

a common pattern for all blood samples from all individuals studied: three different decay parts can be visually identified in the curves, especially when a semi-log representation is used (Panel C). This pattern (Panel D) can be represented by an equation of the form:

$$Cp(t) = A \cdot e^{-\alpha t} + B \cdot e^{-\beta t} + C \cdot e^{-\delta t} \qquad (3)$$

A, B, C, α, β and δ are the parameters that define the intercept and the slope of each of the terms, describing the different parts of the concentration decay curve. These parameters can be estimated by nonlinear regression techniques. These parameters define the equation for a particular drug. The equation defining the curve is called the Unit Disposition Function (UDF), and it is the curve for a dose of one unit of the particular drug. UDF serves as a definition of the kinetic properties of the drug and as a way to compare different drugs.

Volumes of distribution and clearances can also be used as a way to describe the above drug concentration course. These are called compartment models. The values of distribution volumes and clearances are mathematically related to the above parameters in a complex manner. The drug concentration course is envisioned as being the result from injecting the drug into a closed compartment where it immediately gets diluted. As the drug gets diluted, it also simultaneously and irreversibly is cleared from the compartment to the environment. This simple approach is called the one compartment model. This compartment is called the central compartment because it can be connected to other 'peripheral' compartments. They are called multicompartment mammillary models because there is one central compartment from which the other compartments 'receive' the drug. The drug concentration in the central compartment decreases not only due to clearance to the environment but also by disappearing to one or two compartment(s), a process called inter-compartmental or distributional clearance. The drug concentration course of most anaesthetic drugs is best described by a three compartment mammillary model: a central compartment where the drug is administered and from where it is eliminated to the environment, connected to two different peripheral compartments that are not interconnected and are not open to the environment. Once a drug has been administered into the central compartment, elimination to the environment as well as distribution to the peripheral compartments simultaneously occurs. When drug administration ceases, drug flux can be reversed: the drug can return from the peripheral compartment(s) to the central compartment.

The transfer of drug from central compartment to the environment and from central to peripheral compartments can be quantitated by transfer constants that are usually denoted by a letter k and sub-index that defines the direction of drug transfer. For instance, k_{31} is the transfer constant regulating the direction of drug from compartment three, one of the two slow peripheral compartments, to the central compartment, while k_{10} denotes the 'final' elimination from the central compartment to the environment.

Although the physiological meaning is not clear or is even absent, the three compartment model envisions the human body to be a combination of three compartments. The central compartment is the compartment where the drug is injected and where it 'mixes instantaneously'; the fast peripheral compartment could be considered to be composed of well perfused tissues and organs where the drug arrives relatively fast; and the slow peripheral or third compartment could be considered to be composed of poorly perfused tissues, with the drug arriving slowly out of the central compartment. When the gradient is reversed, the drug returns from the slow to the central compartment sluggishly, and usually without having any clinical repercussion. Not all drugs need to be described by a three compartment model. The choice between a one, two, or three compartment model depends on drug characteristics and also on study design. The main point to consider is that enough blood samples have to be drawn to be able to estimate the different parameters of the function that describes the concentration decay curve. If the experiment consists of injecting the drug plus drawing a blood sample five minutes and three hours after injection, it is very likely that the decay would be represented by a straight line, and thus no reliable information about the concentration course can be extracted from what happens between five and 180 minutes. A good example of general study design for PK in anaesthesia can be found in the study of propofol PKPD by Schnider et al [6, 7] or remifentanil PKPD by Minto et al [8, 9].

The use of a compartment model to describe the time course of drug concentrations comes to the clinician in a more physiologically intuitive way. As mentioned before, the equation defining the drug disposition curve (Equation 3) can be represented in other ways using different parameters: equilibration constants, slope and coefficients and also as volumes of distribution and clearances. The parameters of equations that underlie each of these different approaches bear a complex relationship to one another. Software solutions such as PKPD Tools for Excel [10] or convert.xls (available at www.nonmemcourse.com/convert.xls) are very helpful in re-parameterizing. The exponents and coefficients of Equation (3) for example can be converted into volumes of distribution and clearances with these tools. Most publications of PK and PKPD models in anaesthesia literature show the parameters of the model as volumes and clearances terminology.

Variability

Figure 1.4 shows the time course of the plasma concentration of a drug. Panel B shows the plasma decay curves of six different subjects, and Panel D shows all individuals plus the common descriptor of all them, the 'typical individual'. The 'typical individual' or 'population model' represents the sample or population. Between the population model and each one of the individual time courses there are differences. The differences between individuals are the 'inter-individual variability'. Variability can be decomposed into different factors that could potentially influence the PK of a drug. Some of those factors are easily identified with an appropriate study design (age, weight or gender of the subject, concomitant medication or diseases) and can be considered to explain part of the inter-individual variability (see Chapter 2 about PKPD Modelling and Chapter 3 about covariate factors).

Variability is an important issue when it comes to dosing anaesthetic drugs; new methods of data analysis, especially those based on nonlinear mixed effects modelling, permit one to study in detail the expected variability in the response after a dose of any anaesthetic, ultimately with the goal of improving drug titration in such a manner that effects can be individualized.

Pharmacodynamics

Pharmacodynamics (PD) is the part of pharmacology that studies the relation between drug concentration and effect(s). Drug effects can be therapeutic or can be side effects. In our specialty the term 'therapeutic effects' does not apply well, but still we refer to it as such when we define the effect we are looking for: hypnotic effect (unconsciousness, sedation), analgesia, immobility, or potentially dangerous side effects (respiratory depression, bradycardia, arterial hypotension). It is as important to reach the therapeutic effect and intensity of that effect as it is to avoid potentially dangerous side effects.

The Concept of Effect Site

Figure 1.5 represents the time course of drug concentration versus effect. The drug has been administered as a short intravenous infusion. It can be seen that there is a delay between achieving the maximal concentration and the maximal effect. This delay matches our clinical impressions well: after injecting a bolus dose of an anaesthetic drug, it takes a while before the maximal effect is achieved.

When graphically representing plasma drug concentrations versus effect, it can be noted that for a given concentration there can be two different intensities of effect. The type of curve that is generated is called 'hysteresis'. In pharmacology there are two types of hysteresis that relate concentrations to effect: one is clockwise and it corresponds to the phenomenon of

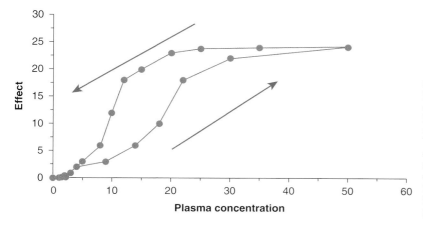

Fig. 1.5 The concept of effect site: hysteresis of plasma concentrations versus effect. As drug concentration starts to increase, the effect increases very slowly until a maximum point has been reached. Thereafter, drug concentrations start to decrease but the effect disappears with a different pattern as compared to the onset of effect. This phenomenon that happens in a counterclockwise pattern is called hysteresis, and it is due to the fact that plasma is not the site of drug effect.

'drug tolerance'. The counterclockwise hysteresis is associated with the inaccurate match between plasma concentrations and effect. Ideally, counterclockwise hysteresis would be absent: if it were possible to measure drug concentrations at the site of drug effect, and if these could be plotted against the measurements of effect, the data points would fall on the same line because every concentration would be associated with only one level of effect. Hysteresis is caused by transport and signal processing delays: blood has to transport the drug to the target organ, where it will have to activate a receptor and trigger a chain of events ranging from subcellular to organ level, ultimately generating the observed effect.

How do we solve the hysteresis problem, i.e. the fact that the same clinical effect can occur in the presence of two different blood or plasma concentrations? As mentioned, we could consider measuring concentrations at the site of drug effect, but this is not yet possible for most of the cases. We could wait for steady state conditions, i.e. a condition where there is equilibrium between drug input and output. This is usually reached after continuous administration of a drug during at least five elimination half-lives. After reaching steady state conditions, we could draw blood samples and assume that there is equilibrium between the concentrations at the effect site and at all organs. However, again this proves to be an impossible approach because it takes too much time to reach such conditions, outlasting surgery itself.

We therefore need another solution: the theoretical 'effect site', a concept that links plasma concentrations to effect measurements. The effect site, also known as the biophase, was initially proposed to explain the relation between concentrations of d-tubocurarine and neuromuscular blockade, first by the Italian pharmacologist G. Segre in 1968 and then, almost simultaneously, by Sheiner [11] and Hull [12]. The effect site is a theoretical mathematical construct that can be considered to be yet another 'special' compartment, linked to the central compartment. After entering the effect site it is assumed that the drug directly and immediately exerts its effect. Another assumption is that the size of the effect site compartment and the amount of drug in it is very small, almost negligible, as compared to the size of the other compartments in the model, so that it has no influence on the PK or the mass balances of the drug. By definition, at steady state, the concentration at the effect site is the same as that in the central compartment because mixing is considered to be instantaneous, because the volume of the effect site is infinitesimally small and because the blood/effect-site partition coefficient is assumed to be one.

The delay between the plasma and effect-site concentration, and thus the clinical effect, is mathematically described by a single parameter, k_{eo}, the effect-site equilibration-rate constant, which is a first-order process. k_{eo} can be expressed as the equilibration half-life between plasma and the effect site according to the following equation:

$$t_{1/2}k_{eo} = ln2/k_{eo} = 0.693/k_{eo} \qquad (4)$$

k_{eo} has units of 1/time (time^{-1}). A large $t_{1/2}k_{eo}$ (small k_{eo} value) implies a longer equilibration between plasma and effect site and a slower onset of effect. Small $t_{1/2}k_{eo}$ means fast onset and large k_{eo}. k_{eo} can be estimated from plasma concentrations and measured effect, or from PK parameters and measured effect. The original paper by Sheiner refers to the constant as k_{e}. Several authors name it k_{e0}, in this book we will refer to it as k_{eo} to be consistent with the original proposal.

So, by definition, one concentration in the effect site, or biophase, is directly linked to one single effect. Different clinical end-points will have different k_{eo} values, e.g. the k_{eo} describing propofol induced arterial hypotension will differ from the propofol k_{eo} for Bispectral Index (BIS) changes, and the k_{eo} for BIS will differ from that for the 95% Spectral Edge of the electroencephalogram.

Sometimes the relations between drug concentration and effect are not as obvious as in the case of anaesthetics. Different approaches have been proposed to establish the link between plasma concentrations and effect in those situations where the effect compartment approach does not help. A common method is the use of 'indirect effect models' [15]. In those models the main assumption is that there are intermediate steps that can be estimated as well. Such steps may include interposed mechanisms, molecular or cellular mediators.

To summarize, the effect site compartment concept is the most commonly used approach to link the plasma concentration of a drug to its effect. It has been a key concept to derive rational dosing that achieves and maintains a defined level of effect. Based on these principles, Target Controlled Infusion (TCI) systems are able to target both plasma and effect site concentrations. The k_{eo} is the mathematical construct that allows PK models to be connected to PD models (see below) and thus allows drug dosing to be linked to clinical effect. It allows us to make estimations or predictions of onset and offset of effect after a given drug dose.

Relation between Effect-site Concentration and Effect

For most anaesthetic drugs, the relationship between effect site concentration (Ce) and clinical effects takes a sigmoidal shape, modelled by the so-called sigmoidal Emax model (Fig. 1.6). As Ce increases from zero, there will initially be no or only a very small increase in effect, but as Ce is further increased, the effect will start to increase rapidly until it reaches a Ce above which the intensity of effect increases no further.

The equation that describes the sigmoid Emax model is known as the Hill equation [13]:

$$E = E_0 + (E_{max} - E_0)\frac{C_e^{\gamma}}{C_e^{\gamma} + IC_{50}^{\gamma}} \qquad (5)$$

Four parameters define the model. E_0 is the baseline effect when no drug has been administered. E_{max} is the maximal effect that could be eventually reached. IC_{50} is the effect site concentration that induces 50% of the maximum effect. Gamma (γ) is the exponent that defines the steepness of the linear part of the curve, and is also referred to as alpha (α) or as the Hill coefficient.

IC_{50} reflects the potency of the drug for a given effect and thus allows drugs from the same drug class to be compared: because the IC_{50} of sufentanil is lower than that of fentanyl and remifentanil (which have a similar IC_{50}) which in turn is lower than that of alfentanil [14], sufentanil is said to be more potent than fentanyl and remifentanil, while the latter two are more potent than alfentanil [14].

Integration of Pharmacokinetics and Pharmacodynamics

PK and PD models and the effect site concept that links them permit us to estimate the onset, intensity, duration and offset of effect after a given dose. To be able to accurately predict the intensity of effect in an individual patient, covariate effects have to be incorporated into the parameters of the PKPD models (see Chapter 4).

Application to Rational Dosing Guidelines

The clinically most useful aspect of PKPD concepts is the ability to predict the 'right dose' that will result in the desired clinical effect at the right time and only during the period that is necessary for every patient. This means that a PKPD model will help the clinician to predict onset, duration and offset of the therapeutic effect. In addition, unwanted side effects have to be avoided or minimized.

Drug concentrations should fall within a therapeutic window, the range of concentrations within which the expected effect is safely attained. Below the therapeutic window, the effect in the patient is not intense enough because the drug is underdosed. Above the therapeutic window, the effect is much more intense than required because the drug has been overdosed and the patient is at risk of developing excessive or significant side effects. Given the special nature of the drugs used in anaesthesia, both under- and overdosing might be a source of serious problems like awareness, unexpected movement causing iatrogenic trauma, excessive haemodynamic depression (hypotension or tissue hypoperfusion), or even death. This is the reason

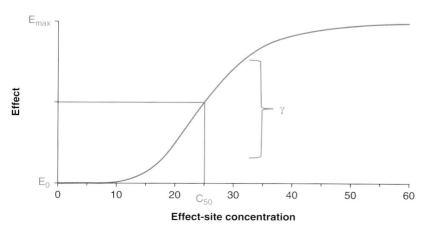

Fig. 1.6 The relation between effect-site concentration and effect. The sigmoid E_{max} model is defined by the effect when no drug is present (E_0), the maximal effect possible (E_{max}), the effect-site concentration that causes 50% of effect between E_{max} and E_0, and the exponent γ defining the steepness of the rectilinear part of the curve.

9

why it is so important to measure effect intensity in every patient. The narrower the range of the therapeutic window, the more challenging drug dosing will be. The clinician will have to weigh onset and offset of effect with the likelihood of overdosing and the probability of developing side effects.

The delay in reaching the maximal effect of the dose, is independent of the dose because even for a minimal dose there will be some degree of intensity of effect, even if it does not reach the therapeutic limit, as displayed in Fig. 1.7. Maximal effect should not be confused with onset of effect. Figure 1.7 shows a therapeutic window that marks the time of peak effect (maximal) and onset and duration, after simulating the time course of effect-site concentrations of propofol after different bolus doses of the drug.

Time to Peak Effect

The effect-site model has been fundamental in PKPD studies of most anaesthetic drugs because it has allowed us to establish a clear relation between dose, plasma concentration, effect-site concentration and effect. A study to characterize the PKPD model of a drug is conducted by accurately administering a certain dose of the drug, by collecting blood samples through an arterial access, and by continuously measuring the effect. This kind of study is usually conducted in a highly controlled environment such as a clinical research laboratory, with volunteers instead of patients, and they carry a significant cost. With so many different models already published, it might be considered that combining the results from different studies to derive new models, for instance the PK results from one model

could be combined with the k_{eo} estimates from another model, could be a good alternative to describe the time course of Ce.

Minto et al proposed the concept of 'Time to Peak Effect' (TPE) to help combine PK parameters with current measures of effect to estimate a k_{eo} value. The requirements for this approach are a PK model plus an accurate measure of the time of maximal intensity of effect after a bolus dose. The bolus should be 'submaximal', meaning that it will not reach or surpass the maximal level of effect. For instance with a high bolus dose of rocuronium that depresses below 0% the TOF ratio, it is not possible to determine the time at which maximal effect is reached because the real induced effect goes beyond the limit of detection of the signal. The time from drug injection until reaching maximal effect is called TPE, and it can be used as an indicator of onset of effect [16].

When PK information is available and TPE is measured, a value for k_{eo} can be estimated. This is very useful because it would significantly simplify the estimation of optimal drug dosing. TPE can be derived from an accurate, already published PK study and from observations of TPE. Indeed, TPE has been used to estimate k_{eo} for different PK models based on measures of effect [17–19]. TPE can also be used as an objective measure of variability in drug effects by studying the correlation between TPE and covariate factors such as ageing or sickness conditions. TPE is unique for a PK model and a measure of effect. The software package PKPD Tools for Excel provides the functions to calculate TPE from PK and k_{eo} as well as the possibility to estimate k_{eo} from a PK model and TPE [10].

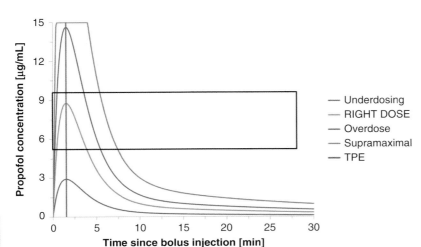

Fig. 1.7 Time to Peak Effect (TPE) and onset of effect. The plot shows the time course of propofol effect site concentrations after four different bolus doses. The black rectangle marks a hypothetical therapeutic window between 5 and 10 µg/mL for induction of a certain clinical endpoint. TPE, maximum effect, can be seen to always set in at 1.53 min after injecting the bolus, independently of the size of the bolus. The first dose does not induce any effect. The second, 'right', dose induces an adequate effect (enters the therapeutic window) 30 sec after the bolus and lasts five min. Note that in the supramaximal dose it is not possible to measure the time to maximum effect.

Estimation of Offset of Effect: Context Sensitive Half-Times

A bolus of an anaesthetic drug has such a fast time course that it is easy to observe when an effect starts and when it wears off. For instance, after a bolus of propofol it is easy to say when the patient falls unconscious and when consciousness is regained, just by observing the reactions of the patient or by using more sophisticated methods such as the EEG. Based on PKPD models, the approximate time of offset of effect can be estimated and the more covariate factors are integrated in the PKPD model, the higher the predictive accuracy of the model will be.

However, often anaesthetic drugs are given not just as boluses but as a continuous infusion, at a variable or fixed rate. The duration of effect of the drug will then depend on for how long the drug has been administered, and this will differ between drugs. Drug concentrations in the blood, or central compartment, decrease because either the drug is being redistributed to peripheral compartments that still have a lower concentration, or because it is irreversibly removed from the central compartment by the liver, the kidney or by plasma and tissue esterase enzymes (e.g. remifentanil). After an initial single bolus or a short infusion, redistribution is the main mechanism that terminates drug effect. However, when longer infusions are used, this mechanism will become less efficient in decreasing central compartment drug concentrations because the drug will also have accumulated in the slower compartments. This will cause the concentration gradient that drives the drug away from the central compartment to the peripheral compartments to decrease: as time goes by and drug delivery continues, redistribution will become less effective as a means to lower drug concentrations in the central compartment. In this context of increasing duration of drug administration, the central compartment will have to 'rely' more and more on 'irreversible elimination to the outside world' rather than on distribution mechanisms to see its drug concentration decrease. In other words, the longer the duration of agent administration, the more metabolism will become responsible for drug elimination from the central compartment and the longer it will take for the drug concentration in the central compartment to decrease. The same will happen to the termination of drug effect, which is directly related to the central compartment concentration via the effect-site

compartment. The rate at which the concentration in the central compartment of a drug decreases is commonly described by the half-time, the time required for the concentration to decrease by 50%. Because the mechanism underlying drug removal from the central compartment progressively changes from the rapid process of drug redistribution to the much slower process of drug elimination, the time for the drug concentration to decrease by 50% after discontinuing its administration will increase as time goes by. Another manner to express this is by saying that the drug elimination half-time is sensitive to the 'context', i.e. the duration of administration, in which the drug has been administered.

Shafer and Varvel applied this concept to study how long it would take for the plasma concentration of fentanyl, alfentanil or sufentanil to fall below 20%, 50% and 80% of the concentration that was present when infusion was stopped. To do so, they used PK models for those three drugs, simulated their plasma concentrations during a continuous infusion, and examined how fast the concentrations decayed when infusions were stopped after different time intervals – and these differed between the different opioids. This principle can also be applied to effect-site concentrations providing estimations of the time course of drug effects after infusions of variable duration. Opioid selection can be rationalized based on differences in context sensitive half-times that describe the concentration decay curves of different drugs after different durations of administration [20].

Figure 1.8 shows the 50% and 80% context sensitive decrement times for propofol and the influence of age on those recovery percentages. Context sensitive decrement times have also been studied for different inhaled anaesthetics using the simulation software GASMAN™ [21].

The integration of full PK and PD information has allowed us to estimate the different effect-site concentration decrement times for almost any drug in anaesthesia. The decrement time concept has been integrated in TCI systems that continuously calculate how long it would take the effect-site concentration to fall to a certain level if the infusion were stopped.

By now, it should have become clear to the reader that rational drug dosing in anaesthesia has to take into account a drug's onset, offset, infusion duration and influence of covariate factors, combined with clinical observation.

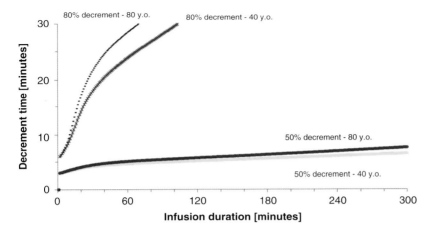

Fig. 1.8 Context sensitive decrement times for propofol. Plot of the time required for the effect site concentration to decrease by 50% (50% context sensitive half-time) and by 80% (80% context sensitive decrement time). The effect of a wide variety of ages has also been incorporated.

Conclusion

The objective of this chapter was to introduce the interested clinician to the concepts needed to understand how modelling and technology can be used to provide us with an accurate prediction of a drug's onset, duration of effect, and termination of effect. The following chapters will describe how characteristics of the individual patient will influence the time course of the effect of a drug, how we can obtain accurate models that relate dose to concentration and effect, how different drugs can potentiate one another's effects, what technical approaches have been taken to measure drug effect, and how to adjust drug dosing to optimally fit the requirements of the procedure and the individual patient.

References

1. Holford NH, Yim DS: Volume of Distribution. Trans. Clin.Pharm. 2016; 24: 74–7.

2. Avram MJ, Krejcie TC: Using front-end kinetics to optimize target-controlled drug infusions. Anesthesiology. 2003; 99: 1078–86.

3. Krejcie TC, Avram MJ: Recirculatory pharmacokinetic modeling: what goes around, comes around. Anesth. Analg. 2012; 115: 223–6.

4. Krejcie TC, Avram MJ: What determines anesthetic induction dose? It's the front-end kinetics, doctor! Anesth.Analg. 1999; 89: 541–4.

5. Holford NH, Yim DS: Clearance. Trans.Clin.Pharm. 2015; 23: 42–5.

6. Schnider TW, Minto CF, Shafer SL, Gambus PL, Andresen C, Goodale DB, Youngs EJ: The influence of age on propofol pharmacodynamics. Anesthesiology. 1999; 90: 1502–16.

7. Schnider TW, Minto CF, Gambus PL, Andresen C, Goodale DB, Shafer SL, Youngs EJ: The influence of method of administration and covariates on the pharmacokinetics of propofol in adult volunteers. Anesthesiology. 1998; 88: 1170–82.

8. Minto CF, Schnider TW, Shafer SL: Pharmacokinetics and pharmacodynamics of remifentanil. II. Model application. Anesthesiology. 1997; 86: 24–33.

9. Minto CF, Schnider TW, Egan TD, Youngs E, Lemmens HJ, Gambus PL, Billard V, Hoke JF, Moore KH, Hermann DJ, Muir KT, Mandema JW, Shafer SL: Influence of age and gender on the pharmacokinetics and pharmacodynamics of remifentanil. I. Model development. Anesthesiology. 1997; 86: 10–23.

10. Minto CF, Schnider TW: PKPD Tools for EXCEL (with XLMEM). 1st(1.02). 1995. Stanford, CA: Anesthesia Department., Stanford University School of Medicine. www.pkpdtools.com

11. Sheiner LB, Stanski DR, Vozeh S, Miller RD, Ham J: Simultaneous modeling of pharmacokinetics and pharmacodynamics: application to d-tubocurarine. Clin.Pharmacol.Ther. 1979; 25: 358–71.

12. Hull CJ, Van Beem HB, McLeod K, Sibbald A, Watson MJ: A pharmacodynamic model for pancuronium. Br.J.Anaesth. 1978; 50: 1113–23.

13. Hill AV: The possible effects of the aggregation of the molecules of hemoglobin on its dissociation curves. J.Physiol. 1910; 40: iv–vii.

14. Gambus PL, Gregg KM, Shafer SL: Validation of the alfentanil canonical univariate parameter as a measure of opioid effect on the electroencephalogram. Anesthesiology. 1995; 83: 747–56.

15. Sharma A, Jusko WJ: Characterization of four basic models of indirect pharmacodynamic responses. J.Pharmacokinet.Biopharm. 1996; 24: 611–35.

16. Minto CF, Schnider TW, Gregg KM, Henthorn TK, Shafer SL: Using the time of maximum effect site concentration to combine pharmacokinetics and pharmacodynamics. Anesthesiology. 2003; 99: 324–33.

17. Cortinez LI, Nazar C, Munoz HR: Estimation of the plasma effect-site equilibration rate constant (ke0) of rocuronium by the time of maximum effect: a comparison with non-parametric and parametric approaches. Br.J.Anaesth. 2007; 99: 679–85.

18. Munoz HR, Leon PJ, Fuentes RS, Echevarria GC, Cortinez LI: Prospective evaluation of the time to peak effect of propofol to target the effect site in children. Acta Anaesthesiol.Scand. 2009; 53: 883–90.

19. Munoz HR, Cortinez LI, Ibacache ME, Altermatt FR: Estimation of the plasma effect site equilibration rate constant (ke0) of propofol in children using the time to peak effect: comparison with adults. Anesthesiology. 2004; 101: 1269–74.

20. Shafer SL, Varvel JR: Pharmacokinetics, pharmacodynamics, and rational opioid selection. Anesthesiology. 1991; 74: 53–63.

21. Eger EI, Shafer SL: Tutorial: context-sensitive decrement times for inhaled anesthetics. Anesth. Analg. 2005; 101: 688–96.

Chapter 2

Pharmacokinetic and Pharmacodynamic Modelling in Anaesthesia

María J. Garrido and Iñaki F. Trocóniz

Introduction

Pharmacokinetic/pharmacodynamic (PK/PD) modelling is a discipline currently under the umbrella of pharmacometrics, and aims to describe, understand and predict the time course of in vivo drug action.

In general PK/PD comprises three major elements: (1) pharmacokinetics (PK), (2) pharmacodynamics (PD), and (3) disease progression [1]. However, given the fact that anaesthesia procedures take place in short periods of time, where the general state of the patient remains unaltered, in this chapter we will limit the focus to the interrelationship between PK and PD.

Drug action in vivo is associated, in addition to the magnitude of drug effects, with the concept of dynamics. In fact, the onset and offset of drug action are important factors always considered when dosing a patient. If we aim to describe the entire course of a particular drug effect, we need to use mathematical models, but if we also want to understand and predict drug effect in new patients and/or under different administration paradigms, we require that those mathematical models resemble the main processes responsible for the clinical outcomes. Therefore PK/PD modelling does not represent just an exercise of applied mathematics. On the contrary, the main challenge is to extract from the available data the relevant underlying mechanisms.

One part of the present chapter is devoted to showing the most used PK/PD model in the specialty of anaesthesia, detailing the mathematical structure and interpreting the parameters that define the model.

One common characteristic of the in vivo response to any drug of any therapeutic area is variability across patients. The magnitude of such variability needs to be quantified accurately, and its causes identified so that the drug will be optimally used in the population it is intended for. In the discipline of pharmacometrics the population approach deals with variability in drug exposure and response and therefore a section in this chapter is devoted to population analysis.

Pharmacokinetic/Pharmacodynamic models

Figure 2.1 represents in a schematic form the processes taking place between drug administration and response, including PK, distribution to the biophase and the different steps between target engagement and measured response. The diagram might discourage anaesthesiologists from developing population PK/PD models because the data required seem overwhelming. We will show later in this section how the complex picture shown in Fig. 2.1 can be simplified on the basis of the rate limiting step concept, making the study of the time course of in vivo drug response tractable [2].

PK principles will be discussed first, followed by PD, and finally how they are integrated [3, 4].

Pharmacokinetics

Prior to drug administration, and in the absence of circadian rhythms and during a short period of time, values of the measured response (i.e. baseline) remain constant, indicating that response, per se, does not vary over time. But as soon as a drug enters the body, the response variable will display a certain profile over time that is influenced by the PK properties of the anaesthetic drug. Therefore, one essential component in understanding the time profiles of a response is PK.

PK can be expressed in different ways: (1) characterization of the time course of the concentration of the active compound(s) [drug and/or metabolite(s)], generally in plasma, or (2) what the body does to the drug.

It has to be emphasized that PK is not just the measurement of plasma or tissue drug levels. Proper PK practice involves a modelling exercise with the aim to get precise PK parameters that accurately represent and quantify the main physiological process responsible for the fate of the drug in the body [3]. Before starting to describe the most commonly used models in anaesthesia, it is important to consider biopharmaceutics and data related aspects.

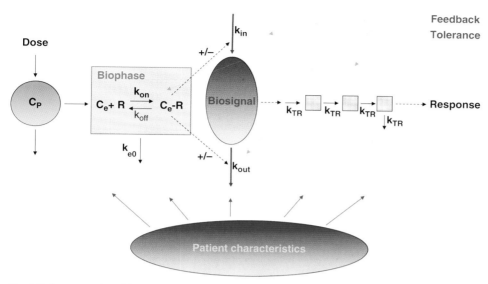

Fig. 2.1 Representation of the main processes involved in the in vivo time course of drug action. The terms C_p, C_e, R and C_e-R represent the plasma and effect-site concentrations, free target receptors, and the concentration–receptor complex, respectively; k_{on} and k_{off} correspond to the association and dissociation binding rate constants, respectively; k_{e0} is the first order rate constant governing the distribution equilibrium between the central and effect site compartment; k_{in} and k_{out} represent rate constants of turnover; and k_{TR} is a first order rate constant controlling signal propagation.

Usually during surgery, anaesthetics are administered intravenously, and in those cases exact information on the infusion rates and the corresponding amount delivered during each infusion have to be carefully recorded. In other areas of anaesthesia practice such as pain control, drugs are also given orally or subcutaneously, and therefore formulation type, mode and route of administration, as well as dose and dosing schedule are important factors to be taken into account.

To perform a proper PK modelling exercise, in addition to the accurate dose- and administration-related aspects commented on above, longitudinal levels of the concentration of drug in plasma are required. Plasma drug concentrations can be obtained either from arterial or venous blood. The operating room setting with an unconscious patient offers the opportunity to gather several early blood samples which, as will be discussed later, has important implications in allowing proper characterization of the onset of drug action. For example, to characterize the PK profile of propofol, arterial blood samples were taken at 0, 1, 2, 4, 8, 16 minutes and beyond after the first bolus injection [5].

Empirical Pharmacokinetic Compartmental Models

The most common approach in PK is to consider the body of the patient to be made of several

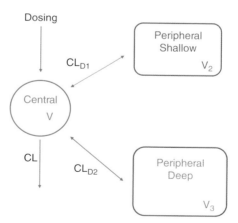

Fig. 2.2 Schematic representation of a three compartment PK model. V, V_2 and V_3, represent the apparent volume of distribution of the central, peripheral shallow and peripheral deep compartments, respectively; CL_{D1} and CL_{D2} are the inter-compartmental distribution clearances, and CL corresponds to the total plasma elimination clearance.

compartments. The three compartment model is one of the most frequently used models in anaesthesia [6]. Figure 2.2 represents schematically the structure of the three compartment model and its parameters. Chapter 1 discusses the compartment approach in more detail.

It is important to point out that besides using volumes and clearances, the primary PK parameters, PK models can be expressed in other parameters such as V, k_{12}, k_{21}, k_{13}, k_{31} and k_{10}. Both parameterizations are mathematically indistinguishable. In fact the above first order rate constants are equal to CL_{D1}/V, CL_{D1}/V_2, CL_{D2}/V, CL_{D2}/V_3 and CL/V, respectively. Primary PK parameters depend only on the physiopathology of the patient, whereas the first order rate constants are secondary PK parameters depending on the primary PK parameters. Therefore, if we want to investigate the influence of patient factors on the PK drug properties, use of volumes and clearances is the best parameterization approach.

It has to be realized that PK (and PD) parameters are not just numbers providing, within a specific mathematical structure, a good fit to the data. It is of great importance to recognize that PK parameters are a reflection of patient physiology.

Physiology-based Pharmacokinetic Models

A more mechanistic representation of the body is provided by the physiological PK models (PBPK), where all compartments do represent real body entities. Predictions of drug concentration over time are carried out using physiological variables such as tissue volumes and blood perfusion values, and a measure of the capacity of the tissue to be filled with drug, named the partition coefficient (KP), defined as the ratio between tissue and plasma concentrations once steady state is achieved.

A schematic representation of a PBPK model is shown in Fig. 2.3. Each of the tissues can be considered either (1) as a single compartment assuming perfusion limited distribution in which tissue drug kinetics can be predicted for a given value of arterial drug concentration, with the use of just KP, φ, the organ perfusion and tissue volume, or (2) as a number of compartments in cases of permeability limited distribution. From a data acquisition perspective, PBPK models are quite demanding because drug concentrations have to be measured in each tissue to compute KP (note that physiological variables such as organ perfusion and real volume values can be obtained from the literature because they are drug independent). Usually, PBPK are developed in laboratory animals and translated to humans assuming that K_p remains equal across different species [13]. Once relevant drug properties are known (i.e. liposolubility, unbound fraction (fu), blood to plasma concentration ratio, elimination pathway, etc.) it would also be possible to use new technologies to provide concentrations. PBPK represents a good tool for hypothesis generation, to explore 'in silico'

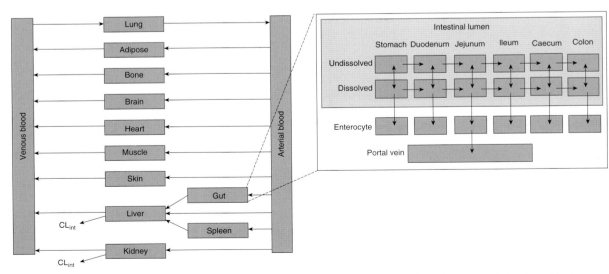

Fig. 2.3 Representation of a physiology-based PK model. Compartments represent real physiological entities, and drug disposition is characterized by the tissue volume, blood flow and partition coefficient defined as the ratio between drug concentrations in tissue and plasma once the distribution equilibrium has been achieved. The inserted graphic provides a granular representation of the intestine. Cl_{int}, intrinsic clearance. *Adapted from: Jones H, Rowland-Yeo K*: Basic concepts in physiologically based pharmacokinetic modeling in drug discovery and development. *CPT Pharmacometrics Syst Pharmacol* 2013; 2(8): e63.

the impact of patient characteristics on drug concentration profiles using the systems pharmacology paradigm, and to predict PK dependent onset of drug action [14, 15].

Pharmacodynamics

PD can be seen as the relationship between drug concentration, generally measured in plasma (C_p), and response. There are several aspects that can complicate the C_p versus response relationship, which will be discussed in later sections. For now we assume that, first, drug concentrations at the site of action are in equilibrium with those in plasma and, second, that all processes taking place from target engagement to clinical response occur so fast that C_p can be related directly to drug effects. Following the simpler description of PK analysis mentioned above, PD could be described as 'what the drug does to the body'.

For the time being, PD models will be constrained to the case of the analysis of continuous response (i.e. bispectral index, other EEG-derived measures, pupil diameter parameters, degree of neuromuscular blockade, heart rate or blood pressure, just to cite some commonly used and analysed clinical end-points in anaesthesia).

Models for Single Agent

Just like the three compartmental model is the most commonly used model in PK analysis, so is the sigmoidal E_{MAX} model (Fig. 2.4a) the most widely used model in PD analysis [16]. This PD model is based on the receptor theory under the following assumptions: (1) more than one molecule of drug can bind to the receptor, (2) there is a single type of drug–receptor complex, (3) the effect is proportional to the drug–receptor complex and (4) the system is in equilibrium (i.e. fast association and dissociation receptor binding processes). A description of the E_{MAX} model is available in Chapter 1.

Figure 2.4b shows some variants of the sigmoidal E_{MAX} model. In the absence of sigmoidicity ($\gamma = 1$) Equation 7 collapses to the E_{MAX} model. When $C_p \ll C_{50}$, or $C_p^\gamma \ll C_{50}^\gamma$, the E_{MAX} and sigmoidal E_{MAX} models simply regress to the linear and exponential models, respectively.

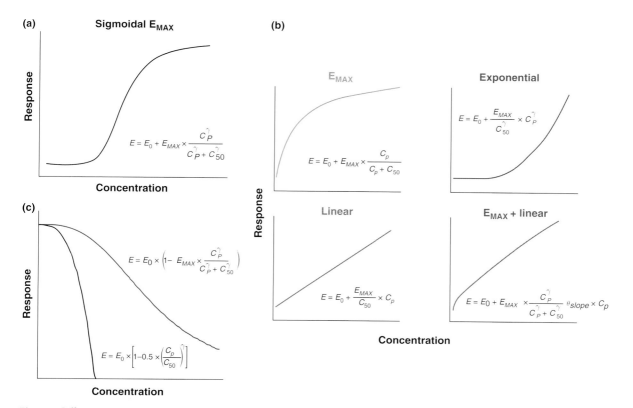

(a) **Sigmoidal E_{MAX}**

$$E = E_0 + E_{MAX} \times \frac{C_P^\gamma}{C_P^\gamma + C_{50}^\gamma}$$

(b)

E_{MAX}

$$E = E_0 + E_{MAX} \times \frac{C_p}{C_p + C_{50}}$$

Exponential

$$E = E_0 + \frac{E_{MAX}}{C_{50}^\gamma} \times C_P^\gamma$$

Linear

$$E = E_0 + \frac{E_{MAX}}{C_{50}} \times C_p$$

E_{MAX} + linear

$$E = E_0 + E_{MAX} \times \frac{C_P^\gamma}{C_P^\gamma + C_{50}^\gamma} {}^\theta slope \times C_p$$

(c)

$$E = E_0 \times \left(1 - E_{MAX} \times \frac{C_P^\gamma}{C_P^\gamma + C_{50}^\gamma}\right)$$

$$E = E_0 \times \left[1 - 0.5 \times \left(\frac{C_P}{C_{50}}\right)^\gamma\right]$$

Fig. 2.4 Different response versus concentration (PD) profiles together with their corresponding mathematical equations and parameters.

In cases where the drug diminishes the baseline response, the following expression (Equation 1) for the sigmoidal E_{MAX} model is used (assuming that the response cannot take negative values) where E_{MAX} is constrained between 0 and 1:

$$E = E_0 \bullet \left(1 - E_{MAX} \bullet \frac{C_P^\gamma}{C_P^\gamma + C_{50}^\gamma}\right) \qquad (1)$$

Figure 2.4c represents a characteristic profile corresponding to Equation 1. When E_{MAX} equals 1, the previous expression allows the response value of 0 to be reached asymptotically. The additional PD profiles shown in Fig. 2.4c correspond to a model which allows a sharp decrease in response until it is abolished within the range of drug concentrations used in clinic [17, 18]. In that model, C_{50} represents C_P eliciting a 50% decrease in effect with respect to E_0.

Models for Drug Combinations

There are fields in medicine such as anaesthesia and analgesia where the administration of two or more drugs to achieve the pharmacological goals represents the rule rather than the exception. There are several types of PD interactions between drugs, which can be summarized as additivity (no interaction), antagonism, allosterism and synergism. The model in Equation 2 represents an empirical flexible model that can be used to describe additivity, antagonism or synergism. In fact, that model satisfactorily described the synergism between propofol (Prop) and remifentanil (Remi) on the BIS response in patients undergoing sedation for a gastrointestinal endoscopic procedure [19].

$$BIS = BIS_0 \times$$

$$\left[1 - E_{MAX} \bullet \frac{\left(\frac{C_{e,Prop}}{C_{50,Prop}} + \frac{C_{e,Remi}}{C_{50,Remi}} + \alpha \bullet \frac{C_{e,Prop}}{C_{50,Prop}} \bullet \frac{C_{e,Remi}}{C_{50,Remi}}\right)^{\gamma_{Prop,Remi}}}{1 + \left(\frac{C_{e,Prop}}{C_{50,Prop}} + \frac{C_{e,Remi}}{C_{50,Remi}} + \alpha \bullet \frac{C_{e,Prop}}{C_{50,Prop}} \bullet \frac{C_{e,Remi}}{C_{50,Remi}}\right)^{\gamma_{Prop,Remi}}}\right]$$

$$(2)$$

The parameter describing the type of interaction in Equation 2 is the parameter α, which can be equal to, greater or lower than 0, depending on the type of interaction occurring between the two drugs: absence of interaction (additivity), synergistic interaction or antagonistic interaction respectively. Usually the values of the steepness parameter γ differ from those of the individual drugs. In those cases the steepness of the

concentration versus response curve resulting from the drug combination ($\gamma_{Prop,Remi}$) can be described as a linear function of γ_{Prop} and γ_{Remi} as follows [20]:

$$\gamma_{Prop,Remi} = R \bullet \gamma_{Prop} + (1 - R) \bullet \gamma_{Remi} \qquad (3)$$

where the variable R is calculated as $r_{Prop}/(r_{Prop} + r_{Remi})$, r_{Prop} and r_{Remi} being the ratio between drug concentration and potency (i.e. $r_{Prop} = C_{e,Prop}/C_{50Prop}$) according to the parameterization originally proposed by Minto et al [21]. The R variable is therefore constrained between 0 and 1, and in the absence of either propofol or remifentanil $\gamma_{Prop,Remi}$ is equal to γ_{Remi} or γ_{Prop}, respectively, and Equation 2 reduces to Equation 1.

In cases where one drug (B) cannot exert a measurable effect when administered alone (perhaps because of very low drug concentrations in plasma) but exacerbates the response elicited by a second compound, the following model resembling an allosteric modulation might be considered (Equation 4), where α is the interaction parameter with a value greater than 0.

$$E = E_0 \times \left(1 - E_{MAX} \bullet \frac{C_P^\gamma}{C_P^\gamma + \left(\frac{C_{50}}{1 + \alpha \times C_B}\right)^\gamma}\right) \qquad (4)$$

The interaction between neuromuscular agents acting as antagonists of the postjunctional acetylcholine nicotinic receptor and the antagonist compounds that inhibit acetylcholinesterase, such as neostigmine or edrophonium, that subsequently increase the presence of the agonist acetylcholine has been modelled using the mechanistic model for competitive interaction [22].

All models mentioned above assume the same type of interaction, regardless of the magnitude of the concentration values and their drug interaction ratio. Surface response models [21] overcome that limitation. However, surface response models can prove cumbersome in the case of three or more interacting drugs. In fact, most published examples deal with only two drugs. Recently Wicha et al proposed a comprehensive framework applied to antibiotics that facilitates quantitative description of the response profiles that are the results of the interaction between two or more drugs [23]. Chapter 3 details the presence of synergy in anaesthetic drug interactions.

Pharmacokinetic/Pharmacodynamic Models

In Fig. 2.4 and Equations 1–4, time is not considered, as the assumption of time invariant PD is implicit. Therefore, to describe the time course of effect, both PK and PD models have to be integrated into a PKPD model, as represented by Fig. 2.5 [3, 4, 16].

Generally, the dynamics of the response are complex and not simply directly related to the time course of drug concentrations in plasma. This discrepancy between the time course of drug exposure and time to obtain a response can sometimes be solved by proper study design, e.g. in the case of drugs with a fast onset of action it is recommended to measure drug concentration in arterial blood rather than in venous blood. Most PK/PD studies in the anaesthesia setting are based on arterial blood sampling.

Still, even when high quality data are obtained, the lack of direct connection between PK and response persists. This phenomenon is called hysteresis. One of the main contributions of PKPD modelling to clinical pharmacology is to provide comprehensive models capable of describing the course of drug effect in relationship to plasma or blood concentrations in those situations.

Models for Delayed Response

In anaesthesia and pain treatment, the observation of a delayed response is very common. Fig. 2.6 shows a delayed response presented either with respect to time (Panel a), or with respect to drug concentrations in plasma (Panel b), where the hysteresis loop becomes apparent. Both panels show how the same drug concentration seems to be able to have more than one effect. There are several mechanisms that

can explain the phenomenon of hysteresis. In anaesthesia the most commonly quoted one is a slow drug distribution between the central compartment (which includes plasma/blood) and the biophase (effect compartment).

As described in Chapter 1 the 'link' model presented schematically in Fig. 2.6c was conceptualized by Sheiner et al in 1979 [25]. The assumptions of the model are: (1) the effect site receives a small amount of drug, (2) drug transfer to and from the effect site follows first order kinetics, (3) at equilibrium, concentrations of drug in the biophase (C_e) equal those in plasma and (4) total drug concentrations in the biophase are in free form (not bound to receptors). k_{eo} is the parameter that controls the time required to achieve distribution equilibrium between the central and effect compartments.

$$\frac{dC_e}{dt} = k_{e0} \bullet (C_P - C_e) \qquad (5)$$

Drug effects are a function of C_e, instead of C_p in Equations 1–4.

Since its first use, the effect compartment model has experienced further developments, for example the need to have different k_{eo} values to describe the time course of BIS at different administration rates [26]. Another example is the discrepancy observed in the impact of chronic administration of phenytoin on the C_{50} of vecuronium (high potency drug) and rocuronium (low potency drug) where an increase and no effect was found, respectively, with respect to naïve patients [7, 27].

The quantitative characterization of spinal anaesthesia represents another interesting and practical application of the PKPD framework that couples compartmental PK models (under certain constraints/assumptions regarding drug disposition in the different segments) with the link model, an approach used by Olofsen et al to describe the effects of levobupivacaine and ropivacaine in humans [28].

The so-called turn-over or indirect response models [29] and those models that account for slow receptor deactivation are used to describe delayed response. The indirect response model has been used to describe the respiratory depressant effects of opioids, based on the main assumption that the studied response (i.e. pO_2, pCO_2) is the result of a balance between the rates of synthesis and degradation, each of them governed by the corresponding rate constant. A drug acts either by inhibiting or stimulating the synthesis or degradation rates, where the relationship between the synthesis or

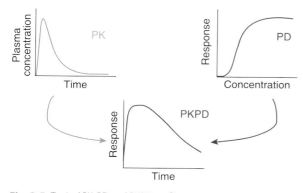

Fig. 2.5 Typical PK, PD and PKPD profiles.

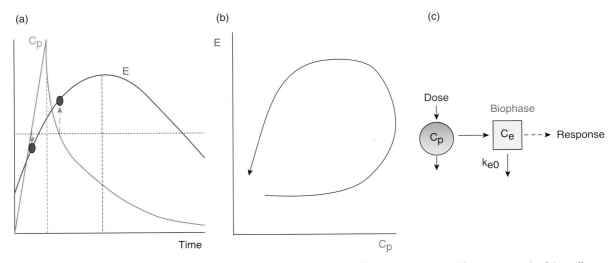

Fig. 2.6 a) Plasma drug concentration (C_p; red) and effect (E, blue) versus time profiles. Points show the different magnitude of drug effects at different times for the same value of C_p; b) counter clockwise hysteresis plot; c) schematic representation of the effect site (link) model. C_e, predicted effect site drug concentrations; k_{e0}, first order rate constant governing the drug distribution disequilibrium between the central and effect site compartments.

degradation rate constant and drug concentrations can be characterized by using the sigmoidal E_{MAX} model or any of its variants. The indirect response models are flexible enough to incorporate complexities such as tolerance and rebound phenomena, as recently shown by Hannam et al [30].

A pharmacological response is the result of the interaction between the drug and its target receptor. Because in anaesthesia rapid onset and offset of drug effect are required, a rapid elimination and reversible drug–receptor binding characteristics are required. On the contrary, in the treatment of chronic pain, sustained analgesic effects are desirable, and in those cases a slower receptor deactivation might be indicated. In the analysis of the migraine effects of the first in class calcitonin gene-related peptide receptor antagonist, Trocóniz et al described the time course of blocked receptors (C_pR) as represented by Equation 6, considering the response is related directly to C_pR [31].

$$\frac{dC_pR}{dt} = k_{on} \bullet C_P \bullet \left[R_{tot} - C_pR \right] - k_{off} \bullet C_pR \qquad (6)$$

Where R_{tot} is the total receptor concentration (arbitrarily set to one), k_{on} is the second order rate constant describing the association between drug and its receptor and k_{off} is the first order rate constant describing the dissociation process of C_pR.

In general, it is difficult to identify and quantify more than one phenomenon responsible for the delayed response (effect-site distribution, turn-over mechanisms, slow receptor deactivation) based upon just data gathered from in vivo studies. A remarkable exception is the description of the antinoceptive effects of buprenorphine in rats and in healthy volunteers by Yassen et al [17, 18].

Models for Non-continuous Responses

The models described so far apply to continuous variables, either PK (i.e. drug concentrations in plasma, or effect site) or PD (i.e. percentage of neuromuscular blockade, drug–receptor complex, BIS, pCO_2). However, on many occasions, the clinical outcome is reported as a non-continuous variable, sometimes as a score category, or as a time to event response, and such data are usually analysed either by logistic regression or survival analysis.

The PK and PK/PD concepts described above for the case of continuous effects apply equally well to non-continuous response analysis. However, in the latter case where the data represent either categories or a time at which a certain event occurs, the model will not predict the value of the effect measured but the probability of being at such category or the probability of survival instead.

Analysis of Ordered Categorical Variables

Ordered categorical data are formed by different scores representing a measurement of the magnitude of the response. In anaesthesia and pain management, ordered categorical variables can be somewhat subjective, either because of the clinicians or the patient. Examples are the Ramsay sedation scale, or scales related to pain relief or pain intensity; the latter includes the use of scores 0, 1, 2 and 3 to denote no, mild, moderate and severe pain, respectively. In the following paragraphs, a modelling framework that allows analysis of ordered categorical covariates is provided [31–33].

The probability [P(Y)] of expressing a certain stage (Y) $\geq m$ (being $m = 0, 1, 2$, or 3) is given by the following expression:

$$P_Y = \frac{e^L}{1 + e^L} \tag{7}$$

Where L stands for logit, and probability of presenting a certain stage (Y) = m, [P(Y=m)], is:

$$P(Y = m) = P(Y \geq m) - P(Y \geq m + 1) \tag{8}$$

The value of the probabilities expressed in Equations 7 and 8 is constrained between 0 and 1. However, L can take any value between $-$ and $+ \infty$, and represents the part of the model in which drug effects are incorporated, and can present the following general form:

$$L = f_{t=0}(m) + h(time) + g(C_e) \tag{9}$$

where h and g correspond to the models for placebo and drug effects, respectively. The description of the stages at the time of administration is given by $f_{t=0}(m)$ and is expressed as $\sum_{k=1}^{m}\beta_k$, where β_k (k=1, …, m) are the parameters defining the baseline probabilities of having an $\geq m$ stage at the start of the study.

Time to Event Modelling

Examples of time to event data in anaesthesia include time of re-medication, time to a nausea episode or time to recovery of consciousness. These events must be analysed through survival analysis. From a modelling point of view in survival analysis the critical point is the search for the best structure of the 'hazard function' (hz). One can think about the hazard rate in a similar way as the logit, with the only limitation that the hazard rate cannot get to negative values. The argument of the

hazard includes baseline components, disease progression and drug effects. The following expression relates the hazard function with the survival probability [S(t)]:

$$S(t) = e^{-Hz} \tag{10}$$

where Hz is the cumulative hazard. In the analgesia literature, time to events modelling has been applied to describe the time to re-medication [31, 32]. Recently, Juul et al proposed a repeated time to event model to predict analgesic consumption during postoperative pain treatment [34].

Data Analysis

In this section of the chapter a brief description of the methodology of analysis is provided in the context of the data driven (top-down) modelling.

One of the main objectives of modelling is to characterize quantitatively the behaviour of the drug in the target population, to identify which are the drug properties in the typical individual, to identify the characteristics, covariate factors, of the patients that are responsible for the differences in drug PK and PK/PD behaviour across subjects, and to quantify the magnitude of the uncertainty that cannot be explained by covariates (inter-individual or inter-patient variability).

Given that one major goal in PK/PD data analysis is to quantify the magnitude of the inter-patient variability, it is not surprising that information from all individuals participating in the study is considered. But there is not just a single manner to analyse data from different individuals. One obvious possibility is to analyse the data on each subject individually and then compute the central tendency (mean, median) and dispersion of the model parameters within the study population, establishing the relationships between model parameters and covariates. This procedure is called the two-step approach. It has the advantage of its simplicity but it also has a number of drawbacks because individuals within the same studied population can be described with different models, or because there is a need to have rich data to get robust estimates of the individual parameters.

Population Approach

Currently the most widely used approach in PK/PD analysis is the population analysis, in which all data from all subjects in the study are included simultaneously, but the individuality is preserved. Each patient contributes to characterize the rest of the population and contributes to generate the typical (and individual) profiles.

This approach is now being applied in all stages of drug development and represents a key pillar in model-based individualization of drug administration. Its goal is to provide a complete quantitative characterization of the PK/PD profile of a drug in the target population. The following three questions need to be answered: (1) what is the typical behaviour? (2) which are the patient characteristics (covariates) affecting PK and PD characteristics of the drug? and (3) what is the degree of unexplained variability in PK and in drug response? [35]. There are currently several software packages that can be used to develop population PK/PD models, with NONMEM [36] and MONOLIX [37] being the most widely used.

Components of a Population and Nomenclature

A population model is composed of two fundamental parts: the structural part and the stochastic part. Fig. 2.7 provides an overview of the elements of a population model [35].

Structural Elements

The structural part of the population model relates to the above first two questions regarding typical characteristics and covariate effects. In the absence of covariate effects, the structural part describes the PK or PK/PD characteristics of the typical individual (represented by the corresponding PK or PK/PD model and the respective model parameters). If a covariate has been identified, for example genotype on CL, the structural part of the model describes the characteristics of the drug for typical poor and fast metabolizing individuals.

Assuming a one compartment PK model after continuous infusion, V and CL represent the parameters of the model. The PK profile for the typical individual is governed by the dosing schedule and the typical parameter values (TPV) that in the population context are defined as fixed effect parameters, as they are equal for all patients in the population. Fixed effects or typical parameters are denoted as THETA (θ).

Covariates – Chapter 4 is fully devoted to the topic of covariate factors. The present section aims to refer only to those aspects more related to PK/PD modelling.

The distribution and elimination characteristics can be different across individuals due to differences in physiopathology which are represented by covariates. The spectrum of possible covariates is very broad.

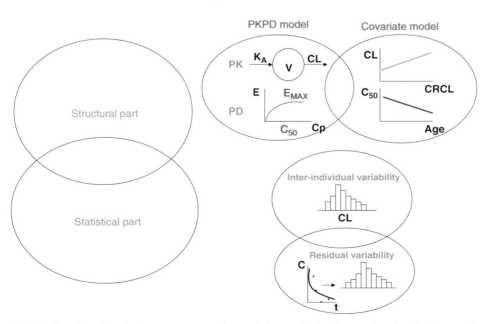

Population model

Fig. 2.7 Overview of the different components of a population model. PK, pharmacokinetics; PD, pharmacodynamics; V, apparent volume of distribution; K_A, first order rate constant of absorption; CL, total plasma clearance; E, drug effects; C_p, plasma drug concentration; E_{MAX}, maximum response magnitude that the drug can elicit; C_{50}, C_p level eliciting half of E_{MAX}; CRCL, creatinine clearance.

For example, there are covariates associated with (1) laboratory values such as ALT, AST, bilirubin, plasma proteins and creatinine clearance, (2) demographic factors such as gender, body weight, age, race, (3) genetics such as polymorphisms of hepatic enzymes or receptors, (4) disease-related factors such as co-medications, markers of severity of the disease and (5) habits, such as diet, exercise and alcohol or caffeine consumption. Covariates can also be classified as continuous and non-continuous. Non-continuous covariates can be either binary (e.g. gender) or categorical [ordered (e.g. alcohol consumption), non-ordered (e.g. race)]. Covariates can vary with time, however within the time frame of an anaesthestic it is considered that they remain constant during the study period.

Equation 11 represents a general expression for a covariate model including both continuous and non-continuous covariates:

$$TVP = \theta_n \bullet \prod_1^m \left(\frac{cov_m}{cov_{m,ref}} \right)^{\theta_{m+n}} \bullet \prod_1^p \theta_{p+m+n}^{cov_p} \qquad (11)$$

where the typical value of a model parameter is described as a function of m continuous (cov_m) and p categorical (cov_p) covariates. θ_n describes the nth typical parameter value for an individual with covariate values (cov_m) equal to the reference values: [($cov_m = cov_{m,ref}$) and ($cov_p = 0$)]. $cov_{m,ref}$ refers usually to the median value across the studied populations. θ_{m+n} and θ_{p+m+n} are parameters quantifying the magnitude of the covariate–parameter relationship.

Stochastic Elements

Inter-patient variability (IIV) and residual error/variability (RV) are the two main stochastic elements. Inter-occasion and inter-study variabilities are also stochastic elements but unlikely to play a relevant role in the field of anaesthesia.

Because differences in physiopathology between patients (represented by covariates) are responsible for the magnitude of IIV, it is important that influential covariates can be identified and incorporated into the PK/PD model to decrease variability, allowing optimal individualization of drug dosing. On the other hand, RV refers to unexplained variability resulting from errors in sampling times, imprecision and inaccuracy of the analytical methods and model misspecifications among others.

IIV and RV are called random effects. Just like in the case of the structural part of a population model where different PK or PKPD are possible, the analysts ('modellers') have to select the models for the random effects.

Because of inter-individual variability and because PK or PK/PD parameters cannot be negative, the exponential model is the most used. The distributions of the parameter and the random effect are log-normal and normal, respectively. The value of a specific parameter (i.e. CL or V) for the ith patient in the studied population (p_i) is therefore expressed as $p_i = \theta \bullet e^{\eta i}$, where η_i is the discrepancy between p_i and the estimate of the typical parameter value θ. For each parameter in the model there is one η value per subject. The set of ηs comprises a random variable with mean and variance of 0 and ω^2, respectively. As any PK or PK/PD model is represented by more than just one parameter, there will be a variance term for each model parameter (i.e. ω^2_V, ω^2_{CL}) that corresponds to the diagonal elements of the variance covariance matrix Ω. The off-diagonal elements represent the covariance between the diagonal elements. That covariance(s), which can be 0, represent the correlation of ηs between two or more parameters.

There are other modelling alternatives to the exponential model for IIV, such as the use of the so-called semi-parametric models, which maintain the assumption of normal distribution of the random effects but use the Box-Cox, Heavy tail or Logit transformations to relate random effects with the individual parameters [38]. In addition, mixture models provide an alternative that considers multi-modal distributions of random effects [39].

Just like with IIV, different models are used to model residual variability. In general, the relationship between observations (y) and model predictions (y_{pred}) is assumed to be one of the following: (1) independent of the magnitude of the predictions (additive error model), (2) proportional to the magnitude of the prediction (proportional error model) and (3) a combination of the additive and proportional models (combined error model). The additive model applies when the entity to be modelled experiences moderate changes during the course of the study, as is usually the case when pharmacological responses are being modelled. The proportional error model is used when the values of the variable differ in several orders of magnitude, as in the case of plasma drug concentrations after intravenous bolus or short infusion administration and short half-lives. The combined error model is recommended in cases when the drug concentrations corresponding to the late sampling times show little change in magnitude.

The following expression corresponds to the proportional error model:

$$y_j = y_{pred,j} \bullet (1 + y_{pred,j} \bullet \varepsilon_j) \qquad (12)$$

where ε_j corresponds to the discrepancies between y and y_{pred} at the jth measurement time. For each observation in the data there is one ε value. The set of εs comprises a random variable with mean and variance of 0 and σ^2, respectively, the latter corresponding to the diagonal element of the variance covariance matrix Σ. The matrix Σ can have more than one diagonal element and eventually covariance in the case of modelling two different entities, for example drug and metabolite concentrations.

Model Building

The objective of a population PK or PK/PD model is to provide accurate and precise estimates of θ, Ω and Σ.

It is important to keep in mind that an adequate and useful population PKPD model is not just the result of the modelling expertise: study design and data (and their organization) play a fundamental role.

In general, the model building process follows three steps as explained below.

Base Population Model

The objective here is to develop a model that does not need to be the one that will finally be selected, but it should be able to properly describe the data by capturing the typical profile(s) and dispersion (variability and noise), and should provide physiologically plausible and precise estimates of the fixed and random effects. The tasks to be performed would be to (1) select between different structural models (i.e. mono- versus two compartments model), (2) identify which of the fixed effect parameters in the model are associated with IIV, and whether or not there is covariance between the off-diagonal elements of the Ω matrix, and (3) select the best residual error model and consider the benefit of performing the analysis using transformed (i.e. logarithmic) data. At this step, covariate effects are not explored, unless a covariate shows such an impact that it has to be included in the model to select the base population model.

Model selection – Selection between models is mainly based on the minimum value of the objective function provided by NONMEM, which is equal to –2X Log likelihood (–2LL); –2LL differences of 3.84, 7.88 and 11 are considered significant at the 5%, 0.5% and 0.1% levels, respectively, for nested models differing in one parameter. For non-nested models the Akaike information criterion can be used to assist during model building [40]. The goodness of fit plot represents another tool commonly used during model building (Fig. 2.8, left).

Covariate Selection

This second step focuses on covariate selection. Often some available covariates show correlations, which are often the case with weight, height and body surface area. In those cases, only the most relevant covariate factors with regard to usual dose-adjustments in the clinical setting are kept for further study of its effects.

Given the fact that, in general, in a clinical trial or study the number of covariates can be high and that several parameters can be affected by the covariate information, efficient covariate selection will benefit from automated procedures. The stepwise covariate model (SCM) building procedure [41] implemented in the Pearl Speaks NONMEM (PsN) software [42] is probably the most frequently used approach to select the group of covariates that statistically (see above) improve the fit. The SCM procedure is based on a forward inclusion followed by a backward deletion approach. During the forward inclusion and the backward deletion approaches the levels of significance used to incorporate the covariate effect in the model are set to 0.05 and 0.001, respectively. When possible it is recommended to perform a science-based covariate grouping before starting the SCM analysis. Covariate grouping means to check out a selection of these covariates and examine whether it makes sense to associate them with each one of the parameters of the model. For example, one should try to link genetic polymorphisms at the level of hepatic enzymes and creatinine clearance to total plasma clearance, and not to the apparent volume of distribution.

Common covariates detected in anaesthesia research are age, weight and gender [43–46], whereas genetic-related effects are less frequently incorporated in population PK/PD models [18, 47].

Model Refinement and Evaluation

Once the population model – including the statistically significant covariates – is in place, some additional checks are convenient to perform in order to evaluate whether or not parameter estimates are meaningful from a physiological perspective, whether the covariates exert an effect on parameters

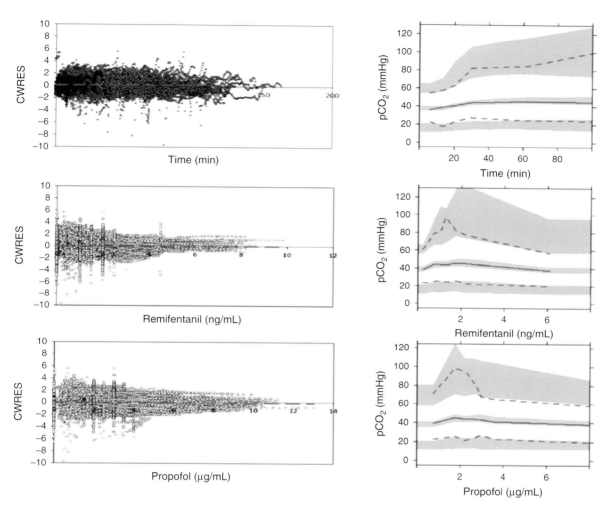

Fig. 2.8 Results from a model evaluation exercise. **Left panels**, conditional weighted residuals (CWRES) versus time (upper), and levels of remifentanil (middle) or propofol (lower). Horizontal lines represent ideal fit (grey solid) and a smoothing (loess) through the points (red dashed line). In the upper panel, red and blue circles correspond to data gathered in presence of propofol or remifentanil alone, respectively. **Right panels**, results from the prediction-corrected visual predictive checks. Shaded areas correspond to the 90% prediction intervals of the corresponding percentiles calculated from 1000 simulated datasets. Lines show the 5th (lower, red dashed), 50th (middle, red solid) and 95th (upper, red dashed) percentiles of the raw data. *Adapted from*: *Hannam JA, Borrat X, Trocóniz IF, Valencia JF, Jensen EW, Pedroso A, Muñoz J, Castellví-Bel S, Castells A, Gambús PL. Modeling respiratory depression induced by remifentanil and propofol during sedation and analgesia using a continuous non-invasive measurement of pCO2. J.Pharmacol.Exp.Ther. 2016 Mar; 356(3): 563–73.*

according to current knowledge of physiology and disease.

The final step refers to model evaluation based on simulation procedures. For example, the precision of the parameters is further evaluated by performing a non-parametric bootstrap analysis. Then the 95% confidence intervals can be compared with those obtained from the COVARIANCE step using the estimates of the standard errors, assuming that the intervals are symmetrically distributed around the point estimate.

Again the PsN software [42] allows one to perform the bootstrap analysis quite efficiently and allows the modeller to keep in the different bootstrap datasets the same characteristics as the original one, for example the number of subjects of a certain ethnicity, or receiving a particular dose level, etc.

The performance of the Model is usually evaluated by Visual, or prediction corrected Visual Predictive Checks (pcVPCs) [48]. To do so requires generating by means of simulation techniques usually a number (e.g. 500, or 1000) of datasets with the same study characteristics as the original. The 2.5th, 50th and 97.5th percentiles of the simulated observations in each dataset are computed for different time intervals and the 95% prediction interval of each calculated percentile is obtained and plotted against the 2.5th, 50th and 97.5th percentiles obtained from the raw data. A model is considered to have a good descriptive capability if the percentiles of the observed time profiles of the drug concentration or response lie within the 95% prediction intervals calculated from the simulations (see Fig. 2.8, right).

Please note that the simulation-based procedure described for model evaluation challenges the model against the raw data used for its development, which represents an internal evaluation. If additional data are available from another cohort of patients, then an external evaluation (in this case prospective validation) can be (and should) be performed, which will increase the validity of the selected model.

It must be kept in mind that most of the population models include covariates. However, if those covariates proved just statistical significance it would be mandatory to conduct an explorative procedure to further explore the clinical significance (i.e. whether or not it would be necessary to modify dose requirements in certain patient populations). Different metrics of interest can be identified, for example Cmax, AUC or steady-state drug concentrations with respect to PK, and maximum effect or time to recover 90% of the baseline value with respect to the pharmacological action. Then, different covariate groups are selected according to the covariates included, and for each group, for instance, 500 individual PK profiles are simulated. Finally, covariate effects are evaluated similarly to drug bioequivalence tests: metrics are compared to the 80–125% range of the distribution obtained from the group with covariate values equal to the median of the patient population studied.

Applications

Once a population PKPD model has been selected and evaluated (and eventually validated), it has to be realized that it represents a very powerful tool to learn and understand how the drug acts in new clinical scenarios. New clinical scenarios we could envision are: (1) different dose levels or administration schedules, (2) other patient populations, or (3) types of surgery that require different degrees of anaesthesia or sedation. Due to the stochastic elements of a population model,

the individual PK and response profiles corresponding to a patient population of interest can be generated under different scenarios and relevant metrics of clinical interest could be compared

If population models for different drugs are available, comparison across drugs can be performed, and the effect of administering them in combination can be explored.

Another very interesting application is the possibility to adapt in real time the patient's dosing requirements with respect to a clinical endpoint or pharmacological target. If a population PK/PD model is available, individual parameters can be obtained based on initial clinical observations, and then the dose can be adjusted appropriately.

References

1. Holford N: Clinical pharmacology = disease progression + drug action. Br.J.Clin.Pharmacol. 2015; 79: 18–27.

2. Verotta D, Sheiner LB: A general conceptual model for non-steady state pharmacokinetic/pharmacodynamic data. J.Pharmacokinet.Biopharm. 1995; 23: 1–4.

3. Tozer TN, Rowland M: *Introduction to Pharmacokinetics and Pharmacodynamics: The Quantitative Basis of Drug Therapy*. Philadelphia, PA: Lippincott Williams & Wilkins, 2006.

4. Holford NH, Sheiner LB: Understanding the dose-effect relationship: clinical application of pharmacokinetic-pharmacodynamic models. Clin. Pharmacokinet. 1981; 6: 429–53.

5. Schnider TW, Minto CF, Gambus PL, Andresen C, Goodale DB, Shafer SL. Youngs EJ: The influence of method of administration and covariates on the pharmacokinetics of propofol in adult volunteers. Anesthesiology. 1998; 88: 1170–82.

6. Hannivoort LN, Eleveld DJ, Proost JH, Reyntjens KM, Absalom AR, Vereecke HE, Struys MM: Development of an optimized pharmacokinetic model of dexmedetomidine using target-controlled infusion in healthy volunteers. Anesthesiology. 2015; 123: 357–67.

7. Fernández-Candil J, Gambús PL, Trocóniz IF, Valero R, Carrero E, Bueno L, Fábregas N: Pharmacokinetic-pharmacodynamic modeling of the influence of chronic phenytoin therapy on the rocuronium bromide response in patients undergoing brain surgery. Eur.J.Clin.Pharmacol. 2008; 64: 795–806.

8. Trocóniz IF, Armenteros S, Planelles MV, Benítez J, Calvo R, Domínguez R: Pharmacokinetic-pharmacodynamic modelling of the antipyretic effect of two oral formulations of ibuprofen. Clin. Pharmacokinet. 2000; 38: 505–18.

9. Anderson BJ, Holford NH: Understanding dosing: children are small adults, neonates are immature children. Arch.Dis.Child 2013; 98: 737–44.

10. Holford N, Heo YA, Anderson B: A pharmacokinetic standard for babies and adults. J.Pharm.Sci. 2013; 102: 2941–52.

11. Allegaert K, Holford N, Anderson BJ, Holford S, Stuber F, Rochette A, Trocóniz IF, Beier H, de Hoon JN, Pedersen RS, Stamer U: Tramadol and o-desmethyl tramadol clearance maturation and disposition in humans: a pooled pharmacokinetic study. Clin. Pharmacokinet. 2015; 54: 167–78.

12. Anderson BJ, Larsson P: A maturation model for midazolam clearance. Paediatr.Anaesth. 2011; 21: 302–8.

13. Björkman S, Wada DR, Stanski DR, Ebling WF: Comparative physiological pharmacokinetics of fentanyl and alfentanil in rats and humans based on parametric single-tissue models. J.Pharmacokinet. Biopharm. 1994; 22: 381–410.

14. Masui K, Upton RN, Doufas AG, Coetzee JF, Kazama T, Mortier EP, Struys MM: The performance of compartmental and physiologically based recirculatory pharmacokinetic models for propofol: a comparison using bolus, continuous, and target-controlled infusion data. Anesth.Analg. 2010; 111: 368–79.

15. Levitt DG, Schnider TW: Human physiologically based pharmacokinetic model for propofol. BMC Anesthesiol. 2005; 5: 4.

16. Holford NH, Sheiner LB: Kinetics of pharmacologic response. Pharmacol.Ther. 1982; 16: 143–66.

17. Yassen A, Olofsen E, Dahan A. Danhof M: Pharmacokinetic-pharmacodynamic modeling of the antinociceptive effect of buprenorphine and fentanyl in rats: role of receptor equilibration kinetics. J. Pharmacol.Exp.Ther 2005; 313: 1136–49.

18. Yassen A, Olofsen E, Romberg R, Sarton E, Teppema L, Danhof M. Dahan A: Mechanism-based PK/PD modeling of the respiratory depressant effect of buprenorphine and fentanyl in healthy volunteers. Clin.Pharmacol.Ther. 2007; 81: 50–8.

19. Borrat X, Trocóniz IF, Valencia JF, Rivadulla S, Sendino O, Llach J, Muñoz J, Castellví-Bel S, Jospin M, Jensen EW, Castells A, Gambús PL: Modeling the influence of the A118G polymorphism in the OPRM1 gene and of noxious stimulation on the synergistic relation between propofol and remifentanil: sedation and analgesia in endoscopic procedures. Anesthesiology. 2013; 118: 1395–407.

20. Jonker DM, Voskuyl RA, Danhof M. Pharmacodynamic analysis of the anticonvulsant effects of tiagabine and lamotrigine in combination in the rat. Epilepsia. 2004; 45: 424–35.

21. Minto CF, Schnider TW, Short TG, Gregg KM, Gentilini A, Shafer SL: Response surface model for anesthetic drug interactions. Anesthesiology. 2000; 92: 1603–16.

22. Verotta D, Kitts J, Rodriguez R, Coldwell J, Miller RD, Sheiner LB: Reversal of neuromuscular blockade in humans by neostigmine and edrophonium: a mathematical model. J.Pharmacokinet.Biopharm. 1991; 19: 713–29.

23. Wicha SG, Chen C, Clewe O, Simonsson USH. A general pharmacodynamic interaction model identifies perpetrators and victims in drug interactions. Nat. Commun. 2017; 8: 2129.

24. Segre G. Kinetics of interaction between drugs and biological systems. Farmaco Sci. 1968; 23: 907–18.

25. Sheiner LB, Stanski DR, Vozeh S, Miller RD, Ham J: Simultaneous modeling of pharmacokinetics and pharmacodynamics: application to d-tubocurarine. Clin.Pharmacol.Ther. 1979; 25: 358–71.

26. Struys MM, Coppens MJ, De Neve N, Mortier EP, Doufas AG, Van Bocxlaer JF, Shafer SL: Influence of administration rate on propofol plasma-effect site equilibration. Anesthesiology. 2007; 107: 386–96.

27. Wright PM, McCarthy G, Szenohradszky J, Sharma ML, Caldwell JE: Influence of chronic phenytoin administration on the pharmacokinetics and pharmacodynamics of vecuronium. Anesthesiology. 2004; 100: 626–33.

28. Olofsen E, Burm AG, Simon MJ, Veering BT, van Kleef JW, Dahan A: Population pharmacokinetic-pharmacodynamic modeling of epidural anesthesia. Anesthesiology. 2008; 109: 664–74.

29. Dayneka NL, Garg V. Jusko WJ: Comparison of four basic models of indirect pharmacodynamic responses. J.Pharmacokinet.Biopharm. 1993; 21: 457–78.

30. Hannam JA, Borrat X, Trocóniz IF, Valencia JF, Jensen EW, Pedroso A, Muñoz J, Castellví-Bel S, Castells A, Gambús PL: Modeling respiratory depression induced by remifentanil and propofol during sedation and analgesia using a continuous non-invasive measurement of pCO_2. J.Pharmacol.Exp.Ther. 2016; 356: 563–73.

31. Trocóniz IF, Wolters JM, Tillmann C, Schaefer HG, Roth W: Modelling the anti-migraine effects of BIBN 4096 BS: a new calcitonin gene-related peptide receptor antagonist. Clin.Pharmacokinet. 2006; 45: 715–28.

32. Mandema JW, Stanski DR: Population pharmacodynamic model for ketorolac analgesia. Clin. Pharmacol.Ther. 1996; 60: 619–35.

33. Fábregas N, Rapado J, Gambús PL, Valero R, Carrero E, Salvador L, Nalda-Felipe MA, Trocóniz IF: Modeling of the sedative and airway obstruction effects of propofol in patients with Parkinson's disease undergoing stereotactic surgery. Anesthesiology. 2002; 97: 1378–86.

34. Juul RV, Rasmussen S, Kreilgaard M, Christrup LL, Simonsson US, Lund TM: Repeated time-to-event analysis of consecutive analgesic events in postoperative pain. Anesthesiology. 2015; 123: 1411–19.

35. Bonate PL: *Pharmacokinetic-pharmacodynamic Modeling and Simulation*. New York: Springer, 2005.

36. Beal S, Sheiner LB, Boeckmann A, Bauer RJ: *NONMEM User's Guides (1989–2015)*. Ellicott City: Icon Development Solutions, 2015.

37. Monolix version 192018R1. Antony, France: Lixoft SAS, 2018. http://lixoft.com/products/monolix/ [last accessed 6 June 2019].

38. Petersson KJ, Hanze E, Savic RM, Karlsson MO: Semiparametric distributions with estimated shape parameters. Pharm.Res. 2009 Sep; 26(9): 2174–85.

39. Carlsson KC, Savić RM, Hooker AC, Karlsson MO: Modeling subpopulations with the $MIXTURE subroutine in NONMEM: finding the individual probability of belonging to a subpopulation for the use in model analysis and improved decision making. AAPS J. 2009 Mar; 11(1): 148–54.

40. Ludden TM, Beal SL, Sheiner LB: Comparison of the Akaike information criterion, the Schwarz criterion and the F test as guides to model selection. J. Pharmacokinet.Biopharm. 1994; 22: 431–45.

41. Jonsson E, Karlsson MO: Automated covariate model building within NONMEM. Pharm.Res. 1998; 15: 1463–8.

42. Lindbom L, Pihlgren P, Jonsson EN: PsN toolkit: a collection of computer intensive statistical methods for nonlinear mixed effect modelling using NONMEM. Comput. Methods. Programs. Biomed. 2005; 79: 241–57.

43. Minto CF, Schnider TW, Egan TD, Youngs E, Lemmens HJ, Gambus PL, Billard V, Hoke JF, Moore KH, Hermann DJ, Muir KT, Mandema JW, Shafer SL: Influence of age and gender on the pharmacokinetics and pharmacodynamics of remifentanil. I. Model development. Anesthesiology. 1997; 86: 10–23.

44. Schnider TW, Minto CF, Shafer SL, Gambus PL, Andresen C, Goodale DB, Youngs EJ: The influence of age on propofol pharmacodynamics. Anesthesiology. 1999; 90: 1502–16.

45. Cortínez LI, Trocóniz IF, Fuentes R, Gambús P, Hsu YW, Altermatt F, Muñoz HR: The influence of age on the dynamic relationship between end-tidal sevoflurane concentrations and bispectral index. Anesth.Analg. 2008; 107: 1566–72.

46. Sarton E, Olofsen E, Romberg R, den Hartigh J, Kest B, Nieuwenhuijs D, Burm A, Teppema L, Dahan A: Sex differences in morphine analgesia: an experimental study in healthy volunteers. Anesthesiology. 2000; 93: 1245–54.

47. Romberg RR, Olofsen E, Bijl H, Taschner PE, Teppema LJ, Sarton EY, van Kleef JW, Dahan A: Polymorphism of mu-opioid receptor gene (OPRM1:c.118A>G) does not protect against opioid-induced respiratory depression despite reduced analgesic response. Anesthesiology. 2005; 102: 522–30.

48. Bergstrand M, Hooker AC, Wallin JE, Karlsson MO: Prediction-corrected visual predictive checks for diagnosing nonlinear mixed-effects models. AAPS J. 2011; 13 (2): 143–51.

Drug Interactions: Additivity and Synergy among Anaesthetic Drugs

Jacqueline A. Hannam and Timothy G. Short

Summary

Modern anaesthesia and sedation consists of giving combinations of hypnotic and analgesic drugs to obtain the desired anaesthetic effect. Understanding how these drugs interact to create the anaesthetic state improves the precision of anaesthetic drug dosing and physiological stability of the patient.

Anaesthetic drugs often interact synergistically, which is important because greater sedative effect occurs at lower doses when combined and concentration-dependent side effects may be reduced if total drug dosage is adjusted appropriately. Propofol and opioids, and volatile anaesthetics and opioids, interact synergistically in suppressing movement and haemodynamic responses to noxious stimulus, but additively for reduction of bispectral index (BIS), and are commonly combined for anaesthesia.

Traditionally, pharmacodynamic interactions have been studied using shifts in dose–response curve or isobolographic analysis. These methods provide useful markers of the magnitude of interaction between various combinations of agents, but do not inform us of the time course of combined drug effect. The adoption of response surface methodology allows continuous prediction of drug effect for any dose combination to be derived in real-time. Interaction models can be incorporated into population models for syringe pump drivers, to guide closed-loop anaesthesia and to display predicted effects of drug combinations. Using measures of depth of hypnotic effect such as the processed EEG or blood pressure to adjust dosage, these population models are surprisingly accurate in individuals and enhance the precision of drug dosage in clinical practice.

The Importance of Drug Interactions in Anaesthesia

Anaesthetic pharmacology teaching has emphasized the actions of individual drugs. However, modern anaesthesia consists of giving combinations of drugs to achieve the desired balance of hypnosis, analgesia, immobility and reflex suppression in our patients. Common drug combinations include a hypnotic such as propofol with an opioid such as fentanyl or remifentanil, or a volatile anaesthetic such as sevoflurane with an opioid analgesic. The individual actions of these drugs have been well described and are familiar to all anaesthetists, but how they interact to produce the anaesthetic state is less well appreciated: combinations can be synergistic in their hypnotic and analgesic effects, but also can increase the incidence of hypotension and respiratory depression. A good understanding of the pharmacology of commonly used drug combinations allows more precise drug dosing and hopefully safer anaesthesia. Modern anaesthetic displays and anaesthesia delivery systems have incorporated these interaction models into their predictions of drug effect.

In this chapter we outline the methods used to study drug interactions, briefly describe the important interactions that occur between commonly used classes of drugs and illustrate how this methodology is incorporated into some practical applications in modern anaesthesia.

Pharmacokinetic Interactions

Interactions may affect a drug's pharmacokinetic (PK) profile, its pharmacodynamic (PD) profile, or both. A PK interaction occurs when a co-administered drug changes the absorption, distribution or elimination of another drug, altering its concentration–time relationship. To describe whether an interaction is due to changes in its PK profile requires the measurement of drug concentrations. Common examples in anaesthesia exist: when midazolam and propofol are combined there is reduced clearance of both drugs, resulting in a 25% increase in propofol concentration and a 27% increase in midazolam concentration in the blood [1, 2]; similarly, alfentanil and sufentanil reduce the clearance of propofol [3].

Pharmacodynamic Interactions

A PD interaction occurs when one drug alters the concentration–effect relationship of another drug. When the two drugs work at the same site on a receptor, then the interaction between the two drugs may be additive or antagonistic, depending on the affinity of each drug for the receptor site and whether it is an agonist or antagonist (efficacy). However, even when drugs have different modes of action, they may also interact, so that the required dose of each drug to produce the same effect is reduced when the combination is given. For example, the dose of propofol to cause hypnosis is reduced by an opioid such as fentanyl, and similarly propofol reduces the dose of fentanyl required to suppress movement to a noxious stimulus.

Most drug combination research in anaesthesia has been based on observational studies of patients without blood sampling, so that the relative contribution of PK and PD interactions to the overall drug effect of the combination has not necessarily been studied.

Methods to Study Drug Interactions

Shift in the Dose–Response Curve

The simplest way to study an interaction is to determine whether one drug alters the dose- or concentration–response curve of a second drug. To do this, a response curve in either the dose or concentration domain is constructed for the first drug when given alone, and this is then repeated in the presence of a fixed dose of the second drug (Fig. 3.1a). If the dose–response curve for the first drug is altered after adding the second drug, then this suggests that the drugs interact. This method has been used extensively for the study of combinations of volatile anaesthetics with opioids and shows a large reduction in the concentration of volatile anaesthetic required to suppress movement to a noxious stimulus (i.e. MAC, the minimum alveolar concentration) and a small reduction in the concentration of volatile anaesthetic required to produce hypnosis (i.e. MACawake). This interaction is often referred to as MAC-reduction. For instance a concentration of remifentanil of 1.25 ng/mL halves the sevoflurane partial pressure required to suppress movement to a noxious stimulus, and is also sufficient to completely eliminate response to a light stimulus such as prodding or shaking [4]. A limitation of this method is that it only describes the interaction for one dose

combination and does not determine whether the interaction is additive or synergistic. It is however a useful method when one of the drugs is not capable of reliably causing the effect under observation in all patients when given alone.

Isobolograms

To determine the nature of a PD interaction, we must first define additivity (or the 'expected' effect) and synergism. The best definition of additivity is that proposed by Loewe [5]. It is based on the concept that a drug cannot interact with itself. If we have a drug that, at a dose of 2 mg, causes 50% of the maximal drug effect (defined as the C_{50}), then it is obvious that two 1 mg doses, or any other combination of doses that equals 2, will also produce the same effect. This can be depicted visually by using an isobologram (Fig. 3.1b). The line connects the dose pairs that together cause the same effect and is called an isoeffect line; if the line is straight then the drugs are additive. Additivity can be defined mathematically as:

$$\frac{a}{A} + \frac{b}{B} = I \qquad (1)$$

where a and b are the doses of two drugs that when given together cause the target effect, A and B are the doses of each drug that when given alone cause the same target effect, and I is the interaction index. $I = 1$ for an additive relationship. If $I < 1$, there is inward bowing of the isobologram curve (i.e. towards the origin of the graph where the concentration of both drugs is zero) and synergy (or supra-additivity) exists. If $I > 1$, there is outward bowing of the isobologram curve and infra-additivity exists. The term infra-additivity is used rather than antagonism to distinguish between those drugs that simply act via different mechanisms, and consequently have contrasting effects, and those that display true pharmacological antagonism in which the dose requirement of one drug is increased by the presence of a second drug (e.g. fentanyl in the presence of naloxone, an opioid antagonist).

Isobolographic methods are robust when both drugs can achieve the target endpoint when given alone, and confidence intervals can be calculated for the line of additivity to assess the precision with which we know the shape of the curve. Multiple isobolograms can be studied for a drug, each determining a different level of effect, but the method suffers from the disadvantage that only one level of effect can be studied at a time. Isobolograms have been drawn for a variety of hypnotic pairs; for instance midazolam–thiopentone and midazolam–propofol combinations have both been found to be synergistic for hypnosis [6, 7].

Response Surface Models

Response surface modelling describes the complete dose–response relationship for a combination of two drugs (Fig. 3.1c). A response surface model incorporates

the shift in dose–response curve and isobologram techniques already mentioned. There are several methods based on a standard sigmoid dose–response curve (or Hill equation, Equation 2) used to describe the PD dose–response relationship for an anaesthetic drug, to two or more drugs [8]:

$$E = E_0 + \left(E_{MAX} \cdot \frac{Ce^{\gamma}}{\left(C_{50}^{\gamma} + Ce^{\gamma}\right)} \right) \quad (2)$$

where E_0 is the baseline response, Ce is the concentration in the effect compartment, C_{50} is the concentration producing 50% of the maximal effect E_{MAX}, and γ relates to the steepness of the curve. E_{MAX}, C_{50} and γ are parameters to be estimated. Although shown here for Ce, this equation can also be used for Cp, concentration in the plasma, or for dose.

Three main methods of deriving a response surface have been used in anaesthesia. They are known as the Minto, Greco and hierarchical methods [9–11]. The Minto and Greco models both normalize the concentration of each drug to account for differences in dose required to achieve the same effect:

$$U_A = Ce/C_{50A} \quad (3)$$

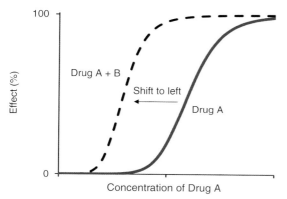

(a) **Shift in dose–response curve**

Effect (%) / Concentration of Drug A

Drug A + B

Shift to left

Drug A

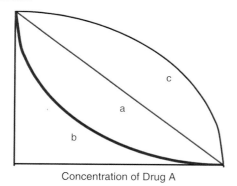

(b) **Isobole**

Concentration of Drug B / Concentration of Drug A

c

a

b

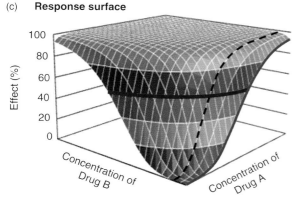

(c) **Response surface**

Effect (%)

Concentration of Drug B

Concentration of Drug A

Fig. 3.1 Different methods for studying drug interactions in anaesthesia.

(a) Shift in dose–response curve. A shift in dose–response curve of drug A in the presence of a constant concentration of drug B indicates an interaction. Shifts to the left (resulting in reduced dose or concentration requirements) indicate synergy. Dose–response curves for both individual drugs (at the outer-faces of the surface) and combinations of dose pairs are displayed on the response-surface (c) as vertical slices (purple lines).

(b) The isobologram. An isobologram shows concentration (or dose) pairs that cause the same effect (often called iso-effect lines, usually these relate to some clinically useful index such as 50% or 95% of the maximal response for the endpoint in question). Additivity is suggested by a linear relationship (a), while supra-additivity [or synergism, (b)] and infra-additivity (c) are displayed by curves bowing towards or away from the origin. Isobolograms are visible on the response-surface (c) as horizontal slices (blue lines).

(c) Response surface. A response surface for the effects of a two-drug combination is shown. All possible concentration combinations of the two drugs and their resulting effects are incorporated into the surface. Bowing of the surface towards the reader (as highlighted by the blue line at the 50% effect level) indicates synergy; a flat surface (i.e. when the isobolograms contained within the surface and depicted by the horizontal lines appear straight or flat) indicates additivity (not shown); and bowing away from the reader indicates infra-additivity (not shown). The two other techniques, shift in dose–response curve (purple line) and the isobologram (blue line), can be seen as individual slices of the surface.

They then introduce an interaction parameter to describe the combined drug effect. The Greco model introduces a first order interaction term (ε):

$$U = (U_A + U_B + \varepsilon \cdot U_A \cdot U_B) \tag{4}$$

The Minto model expresses the drugs as a ratio and introduces a polynomial function containing an interaction term (β) that can be applied to the EC_{50} (or E_{MAX} or γ).

$$U = \frac{(U_A + U_B)}{f(\theta)}, \text{ where } f(\theta) = 1 - \beta \cdot \theta + \beta \cdot \theta^2 \tag{5}$$

Both models then introduce these terms into the standard sigmoid curve equation (Equation 2).

$$E = E_0 + \left(E_{MAX} \cdot \frac{(U)^\gamma}{(1+U)^\gamma} \right) \tag{6}$$

Optimal model parameters are then estimated and additive and non-additive interactions compared to determine statistical significance using log likelihood. The Greco model can also be reduced further to account for interactions where one drug is not capable of reaching the end-point in question at any reasonable dose when given alone (e.g. ablation of movement with an opioid) [12, 13]. The Minto model can also be readily adapted to account for three-drug interactions [10].

The Hierarchical model takes a different approach, which does not require the inclusion of an interaction parameter. The effect of drug A on the chosen end-point, such as ablation of response to a noxious stimulus, is first estimated:

$$E_A = E_0 \cdot \left(1 - \frac{Ce_A^{\gamma_A}}{\left(C_{50A} \cdot E_0\right)^{\gamma_A} + Ce_A^{\gamma_A}} \right) \tag{7}$$

where E_0 in this case is the pre-drug or baseline effect. The effect of drug B on the remaining effect not accounted for by drug A is then estimated:

$$E_{A+B} = \frac{Ce_B^{\gamma_B}}{\left(C_{50B} \cdot E_A\right)^{\gamma_B} + Ce_B^{\gamma_B}} \tag{8}$$

All these models readily allow covariates such as age, weight, body mass index and sex to be incorporated, improving their accuracy and allowing us to individualize both the PK and PD components of drug response for a combination of drugs. Models can be readily created for both continuous variables such as bispectral index (BIS) and also bivariate (dichotomous) responses such as lack of movement to verbal command ('hypnosis') or to a noxious stimulus ('anaesthesia'). It is important to note that all these models are empirical as they do not reflect any true underlying physiological process and also assume that interactions are constant over time. There have been few studies of whether PD interactions vary with the age or sex of a patient.

When drugs are additive, the isobolograms (horizontal lines) within the response surface appear flat. When the interaction is synergistic, the surface takes on a sail-like shape, bowing outwards (i.e. towards the reader, refer to Fig. 3.1), and when the interaction is infra-additive, the surface bows inwards. Response surfaces incorporate earlier study designs using shifts in dose–response curves (refer to Fig. 3.1), which can now be seen as vertical slices of the surface, and isobolograms, which are horizontal lines along the response surface. The parameters of the response surface are estimated simultaneously using all available data points, so that information can be interpolated to inform effect levels or concentration ranges where information is sparse, and outlier data points become less influential. With robust trial design and continuous measures of effect, a response surface can be drawn with data from as few as 20 subjects [14]. These models can then be used to predict effects for all portions of the concentration–response curve for both drugs. They have become incorporated into modern anaesthesia displays and intravenous anaesthesia using twin infusion pumps as described in Chapter 6 of this book. Simulation analysis can be used to estimate the optimal concentration pairs for a certain endpoint, such as those that give the most rapid recovery or least respiratory depression during conscious sedation or total intravenous anaesthesia [15, 16]. The technique was used by LaPierre to identify optimal regions of the propofol–remifentanil response surface that provide reliable loss of responsiveness without ventilatory depression by combining response surface models for the individual end-points [15] (Fig. 3.2).

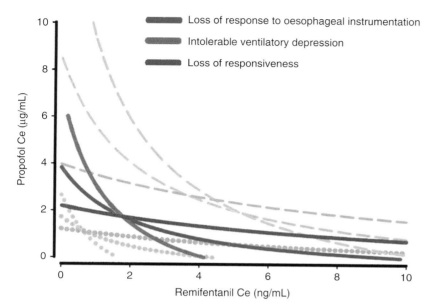

5%, 50% and 95% probability of effect isoboles

— Loss of response to oesophageal instrumentation
— Intolerable ventilatory depression
— Loss of responsiveness

Fig. 3.2 Example of use of isobolograms to delineate optimal drug combinations to achieve maximum clinical effect with least side effects. Isobolograms for the ED$_{50}$ (solid lines), ED$_{5}$ (dotted lines) and ED$_{95}$ (broken lines) for the combination of propofol and remifentanil are displayed for loss of responsiveness to oesophageal instrumentation, severe respiratory depression (respiratory rate less than 5 breaths/minute) and loss of response to shaking and shouting. The study demonstrates the best combination that will provide hypnosis and tolerance to a noxious stimulus whilst minimizing respiratory depression, i.e. concentrations of remifentanil ranging from 0.8 to 1.6 ng/mL paired with propofol concentrations ranging from 1.5 to 2.7 µg/mL. Reprinted with permission from [15].

Interactions among Anaesthetic Agents

We briefly summarize available data on some commonly used anaesthetic drug combinations.

Gamma-aminobutyric Acid and mcg Receptor Acting Drug Interactions

Midazolam combines synergistically with propofol [17, 18] and thiopental for sedation [19] and also markedly reduces the dose of propofol and thiopental required to suppress movement to a noxious stimulus. Both PK and PD explanations have been promoted to explain the interaction, which reduces dose requirements of the two agents by 30–50% [1, 2, 20].

Opioids reduce the dose of midazolam required to cause loss of response to verbal command [21] and act in a markedly synergistic fashion to reduce dose requirements for suppression of movement to a noxious stimulus [18]. Indeed neither opioids nor midazolam reliably suppress movement to a noxious stimulus in all patients when given alone, even at very high doses [6, 11, 12, 18]. The various interactions between these three classes of drugs to achieve hypnosis are displayed in Fig. 3.3. A triple drug interaction model for these three drugs has also been described although synergy for the three drug combination could not be confirmed beyond that demonstrated by the individual drug pairs [10].

The combination of propofol with an opioid is mildly synergistic for suppressing response to verbal command (Fig. 3.4, left pane) and markedly synergistic at suppressing movement to pain (Fig. 3.4, right pane), but additive for BIS. Increasing the opioid dose also increases the steepness of the propofol concentration–response curve for loss of responsiveness to noxious endpoints, and vice versa (see Fig. 3.5 for the impact of propofol on remifentanil pharmacodynamics). This effectively reduces the concentration range over which most patients will become unresponsive, thereby improving the reliability with which we can achieve these end-points. Propofol with an opioid, usually remifentanil, is the preferred combination for modern total intravenous anaesthesia [22] (Fig. 3.5).

Volatile Drug Interactions

Phenylpiperidine opioids such as fentanyl and remifentanil act additively to mildly synergistically to reduce dose requirements of anaesthetic ethers such as isoflurane, sevoflurane and desflurane for loss of consciousness over the lower dose range of opioids, reducing the partial pressure for MACawake by 15% at most [4, 23–25]. The same drugs are markedly synergistic at reducing dose requirements for loss of movement to a noxious stimulus or MAC (Fig. 3.6). It is important to realize opioids differentially affect MACawake, MAC,

33

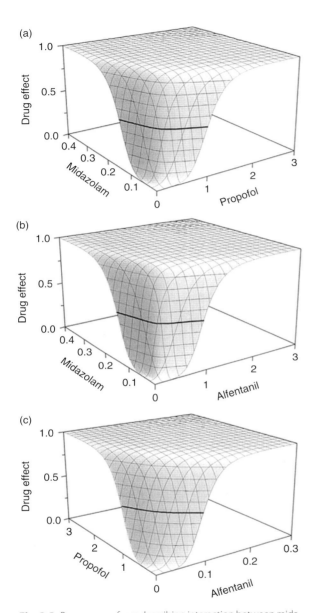

Fig. 3.3 Response surfaces describing interaction between midazolam, propofol and alfentanil for hypnosis

Response surfaces for midazolam–propofol, alfentanil–midazolam, and propofol–alfentanil show the proportion of patients achieving hypnosis, assessed as failure to open eyes to verbal command [10]. Synergy was found for all three drug pairs. Drug effect is plotted against per kg dose (mg) for all drugs. Reprinted with permission from [10].

and MACBAR: a 2 ng/mL remifentanil equivalent reduces MACawake, MAC, and MACBAR (the partial pressure to prevent hypertension and tachycardia after incision in 50% of the population) by 15, 50 and 75%,

respectively [25–27]. These interactions form the basis of modern volatile anaesthesia and enable suppression of movement, reduced cardiovascular responses to noxious stimulation and rapid emergence from anaesthesia. Again, increasing the opioid dose markedly increases the steepness of the dose–response curve [22]. In general, additivity is seen between volatile anaesthetic pairs for MAC [28–30].

NMDA Acting Drug Interactions

Ketamine has a distinct mode of action at NMDA receptors, which contrasts with the above drug combinations that have actions at GABA or opioid receptors. Midazolam has a small (infra-additive) effect on ketamine dose to suppress response to verbal command and no effect on the ketamine dose required to suppress movement to a noxious stimulus [31]. Propofol and ketamine are additive for suppressing response to verbal command and loss of consciousness [32]. Use of this drug combination is common in paediatric and emergency settings, due to its cardiac stability and the low incidence of airway obstruction and apnoea when compared to sedative–opioid drug combinations, and it is useful for minor painful procedures. There is a need for further research into ketamine combinations in anaesthesia using response surface methodology and including its combination with volatile anaesthetics, propofol, and in selected patient groups such as children [33] and the elderly. Nitrous oxide also acts at the NMDA receptor. The interaction between nitrous oxide and sevoflurane for hypnosis is infra-additive [34].

Practical Applications of Interaction Models

Real-Time Display of Anaesthetic Drug Interactions and Simulators

In the last decade, manufacturers have incorporated these models into real-time displays of anaesthetic effect. These displays provide predictions of anaesthetic effect in real-time using the methodology described above. Covariates of age, weight, body mass index and sex together with interactions between the anaesthetic drugs in use are incorporated into these models. Such displays are excellent teaching tools for trainees and also have the ability to improve the precision with which drugs are administered to patients. Most anaesthetics involve drugs from three classes

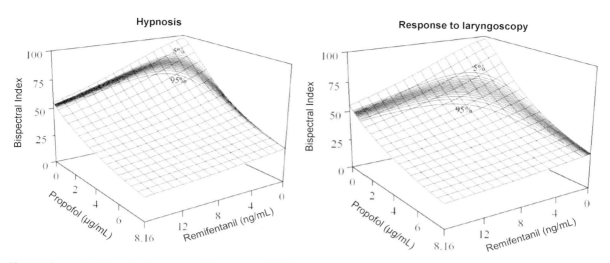

Fig. 3.4 Synergistic interaction between opioids and propofol for hypnosis and immobility after noxious stimulation. Response surface models for propofol with remifentanil for bispectral index (BIS), with the 5 to 95% isobolograms for two bivariate end-points, hypnosis and response to laryngoscopy (a very noxious stimulus), overlaid on the surface. Note that the BIS response surface is drawn with the X and Y axes reversed, that is the BIS decreases with increasing dose, zero effect is in the back top corner of the graph [11]. The interaction for this drug pair is additive for BIS, while for the other end-points synergy is seen. Adapted and reprinted with permission from [11].

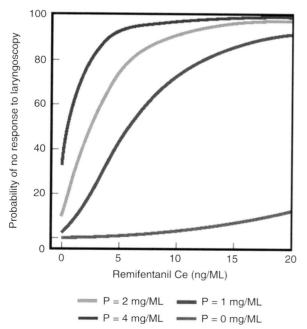

Fig. 3.5 Changes in propofol requirement with increasing dose of remifentanil. The concentration–response curves for ablation of response to laryngoscopy using remifentanil alone and in combination with fixed concentrations of propofol are shown. The graph demonstrates the inability of remifentanil alone to ablate response to this noxious stimulus, the significant reduction in the required concentration of remifentanil for this combination, and the increasing steepness of the relationship as the concentration of propofol is increased [22]. Ce is predicted concentration in the effect site. Adapted and reprinted with permission from [22].

(hypnotics, inhalational anaesthetics and phenylpiperidine opioids). Recently the three drug propofol–remifentanil–sevoflurane interaction has been studied using pooled data from several studies for a derived end-point of response to noxious stimuli [24]. The interactions described are quite robust across studies, lending themselves to incorporation into anaesthetic monitors. The use of interaction models in anaesthetic software for real-time display in the operating room is discussed at length in Chapter 6.

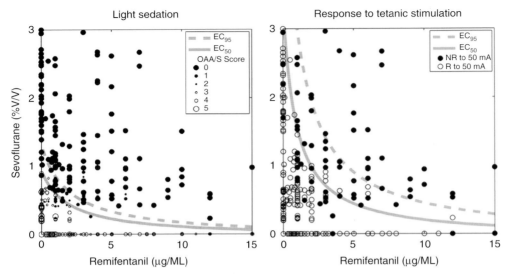

Fig. 3.6 Interaction between remifentanil and sevoflurane for hypnosis and tetanic stimulation. Isobolograms for the combination of sevoflurane and remifentanil at end-points of light sedation, defined as an Observer's Assessment of Alertness/Sedation (OAA/S) score of 1 or less, and loss of response to noxious stimulus (in this case, tetanic stimulation) [4]. Raw data are shown with 50% (EC50) and 95% (EC95) isobolograms for each end-point [sedated or not sedated; responds (R) or doesn't respond (NR) to tetanic stimulation] overlaid. The use of 2.5 ng/mL remifentanil reduces the sevoflurane partial pressure to achieve a 50% probability of being sedated by half but that to achieve a 50% probability of not responding to a tetanic stimulus by almost 75%. These authors were able to use their model to estimate the optimal concentration pairs of remifentanil and sevoflurane to obtain faster recovery times. Adapted and reprinted with permission from [4].

Pharmacodynamic Model, Target-controlled Infusion: The Future

Pharmacodynamic model, target-controlled infusion (PTCI) embraces the earlier concepts of effect-site target-controlled infusion (TCI) of individual drugs, the estimated PD effect on BIS of the individual drugs and also a model of the PD interaction between the two drugs on BIS. Figure 3.7 illustrates the concepts that are included in this complex model and the various personalized covariates that can be introduced. The resulting prediction of combined drug effect is well beyond what can be estimated using mental arithmetic and again carries the promise of being able to improve the precision of anaesthetic drug dosing [35]. This concept could easily be adapted to the three-drug interaction model of propofol, remifentanil and sevoflurane to provide precise administration of these three drugs to patients.

Closed-loop Anaesthesia

The concept of a pair of drugs having a unique pharmacology is implicit in the recently developed dual-drug closed-loop controller for administration of propofol and remifentanil for intravenous anaesthesia [36].

Closed-loop controllers have been shown to reduce both the variability in anaesthetic depth and the variability in blood pressure when compared to anaesthetist administered anaesthesia, and to decrease the variability in wake-up times [36–39], again improving the precision of drug dosage in individuals. To date, those closed-loop controllers reported for administration of two drugs all work by targeting an end-point (usually BIS) within a predefined range, although a closed-loop controller that balances BIS and blood pressure effects for administering propofol alone has been reported [40]. Theoretically this approach benefits from being able to titrate the level of anaesthesia to the varying degree of stimulus that occurs during the various phases of an operation, although to make the most of this feature one would need to include opioid administration within the system.

Conclusions

Currently, no individual drug exists that has all the desired effects to achieve 'anaesthesia' as we currently define it, so the use of drug combinations is routine. A thorough understanding of the pharmacology of commonly used drug combinations is essential to

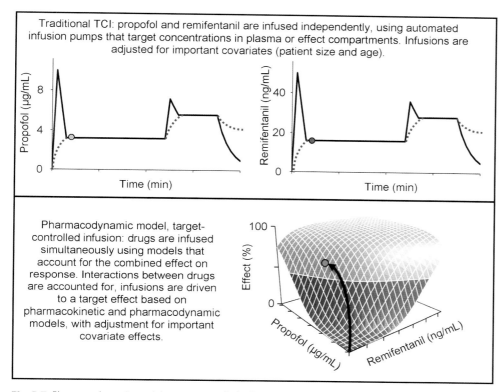

Fig. 3.7 Pharmacodynamic model, target-controlled infusion (PTCI). PTCI embraces the earlier concept of effect-site target-controlled infusion TCI (shown in the upper panel) and includes the estimated pharmacodynamic (PD) effect for both drugs individually and when combined (lower panel). As in Fig. 3.1c, individual drug effect profiles are visible on the outer edges of the surface, with each combination of possible drug concentration pairs represented within the surface. The model incorporates the interaction between the two drugs on the bispectral index (BIS), as well as the important covariates of age, weight and obesity on the pharmacokinetic (PK) component. Important covariates on PD can also be incorporated. This figure demonstrates how these aspects of anaesthetic pharmacology combine. This approach has been used for an BIS endpoint, the resulting prediction of combined drug effect is well beyond what can be estimated using mental arithmetic [35]. Adapted and reprinted with permission from [35].

understanding individual patient responses. These drug combinations should be considered to be a 'new drug', with their own unique pharmacology that does not directly mirror the expected effects of the individual agents. Interaction models are mathematical descriptions of commonly used drug combinations that can be used to estimate the effects of a combination of drugs given to produce anaesthesia. The models are now being incorporated into anaesthetic monitor displays that can predict the effects of a drug combination rather than of just one component of the anaesthetic, as well as closed-loop administration systems that automate drug delivery. They are also being used to drive automated infusions to PD targets as opposed to plasma or effect-site concentrations, and for identification of optimal drug pair concentrations that can be targeted by the anaesthetist with current infusion software. Use of these models will increase the anaesthetist's ability to personalize drug dosage for individuals.

References

1. Lichtenbelt BJ, Olofsen E, Dahan A, van Kleef JW, Struys MMRF, Vuyk J: Propofol reduces the distribution and clearance of midazolam. Anesth. Analg. 2010; 110(6): 1597–606.

2. Vuyk J, Lichtenbelt BJ, Olofsen E, van Kleef JW, Dahan A: Mixed-effects modeling of the influence of midazolam on propofol pharmacokinetics. Anesth. Analg. 2009; 108(5): 1522–30.

3. Mertens MJ, Vuyk J, Olofsen E, Bovill JG, Burm AG: Propofol alters the pharmacokinetics of alfentanil in healthy male volunteers. Anesthesiology. 2001; 94(6): 949–57.

4. Manyam SC, Gupta DK, Johnson KB, White JL, Pace NL, Westenskow DR, et al: Opioid-volatile anesthetic synergy: a response surface model with remifentanil and sevoflurane as prototypes. Anesthesiology. 2006; 105(2): 267–78.

5. Loewe S: The problem of synergism and antagonism of combined drugs. Arzneimittelforschung. 1953; 3(6): 285–90.

6. Short TG, Chui PT: Propofol and midazolam act synergistically in combination. Br.J.Anaesth. 1991; 67(5): 539–45.

7. Kissin I, Vinik HR, Bradley EL, Jr.: Midazolam potentiates thiopental sodium anesthetic induction in patients. J.Clin.Anesth. 1991; 3(5): 367–70.

8. Hill A: The possible effects of the aggregation of the molecules of haemoglobin on its dissociation curves. J. Physiol. 1910; 40(Suppl): i–vii.

9. Greco WR, Park HS, Rustum YM: Application of a new approach for the quantitation of drug synergism to the combination of cis-diamminedichloroplatinum and 1-beta-D-arabinofuranosylcytosine. Cancer Res. 1990; 50(17): 5318–27.

10. Minto CF, Schnider TW, Short TG, Gregg KM, Gentilini A, Shafer SL: Response surface model for anesthetic drug interactions. Anesthesiology. 2000; 92(6): 1603–16.

11. Bouillon TW, Bruhn J, Radulescu L, Andresen C, Shafer TJ, Cohane C, et al: Pharmacodynamic interaction between propofol and remifentanil regarding hypnosis, tolerance of laryngoscopy, bispectral index, and electroencephalographic approximate entropy. Anesthesiology. 2004; 100(6): 1353–72.

12. Mertens MJ, Olofsen E, Engbers FH, Burm AG, Bovill JG, Vuyk J: Propofol reduces perioperative remifentanil requirements in a synergistic manner: response surface modeling of perioperative remifentanil-propofol interactions. Anesthesiology. 2003; 99(2): 347–59.

13. Heyse B, Proost JH, Schumacher PM, Bouillon TW, Vereecke HE, Eleveld DJ, et al: Sevoflurane remifentanil interaction: comparison of different response surface models. Anesthesiology. 2012; 116(2): 311–23.

14. Short TG, Ho TY, Minto CF, Schnider TW, Shafer SL: Efficient trial design for eliciting a pharmacokinetic-pharmacodynamic model-based response surface describing the interaction between two intravenous anesthetic drugs. Anesthesiology. 2002; 96(2): 400–8.

15. LaPierre CD, Johnson KB, Randall BR, White JL, Egan TD, Yang L, et al: An exploration of remifentanil-propofol combinations that lead to a loss of response to esophageal instrumentation, a loss of responsiveness, and/or onset of intolerable ventilatory depression. Anesth.Analg. 2011; 113(3): 441–3.

16. Vuyk J, Lim T, Engbers FH, Burm AG, Vletter AA, Bovill JG: The pharmacodynamic interaction of propofol and alfentanil during lower abdominal surgery in women. Anesthesiology. 1995; 83(1): 8–22.

17. McClune S, McKay AC, Wright PM, Patterson CC, Clarke RS: Synergistic interaction between midazolam and propofol. Br.J.Anaesth. 1992; 69(3): 240–5.

18. Short TG, Plummer JL, Chui PT: Hypnotic and anaesthetic interactions between midazolam, propofol and alfentanil. Br.J.Anaesth. 1992; 69(2): 162–7.

19. Short TG, Galletly DC, Plummer JL: Hypnotic and anaesthetic action of thiopentone and midazolam alone and in combination. Br.J.Anaesth. 1991; 66(1): 13–19.

20. McAdam LC, MacDonald JF, Orser BA: Isobolographic analysis of the interactions between midazolam and propofol at GABA(A) receptors in embryonic mouse neurons. Anesthesiology. 1998; 89(6): 1444–54.

21. Ben-Shlomo I, Abd-el-Khalim H, Ezry J, Zohar S, Tverskoy M: Midazolam acts synergistically with fentanyl for induction of anaesthesia. Br.J.Anaesth. 1990; 64(1): 45–7.

22. Kern SE, Xie G, White JL, Egan TD: A response surface analysis of propofol-remifentanil pharmacodynamic interaction in volunteers. Anesthesiology. 2004; 100(6): 1373–81.

23. Syroid ND, Johnson KB, Pace NL, Westenskow DR, Tyler D, Bruhschwein F, et al: Response surface model predictions of emergence and response to pain in the recovery room: an evaluation of patients emerging from an isoflurane and fentanyl anesthetic. Anesth. Analg. 2010; 111(2): 380–6.

24. Hannivoort LN, Vereecke HEM, Proost JH, Heyse BEK, Eleveld DJ, Bouillon TW, et al: Probability to tolerate laryngoscopy and noxious stimulation response index as general indicators of the anaesthetic potency of sevoflurane, propofol, and remifentanil. Br.J.Anaesth. 2016; 116(5): 624–31.

25. Katoh T, Suguro Y, Kimura T, Ikeda K: Cerebral awakening concentration of sevoflurane and isoflurane predicted during slow and fast alveolar washout. Anesth.Analg. 1993; 77(5): 1012–17.

26. Katoh T, Kobayashi S, Suzuki A, Iwamoto T, Bito H, Ikeda K: The effect of fentanyl on sevoflurane requirements for somatic and sympathetic responses to surgical incision. Anesthesiology. 1999; 90(2): 398–405.

27. Katoh T, Ikeda K: The effects of fentanyl on sevoflurane requirements for loss of consciousness and skin incision. Anesthesiology. 1998; 88(1): 18–24.

28. Murray DJ, Mehta MP, Forbes RB, Dull DL. Additive contribution of nitrous oxide to halothane MAC in infants and children. Anesth.Analg. 1990; 71(2): 120–4.

29. Stevens MD, Wendell C, Dolan MD, William M, Gibbons MD, Robert T, White MSA, Eger MD, Edmond I, Miller MD, Ronald D, et al: Minimum

alveolar concentrations (MAC) of isoflurane with and without nitrous oxide in patients of various ages. Anesthesiology. 1975; 42(2): 197–200.

30. Hendrickx JFA, Eger EI, Sonner JM, Shafer SL: Is synergy the rule? A review of anesthetic interactions producing hypnosis and immobility. Anesth.Analg. 2008; 107(2): 494–506.

31. Hong W, Short TG, Hui TW: Hypnotic and anesthetic interactions between ketamine and midazolam in female patients. Anesthesiology. 1993; 79(6): 1227–32.

32. Hui TW, Short TG, Hong W, Suen T, Gin T, Plummer J: Additive interactions between propofol and ketamine when used for anesthesia induction in female patients. Anesthesiology. 1995; 82(3): 641–8.

33. Coulter FL, Hannam JA, Anderson BJ: Ketofol simulations for dosing in pediatric anesthesia. Paediatr. Anaesth. 2014; 24(8): 806–12.

34. Katoh T, Ikeda K, Bito H: Does nitrous oxide antagonize sevoflurane-induced hypnosis? Br.J.Anaesth. 1997; 79(4): 465–8.

35. Short TG, Hannam JA, Laurent S, Campbell D, Misur M, Merry AF, et al: Refining target-controlled infusion: an assessment of pharmacodynamic target-controlled infusion of propofol and remifentanil using a response surface model of their combined effects on bispectral index. Anesth.Analg. 2016; 122(1): 90–7.

36. Liu N, Chazot T, Hamada S, Landais A, Boichut N, Dussaussoy C, et al: Closed-loop coadministration of propofol and remifentanil guided by bispectral index: a randomized multicenter study. Anesth.Analg. 2011; 112(3): 546–57.

37. Agarwal J, Puri GD, Mathew PJ: Comparison of closed loop vs. manual administration of propofol using the bispectral index in cardiac surgery. Acta Anaesthesiol. Scand. 2009; 53(3): 390–7.

38. Puri GD, Mathew PJ, Biswas I, Dutta A, Sood J, Gombar S, et al: A multicenter evaluation of a closed-loop anesthesia delivery system: a randomized controlled trial. Anesth.Analg. 2016; 122(1): 106–14.

39. Hemmerling TM, Charabati S, Zaouter C, Minardi C, Mathieu PA: A randomized controlled trial demonstrates that a novel closed-loop propofol system performs better hypnosis control than manual administration. Can.J.Anaesth. 2010; 57(8): 725–35.

40. Struys MM, De Smet T, Versichelen LF, Van De Velde S, Van den Broecke R, Mortier EP: Comparison of closed-loop controlled administration of propofol using bispectral index as the controlled variable versus "standard practice" controlled administration. Anesthesiology. 2001; 95(1): 6–17.

Chapter

4

Covariate Analysis in Clinical Anaesthesia

Luis I. Cortinez and Brian J. Anderson

Introduction

The goal of pharmacological treatment is a desired response, known as the target effect (e.g. bispectral index of 50). An understanding of the concentration–response relationship (i.e. pharmacodynamics (PD)) can be used to predict the target concentration (e.g. propofol 4 mg/L) required to achieve this target effect in a typical individual [1]. Pharmacokinetic (PK) knowledge (e.g. clearance, volume) then determines the dose that will achieve the target concentration. Each individual, however, is somewhat different and there is variability associated with all parameters used in PK and PD equations (known as models). Covariate information (e.g. weight, age, pathology, drug interactions, pharmacogenomics) can be used to help predict the dose in a specific patient. The Holy Grail of clinical pharmacology is prediction of drug PK and PD in the individual patient (Fig. 4.1) and this requires knowledge of the covariates that contribute to variability [2]. Adverse effects will also impact on dose.

Quantifying Covariate Effect

Parameter variability has two contributors: between subject variability (BSV; also known as inter-individual variability, IIV) and between occasion variability (BOV, also known as intra-individual variability). The difference between BSV without covariates and with covariates is a measure of the predictable decrease in BSV due to covariates. The variance (ω^2) estimates for the different components contributing to variability of vancomycin pharmacokinetics are shown in Table 4.1 [3]. The ratio of the between-subject variability predictable from covariates ($BSVP^2$) to the total population parameter variability obtained without covariate analysis ($PPVt^2$) gives an indication of how important covariate information is. For example, the ratio of 0.823 achieved for clearance in a study of vancomycin in neonates indicates that 82.3% of the overall variability in clearance is predictable from covariate information. Weight explained 49%, postmenstrual age (PMA) 18% and renal function 34.1% [3].

PHARMACOKINETICS   BIOPHASE   PHARMACODYNAMICS

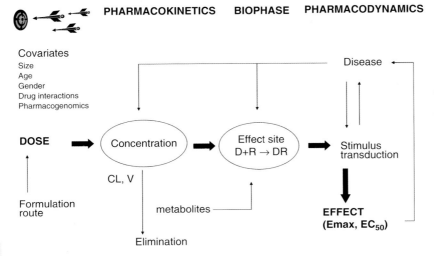

Fig. 4.1 The complex interaction between pharmacokinetics (PK) and pharmacodynamics (PD). Administration of a dose must undergo multiple steps before effect is achieved. Each step in this pathway is associated with variability. In addition, each step experiences either positive or negative feedback from subsequent steps. For example, the drug may impact on the disease, but changes in the disease have multiple effects on PK, PD and the biophase. The use of concentration to describe effect removes variability associated with PK aspects. (Reproduced with permission from Anderson BJ: *Pediatr. Anesth.* 2012; 22: 530–8.)

40

Table 4.1. Effect of covariate analysis on variance of clearance (ω^2) for vancomycin. The impact of each covariate when added sequentially to the model is demonstrated. (Adapted from Anderson BJ et al: Br.J.Clin.Pharmacol. 2007; 63: 75–84.)

Individual covariate alone	PPVt²	BSVR²	BOV²	PPVP²	PPVP²/PPVt²	OBJ
No covariates	0.279	0.279	0	0	0	2835.261
Allometric scaling	0.279*	0.0538	0.0862	0.139	0.498	2632.123
Postmenstrual age	0.279*	0.0452	0.0450	0.189	0.677	2514.865
Renal function	0.279*	0.0362	0.0137	0.230	0.821	2418.198
Ventilation scaling factor	0.279*	0.0356	0.0137	0.230	0.823	2413.725

*=assumed from no covariate model estimate

PPVt² is the total population parameter variance estimated without covariate analysis, which is the sum of PPVP² (the population parameter variance predictable from covariates), BSVR² (the random BSV² estimated on a parameter when covariate analysis is included) and BOV² (the between occasion variance), or mathematically expressed: PPVt²=PPVP²+BSVR²+BOV². The ratio of the between subject variance predictable from covariates (PPVP²) to the total population parameter variance obtained without covariate analysis (PPVt², PPVP²/PPVt²) indicates the fraction of the total variability in the parameter that is predictable from covariates. OBJ is the objective function value, a parameter that measures the goodness of fit.

Major Covariates

Covariate effects will differ depending on the population studied. For example age may have a large effect in those aged less than 1 year or those aged more than 60 years, but minimal effect in young adults. The variability observed for any parameter (e.g. clearance) is contributed to by multiple covariate influences (Fig. 4.2). Covariate effects can be related to known biology (mechanistic), be based on theory or may be related to an observed variable that may or may not reflect physiology to some extent. The latter models are known as empirical. The American Association of Anesthesiologists (ASA) classification, for example, may be used to describe altered propofol disposition in patients when compared to healthy volunteers; this is an empirical model. Allometry (see below), in contrast, could be considered a theoretical model. There is no 'best model' to describe covariates. Theoretical models may fail if assumptions for the theory are not met.

Major Paediatric Pharmacokinetic Covariates

Growth and development are two major aspects of children not readily apparent in adults. How these factors interact is not necessarily easy to determine from observations because they are quite highly correlated. Drug elimination clearance, for example, may increase with weight, height, age, body surface area and creatinine clearance. One approach is to standardize for size before incorporating a factor for maturation [4].

Probability

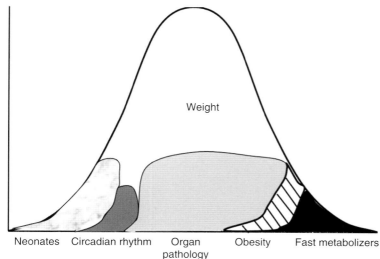

Neonates   Circadian rhythm   Organ pathology   Obesity   Fast metabolizers

Fig. 4.2 Schematic representation of factors contributing to clearance variability in children. Neonates have reduced clearance (e.g. morphine), pharmacogenomic influences may cause increased clearance (e.g. CYP2D6 fast metabolizers of codeine), renal failure may reduce clearance (e.g. aminoglycosides), other drugs may increase clearance (e.g. smoking and theophylline). (Reproduced with permission from Anderson BJ: Pediatr.Anesth. 2012; 22: 530–8).

Size

Size, frequently expressed as weight, is the most common covariate used to determine dose in children [5]. The normal variation of weight with age (from 3rd to 97th percentile) is considerable, being least at 1 year (+25% to –20% at 10 kg) and reaching a maximum at about 13 years (+45% to –26% at 40 kg) [6, 7]. Although total body weight (TBW) is used commonly, it is now more widely recognized that there is a non-linear relationship between weight and drug elimination [8, 9]. Non-linear scaling models include body surface area [10], lean body weight [11], fat free mass [12], normal fat mass [13] and allometric scaling (defined below) [14].

Clearance in children 1–2 years of age, expressed as L/h/kg (the linear per kilogramme model), is frequently greater than that observed in older children and adolescents. This is a size effect and is not due to bigger livers or increased hepatic blood flow in preschool children. This 'artefact of size' disappears when allometric scaling is used to replot the same data

(Fig. 4.3). Allometry is a term used to describe the non-linear relationship between size and function. This non-linear relationship is expressed as:

$$y = a \cdot BodyMass^{PWR} \tag{1}$$

where y is the variable of interest (e.g. basal metabolic rate), a is the allometric coefficient and PWR is the allometric exponent. The value of PWR has been the subject of much debate. Basal metabolic rate (BMR) is the commonest variable investigated and camps advocating for a PWR value of 2/3 (i.e. body surface area) are at odds with those advocating a value of ¾.

Support for a value of ¾ comes from investigations that show that the log of BMR plotted against the log of body weight produces a straight line with a slope of ¾ in all species studied, including humans. Fractal geometry is used to mathematically explain this phenomenon. The ¾ power law for metabolic rates was derived from a general model that describes how essential materials are transported through space-filled fractal

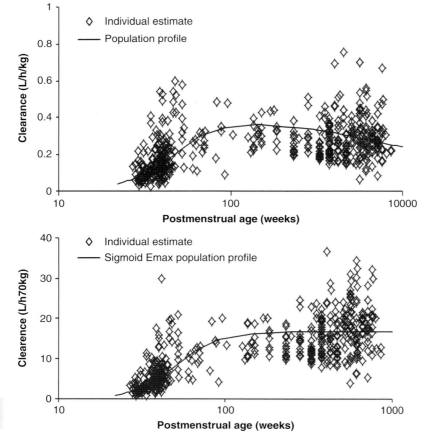

Fig. 4.3 Paracetamol clearance maturation shown as the linear per kilogramme model (upper panel) and using the allometric ¾ power model (lower panel). Data are the same for each graph but clearance units differ. The upper panel using the linear per kilogramme model shows how clearance increases in the first few years of life and then decreases to reach adult rates in teenage years. The lower panel using allometric scaling shows that once clearance maturation matures over the first few years of life, the clearance is constant at all ages until elderly. Data from Anderson BJ et al: *Drug. Metab. Pharmacokinet.* 2009; 24(1): 25–36.

networks of branching tubes [15]. A great many physi-ological, structural and time related variables scale pre-dictably within and between species with weight (W) exponents (PWR) of ¾, 1 and ¼ respectively [16].

These exponents have applicability to PK param-eters such as clearance (CL exponent of ¾), volume (V exponent of 1) and half-time (T$_{1/2}$ exponent of ¼) [16]. The factor for size ($Fsize$) for total drug clearance may be expressed as:

$$Fsize = \left(\frac{W}{70}\right)^{3/4} \qquad (2)$$

Clearance is a metabolic function, and while the pro-cess for drug clearance may differ between animals, the clearance of tramadol plotted against the log of body weight produces a straight line with a slope of ¾ in all species studied (Fig. 4.4) [17].

Maintenance dose is determined by clearance. The difference in drug clearance between an adult and a child is predictable from weight using theory-based allometry:

$$CL_{CHILD} = CL_{ADULT} \times \left(\frac{weight_{CHILD}}{weight_{ADULT}}\right)^{3/4} \qquad (3)$$

Allometric theory predicts maintenance dose per kg is higher in children. For example, remifentanil clearance is increased in neonates, infants and children when expressed per kilogramme [18]. However, remifen-tanil clearance in children aged 1 month–9 years is similar to adult rates when scaled using an allometric exponent of 3/4 [19]. Non-specific blood esterases that metabolize remifentanil are mature at birth [20], and that is when clearance (expressed as per kilogramme) is highest (see Fig. 4.5).

Population analyses of drugs in children using allo-metric models for size report that total body weight contributes more than 50% of clearance variability, e.g. for dexmedetomidine 86% [21], acetaminophen 77% [22], ketamine 54% [23] and levobupivacaine 62% [24]. The contribution that size makes is dependent on the subgroup of the paediatric population studied. For example, weight only contributed 57% of aceta-minophen clearance variability in a neonatal popula-tion. The contribution of size to clearance variability is even less for other drugs in the neonatal period, e.g. tramadol 38% [25], aminoglycosides 47% [26]. The weight range in the neonatal population is smaller (e.g. 0.5–5 kg) than in the entire paediatric population (e.g. 0.5–100 kg) and we might anticipate age to have greater additional impact in the first few years of life because it reflects maturation.

Maturation

Unlike for remifentanil clearance, allometry alone is insufficient to predict clearance in neonates and infants from adult estimates for most drugs [27, 28]. The addi-tion of a model describing maturation is required [29]. The sigmoid hyperbolic or Hill model [30] has been found useful for describing this maturation factor (MF):

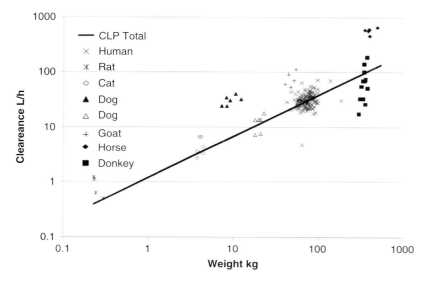

Fig. 4.4 Weight-predicted tramadol total clearance (CLP total) compared to human allometric prediction using a ¾ power exponent (solid line). Clearance can be scaled using allometric theory over four orders of magnitude. (Reproduced with permission from Holford S: *J.Pharmacol. Clin.Toxicol.* 2014; 1: 1023).

43

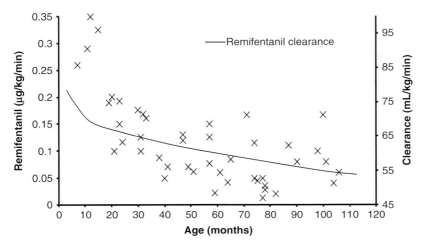

Fig. 4.5 The effect of age on the dose of remifentanil (x) tolerated during spontaneous ventilation under anaesthesia in children undergoing strabismus surgery. Superimposed on this plot is estimated remifentanil clearance (solid curved line) determined using an allometric model. There is a mismatch between clearance and infusion rate for those individuals still in infancy. The higher infusion rates recorded in those infants can be attributed to greater suppression of respiratory drive in this age group than the older children during the study; a respiratory rate of ten breaths per minute in an infant is disproportionately slow compared to the same rate in a 7-year-old child, suggesting excessive dose. (Reproduced with permission from Anderson BJ: *Pediatr. Anesth.* 2010; 20: 223–32).

$$MF = \frac{PMA^{Hill}}{TM_{50}^{Hill} + PMA^{Hill}} \qquad (4)$$

The TM_{50} describes the maturation half-time, while the Hill coefficient relates to the slope of this maturation profile. Maturation of clearance begins before birth, suggesting that PMA would be a better predictor of drug elimination than postnatal age (PNA) [16]. Figure 4.6 shows the maturation profile for dexmedetomidine expressed as both the standard per kilogramme model and using allometry. Clearance is immature in infancy. Clearance is maximal at 2 years of age when expressed using the linear per kilogramme model, decreasing subsequently with age. This 'artefact of size' disappears with use of the allometric model.

The impact of PMA will depend on the speed of maturation and the subpopulation studied; age will contribute more to variability of drugs given to neonates where clearance pathways mature rapidly in the first months of life (e.g. fentanyl CYP3A4) [31] or tramadol (CYP2D6, CYP3A) [25] than those that mature more slowly (acetaminophen, UGT1A6) [9]. PMA only contributed 12% to clearance variability in an acetaminophen neonatal study [32], but 27% of tramadol clearance variability in neonates [25]. Consequently, size, described using weight, is the single most important covariate for determining

acetaminophen clearance in neonates during the initial slow maturation phase (<44 weeks PMA). Age has a greater contribution after this phase so that both age and size contribute 91% of variance of clearance throughout the paediatric age span [33].

Organ Function

Changes associated with normal growth and development can be distinguished from pathological changes describing organ function (OF) [4]. Morphine clearance is reduced in neonates because of immature glucuronide conjugation, but clearance was lower in critically ill neonates than healthier cohorts [34–36], possibly attributable to reduced hepatic function. The impact of organ function alteration may be concealed by another covariate. For example, positive pressure ventilation may be associated with reduced clearance for perfusion limited drugs (e.g. propofol, morphine); reduced hepatic blood flow due to artificial ventilation may be the cause of reduced clearance rather than being critically ill.

Creatinine clearance is commonly used as a measure of renal function and dictates dose of those drugs cleared by that organ. Difficulties arise determining renal function in children. Neonatal creatinine reflects that of maternal function in the first few days of life; creatinine production is reduced because of

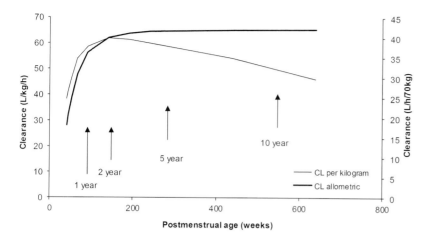

Fig. 4.6 The clearance maturation profile of dexmedetomidine expressed using the per kilogramme model and the allometric ¾-power model. The profiles are similar to those observed for paracetamol (Fig. 4.3). These maturation patterns are typical of many drugs cleared by the liver or kidneys. Clearance is highest in infants when expressed as the linear per kilogramme model. However, use of allometric theory reveals that clearance matures sometime in the first year or so of life and then plateaus. (Data adapted from Potts AL: *Pediatr. Anesth.* 2009; 19: 1119–29, with permission.)

less muscle bulk. Classic methods of creatinine clearance estimation require, in addition to toilet training, complete bladder emptying. Radioisotopes are not ideal in children for repeat studies [37]. A number of formulae have been published that allow estimation of glomerular filtration rate (GFR) from clinical characteristics [38]. These formulae use simple markers such as height, creatinine concentration in plasma and body surface area (BSA). Estimation of GFR is acceptable in adults, but prediction is poor in children with a GFR value less than 40 mL/min [39]. We might expect the maturation of creatinine clearance, a marker for GFR, to reflect the influences of size, maturation and organ function. Estimation methods such as those of Schwartz incorporate a size factor (body length or height) and a scaling factor (k) that is age dependent as follows: k=0.33 in premature neonates; k=0.45 in term infants 0–1 y; k=0.45 in 1–12-y-old; and k=0.7 in 13–21-y-old adolescent males [40–42]. This variable is entered in the following formula:

$$GFR = \frac{k \cdot height}{Serum\ Creatinine} \tag{5}$$

Creatinine clearance estimation over-predicts GFR in children, possibly because of tubular secretion. In premature neonates tubular reabsorption may also create inaccuracies. Dose of renally cleared drugs in premature neonates should be based on size and maturation-based predictions of GFR alone and not

use serum creatinine until creatinine production rate predictions in this age group are better established. A description of GFR maturation from data that ranged from premature neonates (22 weeks PMA) to adulthood (31 years) using an E_{max} model has been published [13].

Modelling Major Pharmacokinetic Covariates in Children

Pharmacokinetic parameters (P) can be described in an individual as the product of size (Fsize), maturation (MF) and organ function (OF) influences where *Pstd* is the value in a standard size adult without pathological changes in organ function [4]:

$$P = Pstd \cdot Fsize \cdot MF \cdot OF \tag{6}$$

This methodology is increasingly used to describe clearance changes with age [29, 43]. An understanding of these principles can be used to predict dose in children using target concentration methodology [5].

Major Adult Pharmacokinetic Covariates

Weight and age are the most relevant covariates used to adjust anaesthetic doses in adult patients (e.g. [44, 45]). Per-kilogramme dosing guidelines are commonly appropriate for normal weight adult subjects.

In the obese, however, linear per-kilogramme schemes using total body weight derived from lean patients can lead to overdose and adverse effects [46–48]. Obesity is highly prevalent in adult patients and will be treated separately in a later section of this chapter. Age, organ function, sex, ethnicity and comorbidity also influence the PK and PD of commonly used anaesthetic drugs.

Age

The average age of the world's population is increasing rapidly and a higher proportion of patients presenting for surgery in the future will be older [49]. Ageing processes are linked mechanistically to body composition changes, decreases in physiological reserve and altered PD responses. These changes are progressive and might affect organ and tissue function. However, much of the age-related decline in OF is secondary to disease rather than normal ageing, since an increased likelihood of underlying comorbidities and polypharmacy are strongly associated with ageing. These characteristics make older patients a very heterogeneous group and a challenging population. In general, drug requirements decrease with ageing due to PK and PD changes.

Ageing is associated with an increase in fat mass (20–40%) and a decrease in body water (10–15%) that may cause an increased plasma concentration of water-soluble drugs and a longer elimination half-life for lipid-soluble drugs. Changes in protein binding with age (e.g. a decrease in albumin and an increase in alpha-1 glycoprotein) may lead to an altered unbound fraction of drugs in the elderly with possible changes in their volumes of distribution and clearances.

Ageing is also commonly associated with a reduction in clearance of drugs. Hepatic clearance is influenced primarily by hepatic blood flow, intrinsic clearance (enzyme activity and liver mass) and protein binding [50]. Liver mass and blood flow decrease by approximately 30–40% in elderly subjects [50, 51]. Similarly, reduced metabolism of drugs can also be associated with ageing. Renal function is progressively reduced in older people. Chronic diseases such as hypertension and diabetes, which are highly prevalent in older subjects, contribute to renal failure.

Ageing is associated with changes that lead to a decrease in cardiovascular reserve. Some of these changes include: conduction system fibrosis, loss of atrial node cells, increased stiffening of connective tissues, myocardial hypertrophy, stiff arteries and veins, decreased response to beta-receptor stimulation and an increase in sympathetic tone at rest. Older people are more susceptible to adverse drug effects and cardiovascular instability [50].

In adult patients, age has also been shown to be an important covariate for anaesthetic drugs. Although it is recognized that biological age is a better covariate than chronological age, most use chronological age as a covariate. For example, age effect in remifentanil pharmacokinetics described by a three-compartment model was represented by a decrease in V1 by approximately 25% and CL1 by 33% from the ages of 20 to 85 years [52]. Propofol elimination clearance decreased linearly in patients older than 60 years; as did V1 similarly [53]. A propofol analysis found that all the model parameters, with the exception of V3, appear to decrease with increasing age [54]. Similarly, paracetamol clearance decreases with increasing age, with changes most marked in frail older patients.

Age as a covariate has been investigated as either a discrete or continuous variable. The simplest method is to simply add an additional factor (F_{AGE}) to the mathematical formula for those patients older than a certain age (e.g. 70 years), but a continuous variable may be more appropriate because changes rarely suddenly begin at a specified age:

$$F_{AGE} = 1 + SLOPE(AGE - 50) \tag{7}$$

Where SLOPE is a parameter describing changes about a median age (e.g. 50 years). The use of an exponential function avoids a negative F_{AGE}:

$$F_{AGE} = EXP(SLOPE(AGE - 50)) \tag{8}$$

This F_{AGE} can then be used as a covariate for the estimation of the PK parameter (P, e.g. CL or V) as in Equation 6.

Organ Dysfunction

Organ dysfunction is an important covariate in adults. Renal, hepatic and cardiac function can all impact on drug clearance. Collinearity between organ function and age or disease is common and so reduced function may be marked by a surrogate e.g. age. While hepatic and renal disease and their impact on clearance are well documented, cardiac function may have more subtle effects, impacting on initial volume of distribution [55] or plasma to effect-site equilibration rate ($T_{1/2}k_{eo}$) [55–57] and clearances (particularly for those drugs that are perfusion limited) [54, 57]. For example, a reduction in mean arterial blood pressure is associated with propofol PK alterations that increase the blood propofol concentration [58].

Liver Function

The liver is the most important organ involved in biotransformation and elimination of drugs [59]. Liver failure may alter absorption, distribution, metabolization and elimination (ADME) processes. A sensitive marker of liver function that could be used to characterize PK effects is not available. Hepatic dysfunction using clinical scoring systems (e.g. Child–Pugh or MELD classification) may be hard to quantify and relate to altered drug disposition because the impact of dysfunction is multipronged: alteration in hepatic blood flow, reduced hepatocellular mass, reduced synthetic ability, reduced plasma protein concentrations and binding, and reduced clearance for some pathways. Each patient may have an individual pattern of dysfunction and different drugs are affected differently depending on their clearance mechanism [60]. Clearance of dexmedetomidine, a highly selective α-2 adrenergic agonist that is extensively metabolized in the liver [61, 62], decreased by 33% with obstructive jaundice [63]. In contrast, cirrhotic patients had a similar propofol clearance but a greater volume of distribution than healthy patients [64].

Hepatic elimination of drugs (CL_H) depends on liver blood flow (Q_H), intrinsic clearance (CLint) and the fraction of unbound drugs in the blood (fu) [59]:

$$CL_H = Q_H \times \frac{fu \times CLint}{Q_H + fu \times CLint} \qquad (9)$$

The efficiency of the liver to eliminate a drug from the circulation is expressed by the hepatic extraction ratio (EH) as high (EH>0.7), intermediate (0.3<EH<0.7) or low (EH<0.3). Hepatic elimination of highly extracted drugs (perfusion limited clearance) is affected by changes in liver blood flow, and is relatively insensitive to changes in plasma protein binding or enzymatic activity, whereas poorly extracted drugs are mostly influenced by plasma protein binding and enzyme activity (capacity limited clearance). Drugs with high capacity clearance pathways (e.g. glucuronidation) are less affected by hepatic dysfunction than those with capacity limited clearance. Clearance estimation of drugs that are highly bound to albumin or alpha1-acid glycoprotein in patients with severe liver failure should always account for the potential increase in the unbound fraction (fu) to correctly interpret clearance

estimations, since a decrease in plasma protein binding is frequently observed in chronic hepatic disease. A potential decrease in the liver metabolic capacity might be masked by an increase in *fu* if only total plasma clearance is considered [59].

Renal Function

Renal dysfunction impacts on both those drugs dependent on the kidney for clearance and unmetabolites that may be cleared by the renal system [65]. Morphine, for example, is metabolized predominantly by hepatic glucuronide conjugation, but the water soluble active metabolites (morphine 3-glucuronide, morphine 6-glucuronide) are cleared by the kidneys [66]. Accumulation of the active metabolite, morphine-3-gluronide, in patients with renal failure can cause respiratory depression [67].

Renal clearance of drugs is determined by glomerular filtration, tubular secretion and tubular reabsorption. GFR has been shown to be a sensitive marker to assess kidney function and is widely used to adjust dose in patients with renal compromise. There are several methods to measure or estimate GFR [68]. The Cockroft–Gault equation can be used to estimate creatinine clearance (CrCL) and to guide dose in adult patients:

$$CrCL = \frac{(140 - AGE) \cdot Wt \cdot Constant}{SeCr \ (mcmo/L)} \qquad (10)$$

The constant is 1.23 for males and 1.04 for females. Additional constants can be added to account for race. Such adjustments simply allow for differences in creatinine production rate (CPR) between races and sexes. The standard adult CPR is 0.516 mmol/h in a 70 kg, 40-year-old male [49]. The increase of CPR with age in adolescents is assumed to be a consequence of increasing muscle bulk as opposed to the decrease in muscle bulk that occurs with older age in adults.

The volume of distribution of many drugs is increased in end stage renal disease due to fluid overload, decreased protein binding or altered tissue binding [68]. An increase in volume of distribution normally requires a larger loading dose to reach the target concentration more rapidly.

Drug Interactions

Drug interactions may involve either PK interactions, PD interactions or even both [69]. These are discussed in Chapter 3.

Some Additional Covariates

Disease Progression

Pathological states may resolve, worsen or remain static and the interpretation of the impact of medication on these changes can be complex [70]. Pain, for example, is not constant over time. It may wax and wane. A cyclic function has been used for interpreting fever response to ibuprofen in children [71], but not yet for pain response. Pain scores in children after tonsillectomy decrease after only three days, but are often worse on the second or third day [72–74]. Subsequent pain resolves over two weeks, and a variant of the Hill equation (Equation 4) has been used to model this resolution [75].

Assessment of the impact of any analgesic intervention in children should take into account changes with pain over time. Functions describing these changes have been incorporated into disease progression models. Disease status (or pain) usually has a baseline (S_0) from which it decreases over time. A simple model to describe the natural history of pain could be a linear decrease with time, where α describes the slope of pain decrease, e.g.

$$Pain(t) = S_0 - \alpha \cdot t \tag{11}$$

Response to treatment is then a sum of the natural history of the pain resolution and the drug effect:

$$Effect(t) = S_0 - (natural\ history + drug\ effect) \tag{12}$$

Placebo and Nocebo

Placebo and nocebo effects may be transient yet substantial, and few reports of pharmacological effect acknowledge their impact. An attempt to determine paracetamol analgesic effect in children after tonsillectomy, in which placebo was unaccounted for, overestimated the drug's analgesic effect [76]. An additional function describing placebo effects was required in order to define more clearly the analgesic effect from medication [75]. The placebo effect can be difficult to quantify in a clinical study. It may be present in paediatric studies in almost all children studied, but quantification of this effect is greatly improved if some children are given a placebo drug [75]. Use of placebo in children can be difficult to justify ethically [77].

Placebo mechanisms can affect therapeutic outcomes and potentially be exploited clinically to improve clinical outcomes in paediatric populations

[78]. Placebo effect is rarely considered in paediatric analgesic studies [79], even though placebo responses might be more pronounced in children than in adults [80]. Certainly, the placebo effect accounted for a mean pain reduction of 5.6 units (VAS, 0–10) at three hours in a study investigating paracetamol analgesia after tonsillectomy [75]. This placebo effect is greater than that described in adults given naproxen analgesia following wisdom tooth extraction. Those adults only reported a maximum reduction in baseline pain attributable to placebo of 20% [81].

The placebo response in the paediatric study reflected a combination of placebo effect, natural pain resolution, behavioural pain coping mechanisms and our inability to discriminate pain from emergence phenomena in the early postoperative period [82]. Following emergence from anaesthesia, children were reunited with family, given access to movies and allowed flavoured ice. These are all important contributors to the relief of pain that was described as the placebo response. This response can be augmented by verbally induced expectations, conditioning and learning mechanisms, and the child–parent–physician interactions [78].

The same factors that may be used to augment the placebo response can also induce a nocebo response. The nocebo effect is the development of aversive effects also following any treatment or situation that normally has no therapeutic effect for the treated condition [83]. Virtually all treatment, pharmacological or not, will carry a placebo or nocebo effect related to the conditioned response to a similar situation and the expectation of the patient [84]. There are currently few studies in children that monitor nocebo effect, although the nocebo effect in epilepsy treatment in children [85] and in adult patients suffering undergoing interventional pain management has been reported [86]. Differentiating this placebo or nocebo response from drug effect can be difficult. Ethical considerations often preclude a group of children randomized to receive a placebo drug [77]. The continuing use of placebo controls has been strongly argued against in the literature [77, 87].

Functions that have been used to quantify the placebo effect include:

1) the exponential function:

$$Placebo = P_{MAX} \cdot (1 - e^{-kpl \cdot t}) \tag{13}$$

where t is time, P_{MAX} is the maximum placebo effect and kpl is the rate constant for onset of placebo effect.

2) The inverse Bateman function:

$$Placebo = P_{MAX} \cdot (1 - (e^{-kon \cdot t} - e^{-koff \cdot t})) \qquad (14)$$

where P_{MAX} is the maximum placebo effect and kon and $koff$ are the rate constants for onset and offset of placebo effect, respectively.

3) The Weibull function

$$Placebo = P_{MAX} \cdot \left(1 - e^{-\left(t/\lambda\right)^k}\right) \qquad (15)$$

where P_{MAX} is the maximum placebo effect and λ and k are the scale and shape parameters of the Weibull function.

The shape of the curve described by these functions depends on the variables estimated for each function. Some typical examples of such curves for placebo effects are shown in Fig. 4.7. Nocebo effects could be described by the inverse of these curves.

Consequently, the observed effect is further complicated by placebo (or nocebo):

$$Effect(t) = S_0 - (natural\ history + drug\ effect + \\ placebo\ effect) \qquad (16)$$

Drop Outs

Patients who receive rescue medication and are withdrawn from a study may introduce bias because the remaining study patients are those who do not have such severe pain; the reason for their reduced analgesia may not be solely pharmaceutical [88]. Failure to account for drop out in pain studies means that we consider all study attrition to be random, when in fact attrition usually occurs because of some factor (such as inadequate pain control or unpleasant drug effects) and may not be equally distributed among study groups. The rate of loss of study subjects (i.e. drop outs) can be explained as a hazard (h), with contributing factors explaining attrition included. For example, the time to request of rescue medication can be described using a time-to-event model where the hazard of requesting rescue medication is modelled as:

$$h(t) = h_0 \cdot e^{COV} \qquad (17)$$

where $h(t)$ is the hazard at time t, h_0 is the hazard without influence of covariates, and COV is the influence of covariates on the hazard. The hazard without influence of covariates (h_0) can be described using different hazard distributions such as the exponential, Weibull and Gompertz functions [89].

Introduction of a hazard model in an investigation of combined paracetamol and diclofenac analgesia after tonsillectomy helped to correct bias in model predictions of pain score introduced by study drop out. Those patients with severe pain, for example, were more likely to drop out of the study [90].

Coexisting Morbidity

Patients commonly present for anaesthesia with conditions that require investigation or surgical intervention;

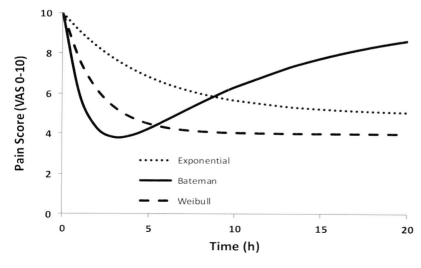

Fig. 4.7 Examples of three functions (exponential decay, Bateman and Weibull) that could be used to describe placebo effect for pain relief. The y-axis uses a visual analogue scale (VAS) where a score of 10 is the worst pain imaginable. The Bateman function demonstrates a placebo effect that wears off with time. Nocebo effects can be imagined as the inverse of these curves.

they also present with diseases unrelated to the need for surgery. The impact of disease on therapy (and vice versa) has been known for centuries. Pythagoras (510 BC) observed haemolytic anaemia after fava bean ingestion and this observation was later attributed to glucose-6-phosphate dehydrogenase (G-6-PD) deficiency only last century.

Disorders affect all ages. In the very young, congenital malformations (e.g. duodenal atresia) or disease characteristics (e.g. necrotizing enterocolitis) contribute to absorption variability. Perinatal circulatory changes (e.g. ductus venosus, ductus arteriosus) alter drug disposition [91]. Induction of anaesthesia may be slowed by right-to-left shunting of blood in neonates suffering cyanotic congenital cardiac disease or intrapulmonary conditions.

The environment in which children live can have subtle effects. Opioid administration was reduced in otherwise healthy children with altitude-induced chronic hypoxia when compared to non-hypoxic children undergoing similar operations under similar anaesthetic regimens [92]. Similar findings have been reported in obese children suffering obstructive sleep apnoea who have increased sensitivity to opioids [93]. Opioid sensitivity may be affected in disease states because there are specific transport systems that mediate active transport. Pathological central nervous system (CNS) conditions can cause blood–brain barrier (BBB) breakdown and alter functioning of its transport systems. Fentanyl is actively transported across the BBB by a saturable ATP-dependent process, while ATP-binding cassette proteins such as P-glycoprotein actively pump out opioids such as fentanyl and morphine [94]. P-glycoprotein modulation significantly influences opioid brain distribution and onset time, magnitude and duration of analgesic response [95]. Modulation may occur due to disease processes, fever or other substances (e.g. verapamil, magnesium) [94].

The influence of coexisting morbidity on the PK effect of anaesthetic drugs in adult patients is well recognized. For example ASA III patients had a smaller central volume of distribution and a reduced clearance for propofol compared to ASA I patients [96]. Similarly, in a pooled analysis of 21 propofol datasets, patients were found to have decreased propofol elimination and distribution clearances (CL, Q2, Q3) using a three compartment model, and slow peripheral volume of distribution (V3) compared with healthy volunteers [54]. The use of such empirical models describes an observed difference between patients and healthy volunteers; the cause is uncertain and might be related to concomitant medication, comorbidity or the anaesthetic technique applied. Another study in critically ill patients showed that fentanyl PK was strongly influenced by severe liver disease and congestive heart failure [97]. In that same study severity of illness as a covariate did not improve the model fit after liver and heart diseases were included. The expected PK and PD alterations of coexisting morbidity should consider not only the severity of the disease and its pathophysiological implications, but the possible effect of drug interactions from concomitant medications used.

Circadian Rhythms

Drugs can show time-of-day variation in their effect, and some are dosed according to a circadian schedule [98]. This effect can be due to either PK or PD changes over the day since the circadian system influences multiple biochemical and physiological variables which include changes in body temperature, hormone secretion, metabolism and our immune systems [99]. Local anaesthetic action is longest during the afternoon [100–102] and neuromuscular blockade by rocuronium lasts one-third longer in the morning compared to the afternoon [103]. Chronotherapeutic dosing of 5-fluorouracil, with peak delivery at 0400 h, is more effective and less toxic than when administered as a constant infusion [104]. Both absorption and bioavailability differences at different times of the day have been described for paracetamol [105], indomethacin [106, 107], diclofenac [108] and ketoprofen [109] in adults.

The Burgeoning Obesity Problem

Volume (determining loading dose) and clearance (determining maintenance dose) of some drugs are known to be changed in obesity [110]. Although body fat has minimal metabolic activity, fat mass contributes to overall body size and may have an indirect influence on both metabolic and renal clearance from the secondary increase in lean tissues needed to support the increase in fat weight. In addition, an increase in abdominal visceral fat can produce an excessive secretion of hormones and inflammatory bio-active peptides, with a variety of potential effects in organ systems and circulation. On the other hand, the volume of distribution of a drug depends on its physicochemical properties [111]. There are drugs whose apparent volume of distribution may be independent of fat mass (e.g. digoxin) or be extensively determined by it (e.g. diazepam).

A number of size descriptors (Fig. 4.8) have been put forward for use in the obese patient e.g. total body weight (TBW), lean body weight (LBW), ideal body weight (IBW), body mass index (BMI), fat free mass (FFM) and normal fat mass (NFM). These size descriptors invariably demonstrate nonlinear relationships between weight and clearance. **The best size descriptor accounting for obesity remains unknown** [112]. LBW is often advocated for use in the obese, but that descriptor may not apply for all drugs [113, 114]. For example, for propofol, commonly used to maintain anaesthesia in the paediatric patient, the infusion rate is dependent on clearance. An incorrect estimate of clearance may lead to inadequate anaesthesia, and awareness. Propofol clearance in obese children [115] and adults, [54, 116] and in non-obese adults and children [53, 117], is best predicted using TBW as the size descriptor with theory-based allometry. But for remifentanil, another commonly used drug, lean body weight appears to be the better size descriptor [45, 48].

The use of NFM [118] with allometric scaling as a size descriptor may prove versatile [13, 119–121]. That size descriptor uses the idea of FFM (which is similar to LBW but excludes lipids in cell membranes, CNS and bone marrow) plus a 'bit more'. The 'bit more' will differ for each drug and the maximum 'bit more' added to fat free mass would equal TBW.

$$FFM = WHS_{max} \cdot HT^2 \cdot \left[\frac{TBW}{\left(WHS_{50} \cdot HT^2 + TBW\right)} \right]$$

(18)

Where WHS_{max} is the maximum FFM for any given height (HT, m) and WHS_{50} is the TBW value when FFM is half of WHS_{max}. For men, WHS_{max} is 42.92 kg/m^2 and WHS_{50} is 30.93 kg/m^2 and for women WHS_{max} is 37.99 kg/m^2 and WHS_{50} is 35.98 kg/m^2 [12].

NFM is then defined as:

$$NFM = FFM + Ffat \cdot (TBW - FFM)$$

(19)

The parameter *Ffat* is estimated and accounts for different contributions of fat mass. If *Ffat* is estimated to be zero, then FFM alone predicts size, while if *Ffat* is 1, then size is predicted by TBW. This parameter is drug specific and also specific to the PK parameter such as clearance or volume of distribution. *Ffat* has a value of 0.211 for GFR which implies that 21% of fat mass is a size driver for kidney function in addition to FFM [13]. Size based on NFM assumes that FFM is the primary determinant of size with an extra *Ffat* factor (which may be positive or negative) that determines how fat mass contributes to size. A negative value for *Ffat* might suggest organ dysfunction, which is not an uncommon scenario in the morbidly obese. A negative *Ffat* has been described for the drug dexmedetomidine [122].

Pharmacodynamic Variability

Pharmacodynamic (concentration–effect) variability also exists. Receptor sensitivity variability (5–50%) and efficacy variability (30%) exist. Variability also exists due to distribution from the blood to the site of action and depends largely on changes in perfusion of target tissue (5–60%), the link between PK and PD. However, the observed response may not be a direct consequence of drug–receptor binding itself, but it may rather have been mediated through intermediate physiological

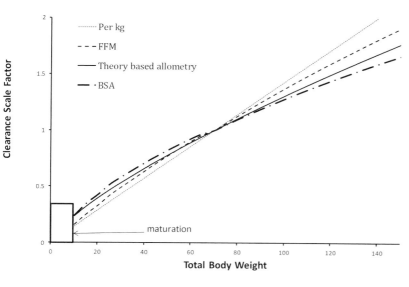

Fig. 4.8 Body size metrics used to describe clearance changes with weight for individuals of average height for weight. The clearance scale factor shows how clearance would differ with weight. A nonlinear relationship exists between weight and clearance using theory-based allometry. The per kg method increasingly overestimates clearance in adults and underestimates clearance in children. The BSA method overestimates clearance in children compared to theory-based allometry. Scaling with fat free mass (FFM) lies between the per kg method and theory-based allometry. An additional function is required to describe maturation (not shown). (Reproduced with permission from Anderson BJ: *Arch.Dis.Child.* 2013; 98: 732–6).

mechanisms (e.g. antipyretics, angiotensin converting enzyme inhibitors). A typical value for this variability is 30% [123].

Age may also be a marker for PD changes. Age was a significant covariate of remifentanil EC_{50} and k_{eo}, with both decreasing with increasing age by approximately 50% over the age range studied [52]. Similar results are reported for propofol in the elderly patient. The EC_{50} values for loss of consciousness were 2.35, 1.8 and 1.25 µg/mL in volunteers of 25, 50 and 75 years old, respectively [124].

The minimum alveolar concentration (MAC) is commonly used to express anaesthetic vapour potency. The MAC values for most vapours in neonates are less than those in infants [125]. MAC increases with age in preschool children, and thereafter decreases again through childhood [126, 127]. The MAC of isoflurane in preterm neonates < 32 weeks' gestation was 1.28% (SD 0.17), and in preterm neonates 32–37 weeks' gestation was 1.41% (SD 0.18) which in turn is less than in full-term neonates [126]. Similar data are reported for halothane (Fig. 4.9) and sevoflurane [127–129].

Changes in regional blood flow may influence the amount of drug that reaches the brain. Volatile anaesthetics possibly act partly through gamma-aminobutyric acid ($GABA_A$) receptors [130] and receptor numbers or developmental shifts in the regulation of chloride transporters in the brain may change with age [131], altering the response to these anaesthetics. $GABA_A$ receptor binding in human neonates is strikingly different from that in older children and adults [132]. Midazolam also acts through the GABA neurotransmitter. Data from rodents from immediate neonates to PNA 40 days have shown developmental

PD changes for sedation that mimic those observed in human childhood [133]. Genetic polymorphisms affecting P-glycoprotein-related genes influencing drug movement across the BBB also contribute to differences in CNS-active drug sensitivity [134].

The between-subject PD variability associated with the inhalation agents is considerably less than that reported with intravenous anaesthetic drugs. Steeper concentration–response curves (with perhaps the exception of ketamine [135]) are also described [136, 137]. Within a population, MAC may vary by as little as 10–15% among individuals [138]. This small variability about MAC can be compared to the three- to five-fold variability described for plasma opioid concentration that blocks a defined response to stimulus in 50% of patients [139]. It seems odd that there is such a discrepancy between variability of MAC and EC_{50}. The imprecision and bias of the EC_{50} estimate using population modelling may be contributed by our inability to often measure effect intensity of more than 75% of E_{MAX} [140]. However MAC is commonly estimated using modifications of the 'up and down' technique of Dixon [141]. That methodology uses few subjects and may result in less observed variability. Improvements to the original methodology reveal that variability is considerably greater than originally reported [142]. The small MAC variability reported in early studies did not lend itself to investigation of covariate effects, which surely exist.

Response may also vary due to pharmacogenomic changes that affect opioid receptors and pain perception and processing [143–145]. Some patients may truly have a 'low pain threshold'. Of less clinical importance, desflurane requirements have been postulated to be increased in those with red hair compared to those with dark hair: attributed to those homozygous or compound heterozygous for mutations on the melanocortin-1 receptor gene [146]. This observation remains debated [147]. Although phenotypic expression of hair colour poses no greater operative risk to patients [148], it may be another marker of variability that contributes to the pharmacological uniqueness of each child.

Opioid dosing is commonly reduced in children with cognitive impairment [149], an observation supported by lower BIS scores in this cohort when given similar doses to healthy comparators [150]. Behavioural predispositions such as preoperative anxiety also increase propofol induction dose [151].

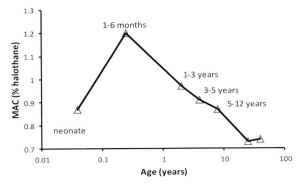

Fig. 4.9 Halothane minimum alveolar concentration (MAC) changes with age. MAC is greatest in infancy. (Data from Gregory GA et al: *Anesthesiology.* 1969; 30: 488–91 and Lerman J et al: *Anesthesiology.* 1983; 59: 421–4.)

Does Sex Matter?

Sex-specific differences in drug response have been reported. Molecular factors influencing these differences include: drug transporters, drug metabolizing enzymes (phase I and phase II) and protein binding. Physiological factors include differences in body size and composition, gastrointestinal physiology and renal excretion of drugs [152]. Clinically significant differences in therapeutic response based on these factors are, however, rare [152, 153]. Some differences may be attributed to PK rather than PD factors. Standardizing PK parameters using more comprehensive size descriptors capable of describing gender-specific differences in body composition is desirable in future studies to improve our understanding of dose adjustment according to sex.

Female patients given propofol woke up faster than men [154–156]. Differences in propofol kinetics, which might explain the faster emergence in women, have been reported. One study found that women have larger slow peripheral volume (V3) and elimination clearance (CL) but lower rapid distribution clearance (Q2) than men using a three compartment model [157]. Another study described a smaller V1 for women compared with men and higher CL for the age range 22 to 69 years [54]. Similarly, a recent study showed that faster awakening of women from propofol anaesthesia was mainly explained by a faster decline of propofol plasma concentrations but that analysis also suggested that women were more sensitive to propofol than men [158].

Sex differences in opioid-induced analgesia have also been described in several studies [159]. In adult subjects differences in morphine consumption have been shown to be due to PD reasons. Compared with men, women showed greater morphine potency but slower onset and offset of analgesic effect [160]. Similarly, it has been also shown that women are more sensitive than men to opioid-induced respiratory depression and other adverse effects [161].

Sex differences depend on many variables which include those specific to the drug, such as the dose or time of administration, and those particular to the subject, such as, genetics, age or hormonal factors [161].

Does Race Have Impact?

Pain differences exist between peoples of different races and ethnicities. The contribution of culture, geography [92, 162] and genetics as covariates remains to be teased apart. The incidence of adverse effects after morphine is greater in Latino than non-Latino children. Neither differences in morphine or metabolite concentrations, nor genetic polymorphisms examined explained these findings [146]. Caucasian children had a higher incidence of opioid related adverse effects but less pain than African American children [163]. The latter had higher morphine clearance, and although UGT2B7 genetic variations (2161C>T and 802C>T) were not associated with observed racial differences in morphine's clearance, the wild type of the UGT2B7 isozyme was more prevalent in the African Americans [164].

Although neither race nor ethnicity is a true biological construct, race is often used as entho-variance and is based on self-identification. Modelling can be done similar to that used for sex.

Contribution from the Genes

Genetic influences may have a profound effect on metabolic clearance pathways [165, 166]. Reduced succinylcholine clearance by butyrylcholinesterase and reduced isoniazid acetylation activity are well known examples. Single nucleotide changes or polymorphisms (SNPs) in the DNA sequence of CYP enzymes usually decrease but may also increase metabolic activity for a specific drug or drug substrate [167]. The CYP2D6 drug-metabolizing enzyme is responsible for clearance of a number of drugs including amitriptyline, codeine, tramadol and hydrocodone [168]. For the 2% to 10% of the population who are CYP2D6 poor metabolizers, codeine causes limited opioid effects. However, individuals with duplicated active CYP2D6 genes are classified as ultra-extensive metabolizers and the rapid metabolism of codeine into morphine can result in narcosis, apnoea and death [169].

Single nucleotide polymorphisms for the enzyme responsible for metabolizing catecholamines (catechol-O-methyl transferase, COMT) have been described and distinct haplotypes categorized (low, average and high pain sensitivity). Haplotypes have also been associated with catecholamine synthesis [e.g. cofactor tetrahydrobiopterin (BH4) synthesis and metabolism] that are associated with chronic pain. BH4 blocking drugs may prove useful as a novel analgesic. In addition, haplotypes for the B_2 adrenergic receptor, based on eight single nucleotide polymorphisms, have been identified. Anxious patients can be assumed to have higher concentrations of circulating catecholamines. The extremely anxious patient may require a greater anaesthesia induction dose of propofol than less anxious patients [170]. Increased circulating catecholamines may also contribute to perceived pain.

It is not surprising that inflammatory cytokines (interleukins, tumour necrosis factor) have impact on the pain response. The inflammatory response mediated after surgery has impact on pain [171]. Polymorphism in the interleukin-1 receptor antagonist gene is associated with serum interleukin-1 receptor antagonist concentrations and postoperative opioid consumption [172].

Morphine works through the μ-opioid receptor, a protein coded for by the OPRM1 gene on chromosome 6q24-q25. Polymorphisms of this gene (e.g. A118 G) may increase this receptor's affinity for morphine and its metabolite morphine 6-glucuronide [173] but their clinical impact continues to be debated [174, 175]. A number of other genetic variations may also influence the μ-opioid receptor. The melanocortin-1 receptor that serves a role in skin pigmentation may influence morphine 6-glucuronide effects as well as the κ-opioid receptor in females [176]. Signal transmission from opioid receptors requires involvement of ion channels (K, Na, Ca) and polymorphisms of these channels have also been noted to have an influence on pain sensitivity. Mutations in voltage gated transient receptor potential channels have been identified and may modulate the effects of analgesics [177]. Efflux transporters like the P-glycoproteins are also associated with polymorphisms and may affect transport into or out of the brain [178].

It would be nice to adjust dose further based on individual characteristics [179], but it remains uncertain how much an understanding of pharmacogenomics will play in dose individualization. If a single genetic variant were responsible for major PK or PD differences, then dose individualization would be easier. The drug irinotecan, used to treat cancer, has an active metabolite that is metabolized by a glucuronide (UGT1A1), a pathway similar to that involved in morphine clearance (UGT2B7). A variant allele UGT1A1*28 has been identified that is associated with severe neutropenia and diarrhea. Genetic testing in patients to identify this allele (present in 10% of Caucasians) has been shown to be beneficial [180]. However, there appears a multiplicity of genetic influences on both morphine PK and PD and the impact from interaction of these variants is not fully understood. Pain response is further complicated by numerous other factors (e.g. psychosocial, race, environment, underlying pathology, age).

Adverse Effects

Adverse effects may also be related to covariates. Age is an important covariate in children. Neonates and young children may suffer permanent effects resulting from a stimulus applied at a sensitive point in development. For example, congenital hypothyroidism, if left untreated, causes lifelong phenotypic changes. Tetracyclines cause staining of developing teeth. There are concerns that neonatal exposure to some anaesthetic agents (e.g. ketamine, midazolam) may cause widespread neuronal apoptosis and long-term memory deficits [181–183]. Oxyhaemoglobin desaturation was directly correlated with younger chronological age in term infants given chloral hydrate [184]. But in other respects, the very young may be less susceptible to adverse effects. The susceptibility of neonates to cardiotoxicity from bupivacaine may be reduced due to differences in the mechanisms regulating intracellular calcium [185].

The 'right' dose of a drug is a balance between beneficial and adverse effects. Anaesthesia generally involves monitoring and possibly treating immediate adverse effects such as hypotension, respiratory depression or postoperative nausea and vomiting. Therapeutic use of drugs balances beneficial effects against adverse effects. A dose–response curve for intravenous morphine and vomiting was investigated in children having day-stay tonsillectomy. Doses above 0.1 mg/kg were associated with a greater than 50% incidence of vomiting [186]. These data are similar to those in children undergoing inguinal herniorrhaphy [187]. However, age-related changes have not been investigated in children. While it is recognized that postoperative nausea and vomiting may increase after puberty, changes in other age groups are seldom reported. Other covariates such as the type of surgery (e.g. strabismus correction, tonsillectomy) are also implicated in the incidence of postoperative nausea and vomiting; these may be more significant than age.

PK/PD modelling has demonstrated that remifentanil concentrations well tolerated in the steady state will cause a clinically significant hypoventilation following bolus administration, confirming the acute risk of bolus administration of fast-acting opioids in spontaneously breathing patients [188]. A relationship between hypotension and remifentanil has also been described in children [189], but not in adults. Covariates such as hypertension in adults and its effect on the concentration–blood pressure response curve are unknown.

Gains in therapeutic effect must be balanced by the adverse effect profile of a drug. The middle ground sought is a compromise between these two effects (Fig. 4.10) and will differ for each individual child. Opioid dose, for example, is a balance between sufficient analgesia and an acceptably low risk of postoperative nausea and vomiting and sedation (or respiratory depression). Children using PCA devices invariably achieve such a compromise, albeit with the added safety features inherent within the device delivery programme.

Conclusions

The Holy Grail of clinical pharmacology is prediction of drug PK and PD in the individual patient and this requires knowledge of the covariates that contribute to variability [2]. The specialty of anaesthesia has embraced population modelling with its ability to explore covariate effects. Major covariates such as age and weight are programmed into infusion pumps that administer propofol and remifentanil. Effect monitoring using modified electroencephalographic signals can become part of a feedback loop. A greater understanding of covariate effects will allow better dose individualization of other drugs within our armamentarium.

References

1. Holford NHG: The target concentration approach to clinical drug development. Clin.Pharmacokinet. 1995; 29 (5): 287–91.

2. Benet LZ: A Holy Grail of clinical pharmacology: prediction of drug pharmacokinetics and pharmacodynamics in the individual patient. Clin. Pharmacol.Ther. 2009; 86 (2): 133–4.

3. Anderson BJ, Allegaert K, Van den Anker JN, Cossey V, Holford NH: Vancomycin pharmacokinetics in preterm neonates and the prediction of adult clearance. Br.J.Clin.Pharmacol. 2007; 63 (1): 75–84.

4. Tod M, Jullien V, Pons G: Facilitation of drug evaluation in children by population methods and modelling. Clin.Pharmacokinet. 2008; 47 (4): 231–43.

5. Anderson BJ, Holford NH: Understanding dosing: children are small adults, neonates are immature children. Arch.Dis.Child. 2013; 98 (9): 737–44.

6. Lack JA, Stuart Taylor ME: Calculation of drug dosage and body surface area of children. Br.J.Anaesth. 1997; 78 (5): 601–5.

7. Sumpter AL, Holford NH: Predicting weight using postmenstrual age – neonates to adults. Paediatr. Anaesth. 2011; 21 (3): 309–15.

8. Anderson BJ, Meakin GH: Scaling for size: some implications for paediatric anaesthesia dosing. Paediatr.Anaesth. 2002; 12 (3): 205–19.

9. Anderson BJ, Holford NH: Mechanistic basis of using body size and maturation to predict clearance in humans. Drug.Metab.Pharmacokinet. 2009; 24 (1): 25–36.

10. Du Bois D, Du Bois EF: Clinical calorimetry: tenth paper. A formula to estimate the approximate surface area if height and weight be known. Arch.Intern.Med. 1916; 17: 863–71.

11. James W. Research on Obesity. London: Her Majesty's Stationary Office, 1976.

12. Janmahasatian S, Duffull SB, Ash S, Ward LC, Byrne NM, Green B: Quantification of lean bodyweight. Clin. Pharmacokinet. 2005; 44 (10): 1051–65.

13. Rhodin MM, Anderson BJ, Peters AM, Coulthard MG, Wilkins B, Cole M, et al: Human renal function maturation: a quantitative description using weight and postmenstrual age. Pediatr.Nephrol. 2009; 24 (1): 67–76.

14. West GB, Brown JH: The origin of allometric scaling laws in biology from genomes to ecosystems: towards a

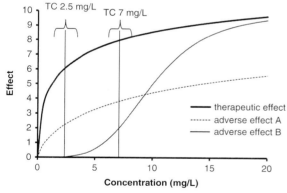

Fig. 4.10 Dose is not determined solely by PK and PD. Adverse effects also influence dose. This figure demonstrates the interplay between beneficial and adverse effects of a drug. The higher target concentration of 7 mg/L for a theoretical drug achieves a better effect, but at the expense of increased adverse effects. The lower concentration of 2.5 mg/L may be satisfactory and have fewer adverse effects. However, each individual will have different concentration–response relationships. This scenario is typical for patient controlled analgesia (PCA) devices where the patient determines a satisfactory target concentration and consequent analgesic level that is balanced against acceptable adverse effects (e.g. postoperative nausea or sedation). Some patients may opt for a target of 2.5 mg/L; they achieve some analgesia but minimal adverse effects. This is satisfactory for them because the adverse effects are insufferable. Others may opt for a higher target concentration and better analgesia; adverse effects may either not trouble them or be balanced against the benefits of pain relief. (Reproduced with permission from Anderson BJ: Pediatr.Anesth. 2012; 22: 530–8).

quantitative unifying theory of biological structure and organization. J.Exp.Biol. 2005; 208 (Pt 9): 1575–92.

15. West GB, Brown JH, Enquist BJ: A general model for the origin of allometric scaling laws in biology. Science. 1997; 276 (5309): 122–6.

16. Anderson BJ, Holford NH: Mechanism-based concepts of size and maturity in pharmacokinetics. Annu.Rev. Pharmacol.Toxicol. 2008; 48: 303–32.

17. Holford S, Allegaert K, Anderson BJ, Kukanich B, Sousa AB, Steinman A, et al: Parent-metabolite pharmacokinetic models for tramadol – tests of assumptions and predictions. J.Pharmacol.Clin. Toxicol. 2014; 2 (1): 1023.

18. Ross AK, Davis PJ, Dear Gd GL, Ginsberg B, McGowan FX, Stiller RD, et al: Pharmacokinetics of remifentanil in anesthetized pediatric patients undergoing elective surgery or diagnostic procedures. Anesth.Analg. 2001; 93 (6): 1393–401.

19. Rigby-Jones AE, Priston MJ, Sneyd JR, McCabe AP, Davis GI, Tooley MA, et al: Remifentanil-midazolam sedation for paediatric patients receiving mechanical ventilation after cardiac surgery. Brit.J.Anaesth. 2007; 99 (2): 252–61.

20. Welzing L, Ebenfeld S, Dlugay V, Wiesen MH, Roth B, Mueller C: Remifentanil degradation in umbilical cord blood of preterm infants. Anesthesiology. 2011; 114 (3): 570–7.

21. Potts AL, Larsson P, Eksborg S, Warman G, Lonnqvist P-A, Anderson BJ: Clonidine disposition in children; a population analysis. Pediatr.Anesth. 2007; 17 (10): 924–33.

22. Anderson BJ, van Lingen RA, Hansen TG, Lin YC, Holford NH: Acetaminophen developmental pharmacokinetics in premature neonates and infants: a pooled population analysis. Anesthesiology. 2002; 96 (6): 1336–45.

23. Herd D, Anderson BJ: Ketamine disposition in children presenting for procedural sedation and analgesia in a children's emergency department. Paediatr.Anaesth. 2007; 17 (7): 622–9.

24. Chalkiadis GA, Anderson BJ: Age and size are the major covariates for prediction of levobupivacaine clearance in children. Paediatr.Anaesth. 2006; 16 (3): 275–82.

25. Allegaert K, van den Anker JN, de Hoon JN, van Schaik RH, Debeer A, Tibboel D, et al: Covariates of tramadol disposition in the first months of life. Brit.J.Anaesth. 2008; 100 (4): 525–32.

26. Allegaert K, Anderson BJ, van den Anker JN, Vanhaesebrouck S, de Zegher F: Renal drug clearance in preterm neonates: relation to prenatal growth. Ther. Drug.Monit. 2007; 29 (3): 284–91.

27. Johnson TN: The problems in scaling adult drug doses to children. Arch.Dis.Child. 2008; 93 (3): 207–11.

28. Edginton AN, Schmitt W, Voith B, Willmann S: A mechanistic approach for the scaling of clearance in children. Clin.Pharmacokinet. 2006; 45 (7): 683–704.

29. Holford N, Heo YA, Anderson B: A pharmacokinetic standard for babies and adults. J.Pharm.Sci. 2013; 102 (9): 2941–52.

30. Hill AV: The possible effects of the aggregation of the molecules of haemoglobin on its dissociation curves. J. Physiol. 1910; 14: iv–vii.

31. Saarenmaa E, Neuvonen PJ, Fellman V. Gestational age and birth weight effects on plasma clearance of fentanyl in newborn infants. J.Pediatr. 2000; 136 (6): 767–70.

32. Allegaert K, Palmer GM, Anderson BJ: The pharmacokinetics of intravenous paracetamol in neonates: size matters most. Arch.Dis.Child. 2011; 96 (6): 575–80.

33. Anderson BJ, Pons G, Autret-Leca E, Allegaert K, Boccard E: Pediatric intravenous paracetamol (propacetamol) pharmacokinetics: a population analysis. Paediatr.Anaesth. 2005; 15 (4): 282–92.

34. Pokela ML, Olkkola KT, Seppala T, Koivisto M: Age-related morphine kinetics in infants. Dev.Pharmacol. Ther. 1993; 20 (1–2): 26–34.

35. Peters JW, Anderson BJ, Simons SH, Uges DR, Tibboel D: Morphine metabolite pharmacokinetics during venoarterial extra corporeal membrane oxygenation in neonates. Clin.Pharmacokinet. 2006; 45 (7): 705–14.

36. Anand KJ, Anderson BJ, Holford NH, Hall RW, Young T, Shephard B, et al: Morphine pharmacokinetics and pharmacodynamics in preterm and term neonates: secondary results from the NEOPAIN trial. Brit.J.Anaesth. 2008; 101 (5): 680–9.

37. Schwartz GJ, Work DF: Measurement and estimation of GFR in children and adolescents. CJASN. 2009; 4 (11): 1832–43.

38. Paap CM, Nahata MC: Prospective evaluation of ten methods for estimating creatinine clearance in children with varying degrees of renal dysfunction. J. Clin.Pharm.Ther. 1995; 20 (2): 67–73.

39. Cole M, Price L, Parry A, Keir MJ, Pearson AD, Boddy AV, et al: Estimation of glomerular filtration rate in paediatric cancer patients using 51CR-EDTA population pharmacokinetics. Br.J.Cancer. 2004; 90 (1): 60–4.

40. Schwartz GJ, Haycock GB, Edelmann CM, Jr., Spitzer A: A simple estimate of glomerular filtration rate in children derived from body length and plasma creatinine. Pediatrics. 1976; 58 (2): 259–63.

41. Schwartz GJ, Feld LG, Langford DJ: A simple estimate of glomerular filtration rate in full-term infants during the first year of life. J.Pediatr. 1984; 104 (6): 849–54.

42. Brion LP, Fleischman AR, McCarton C, Schwartz GJ: A simple estimate of glomerular filtration rate in low birth weight infants during the first year of life:

noninvasive assessment of body composition and growth. J.Pediatr. 1986; 109 (4): 698–707.

43. Standing JF: Understanding and applying pharmacometric modelling and simulation in clinical practice and research. Br.J.Clin.Pharmacol. 2017; 83 (2): 247–54.

44. Eleveld DJ, Colin P, Absalom AR, Struys M: Pharmacokinetic-pharmacodynamic model for propofol for broad application in anaesthesia and sedation. Br.J.Anaesth. 2018; 120 (5): 942–59.

45. Eleveld DJ, Proost JH, Vereecke H, Absalom AR, Olofsen E, Vuyk J, et al: An allometric model of remifentanil pharmacokinetics and pharmacodynamics. Anesthesiology. 2017; 126 (6): 1005–18.

46. Cheymol G: Effects of obesity on pharmacokinetics implications for drug therapy. Clin.Pharmacokinet. 2000; 39 (3): 215–31.

47. Cortinez LI, Anderson BJ, Holford NH, Puga V, de la Fuente N, Auad H, et al: Dexmedetomidine pharmacokinetics in the obese. Eur.J.Clin. Pharm. 2015; 71(12): 1501–8.

48. Egan TD, Huizinga B, Gupta SK, Jaarsma RL, Sperry RJ, Yee JB, et al: Remifentanil pharmacokinetics in obese versus lean patients. Anesthesiology. 1998; 89 (3): 562–73.

49. Coldrey JC, Upton RN, Macintyre PE: Advances in analgesia in the older patient. Best practice and research. Clin.Anaesth. 2011; 25 (3): 367–78.

50. McLean AJ, Le Couteur DG: Aging biology and geriatric clinical pharmacology. Pharmacol. Rev. 2004; 56 (2): 163–84.

51. Le Couteur DG, McLean AJ: The aging liver. Drug clearance and an oxygen diffusion barrier hypothesis. Clin.Pharm. 1998; 34 (5): 359–73.

52. Minto CF, Schnider TW, Egan TD, Youngs E, Lemmens HJ, Gambus PL, et al: Influence of age and gender on the pharmacokinetics and pharmacodynamics of remifentanil. Anesthesiology. 1997; 86: 10–23.

53. Schuttler J, Ihmsen H: Population pharmacokinetics of propofol: a multicenter study. Anesthesiology. 2000; 92 (3): 727–38.

54. Eleveld DJ, Proost JH, Cortinez LI, Absalom AR, Struys MM: A general purpose pharmacokinetic model for propofol. Anesth.Analg. 2014; 118 (6): 1221–37.

55. Upton RN, Ludbrook GL: A physiological model of induction of anaesthesia with propofol in sheep. 1. Structure and estimation of variables. Br.J.Anaesth. 1997; 79 (4): 497–504.

56. Cortinez LI, Troconiz IF, Fuentes R, Gambus P, Hsu YW, Altermatt F, et al: The influence of age on the dynamic relationship between end-tidal sevoflurane concentration and bispectral index. Anesth.Anal. 2008; 107: 1566–72.

57. Minto CF, Schnider TW, Egan TD, Youngs E, Lemmens HJ, Gambus PL, et al: Influence of age and gender on the pharmacokinetics and pharmacodynamics of remifentanil. I. Model development. Anesthesiology. 1997; 86 (1): 10–23.

58. Vuyk J, Lichtenbelt BJ, Olofsen E, van Kleef JW, Dahan A: Mixed-effects modeling of the influence of midazolam on propofol pharmacokinetics. Anesth. Analg. 2009; 108 (5): 1522–30.

59. Verbeeck RK: Pharmacokinetics and dosage adjustment in patients with hepatic dysfunction. Eur.J.Clin.Pharm. 2008; 64 (12): 1147–61.

60. Blaschke TF: Protein binding and kinetics of drugs in liver diseases. Clin.Pharmacokinet. 1977; 2 (1): 32–44.

61. Kaivosaari S, Toivonen P, Aitio O, Sipila J, Koskinen M, Salonen JS, et al: Regio- and stereospecific N-glucuronidation of medetomidine: the differences between UDP glucuronosyltransferase (UGT) 1A4 and UGT2B10 account for the complex kinetics of human liver microsomes. Drug.Metab.Dispos. 2008; 36 (8): 1529–37.

62. Kohli U, Pandharipande P, Muszkat M, Sofowora GG, Friedman EA, Scheinin M, et al: CYP2A6 genetic variation and dexmedetomidine disposition. Eur.J.Clin.Pharm. 2012; 68 (6): 937–42.

63. Song JC, Gao H, Qiu HB, et al. The pharmacokinetics of dexmedetomidine in patients with obstructive jaundice: A clinical trial. PLoS One 2018; 13: e0207427.

64. Servin F, Cockshott ID, Farinotti R, Haberer JP, Winckler C, Desmonts JM: Pharmacokinetics of propofol infusions in patients with cirrhosis. Br.J.Anaesth. 1990; 65 (2): 177–83.

65. Elston AC, Bayliss MK, Park GR: Effect of renal failure on drug metabolism by the liver. Br.J.Anaesth. 1993; 71 (2): 282–90.

66. Chauvin M, Sandouk P, Scherrmann JM, Farinotti R, Strumza P, Duvaldestin P: Morphine pharmacokinetics in renal failure. Anesthesiology. 1987; 66 (3): 327–31.

67. Hannam JA, Anderson BJ: Contribution of morphine and morphine-6-glucuronide to respiratory depression in a child. Anaesth.Intensive.Care. 2012; 40 (5): 867–70.

68. Verbeeck RK, Musuamba FT: Pharmacokinetics and dosage adjustment in patients with renal dysfunction. Eur.J.Clin.Pharm. 2009; 65 (8): 757–73.

69. Hannam JA, Anderson BJ: Pharmacodynamic interaction models in pediatric anesthesia. Paediatr. Anaesth. 2015; 25: 970–80.

70. Chan PL, Holford NH: Drug treatment effects on disease progression. Annu.Rev.Pharmacol.Toxicol. 2001; 41: 625–59.

71. Brown RD, Kearns GL, Wilson JT: Integrated pharmacokinetic-pharmacodynamic model for acetaminophen, ibuprofen, and placebo antipyresis

in children. J.Pharmacokinet.Biopharm. 1998; 26 (5): 559–79.

72. Lavy JA: Post-tonsillectomy pain: the difference between younger and older patients. Int.J.Pediatr. Otorhinolaryngol. 1997; 42 (1): 11–15.

73. Murthy P, Laing MR: Dissection tonsillectomy: pattern of post-operative pain, medication and resumption of normal activity. J.Laryngol.Otol. 1998; 112 (1): 41–4.

74. Stewart DW, Ragg PG, Sheppard S, Chalkiadis GA: The severity and duration of postoperative pain and analgesia requirements in children after tonsillectomy, orchidopexy, or inguinal hernia repair. Pediatr.Anesth. 2012; 22 (2): 136–43.

75. Anderson BJ, Woollard GA, Holford NH: Acetaminophen analgesia in children: placebo effect and pain resolution after tonsillectomy. Eur.J.Clin. Pharmacol. 2001; 57 (8): 559–69.

76. Anderson BJ, Holford NH, Woollard GA, Kanagasundaram S, Mahadevan M: Perioperative pharmacodynamics of acetaminophen analgesia in children. Anesthesiology. 1999; 90 (2): 411–21.

77. Anderson B, Cranswick N: The placebo (I shall please)– is it so pleasing in children? Paediatr.Anaesth. 2005; 15 (10): 809–13.

78. Simmons K, Ortiz R, Kossowsky J, Krummenacher P, Grillon C, Pine D, et al: Pain and placebo in pediatrics: a comprehensive review of laboratory and clinical findings. J.Pain. 2014; 155 (11): 2229–35.

79. Weimer K, Gulewitsch MD, Schlarb AA, Schwille-Kiuntke J, Klosterhalfen S, Enck P: Placebo effects in children: a review. Pediatr.Res. 2013; 74 (1): 96–102.

80. Krummenacher P, Kossowsky J, Schwarz C, Brugger P, Kelley JM, Meyer A, et al: Expectancy-induced placebo analgesia in children and the role of magical thinking. J.Pain. 2014; 15 (12): 1282–93.

81. Bjornsson MA, Simonsson US: Modelling of pain intensity and informative dropout in a dental pain model after naproxcinod, naproxen and placebo administration. Br.J.Clin.Pharmacol. 2011; 71 (6): 899–906.

82. Johr M: Postanaesthesia excitation. Paediatr.Anaesth. 2002; 12 (4): 308–12.

83. Benedetti F: Placebo and endogenous mechanisms of analgesia. Handb.Exp.Pharmacol. 2007; 177: 393–413.

84. Marchand S, Gaumond I: Placebo and nocebo: how to enhance therapies and avoid unintended sabotage to pain treatment. Pain.Manag. 2013; 3 (4): 285–94.

85. Zaccara G, Giovannelli F, Schmidt D: Placebo and nocebo responses in drug trials of epilepsy. Epilepsy. Behav. 2015; 43: 128–34.

86. Manchikanti L, Pampati V, Damron K: The role of placebo and nocebo effects of perioperative administration of sedatives and opioids in interventional pain management. Pain.Physician. 2005; 8 (4): 349–55.

87. Rothman KJ, Michels KB: The continuing unethical use of placebo controls. N.Engl.J.Med. 1994; 331 (6): 394–8.

88. Sheiner LB: A new approach to the analysis of analgesic drug trials, illustrated with bromfenac data. Clin. Pharmacol.Ther. 1994; 56 (3): 309–22.

89. Anderson BJ, Hannam JA: Considerations when using pharmacokinetic/pharmacodynamic modeling to determine the effectiveness of simple analgesics in children. Expert.Opin. Drug.Metab.Toxicol. 2015; 11 (9): 1393–408.

90. Hannam J, Anderson BJ: Explaining the acetaminophen-ibuprofen analgesic interaction using a response surface model. Paediatr.Anaesth. 2011; 21 (12): 1234–40.

91. Gal P, Gilman JT: Drug disposition in neonates with patent ductus arteriosus. Ann.Pharmacother. 1993; 27 (11): 1383–8.

92. Rabbitts JA, Groenewald CB, Rasanen J: Geographic differences in perioperative opioid administration in children. Pediatr.Anesth. 2012; 22 (7): 676–81.

93. Klockars JG, Hiller A, Munte S, van Gils MJ, Taivainen T: Spectral entropy as a measure of hypnosis and hypnotic drug effect of total intravenous anesthesia in children during slow induction and maintenance. Anesthesiology. 2012; 116 (2): 340–51.

94. Henthorn TK, Liu Y, Mahapatro M, Ng KY: Active transport of fentanyl by the blood-brain barrier. J. Pharmacol.Exp.Ther. 1999; 289 (2): 1084–9.

95. Hamabe W, Maeda T, Kiguchi N, Yamamoto C, Tokuyama S, Kishioka S: Negative relationship between morphine analgesia and P-glycoprotein expression levels in the brain. J.Pharmacol.Sci. 2007; 105 (4): 353–60.

96. Wietasch JK, Scholz M, Zinserling J, Kiefer N, Frenkel C, Knufermann P, et al: The performance of a target-controlled infusion of propofol in combination with remifentanil: a clinical investigation with two propofol formulations. Anesth.Analg. 2006; 102 (2): 430–7.

97. Choi L, Ferrell BA, Vasilevskis EE, Pandharipande PP, Heltsley R, Ely EW, et al: Population pharmacokinetics of fentanyl in the critically ill. Crit.Care.Med. 2016; 44 (1): 64–72.

98. Potts AL, Cheeseman JF, Warman GR: Circadian rhythms and their development in children: implications for pharmacokinetics and pharmacodynamics in anesthesia. Pediatr.Anesth. 2011; 21 (3): 238–46.

99. Brainard J, Gobel M, Bartels K, Scott B, Koeppen M, Eckle T: Circadian rhythms in anesthesia and critical

care medicine: potential importance of circadian disruptions. Semin.Cardiothorac.Vasc.Anesth. 2015; 19 (1): 49–60.

100. Reinberg A, Reinberg MA: Circadian changes of the duration of action of local anaesthetic agents. Naunyn-Schmiedebergs Arch.Pharmacol. 1977; 297 (2): 149–52.

101. Lemmer B, Wiemers R: Circadian changes in stimulus threshold and in the effect of a local anaesthetic drug in human teeth: studies with an electronic pulptester. Chronobiol.Intern. 1989; 6 (2): 157–62.

102. Debon R, Chassard D, Duflo F, Boselli E, Bryssine B, Allaouchiche B: Chronobiology of epidural ropivacaine: variations in the duration of action related to the hour of administration. Anesthesiology. 2002; 96 (3): 542–5.

103. Cheeseman JF, Merry AF, Pawley MD, de Souza RL, Warman GR: The effect of time of day on the duration of neuromuscular blockade elicited by rocuronium. Anaesthesia. 2007; 62 (11): 1114–20.

104. Levi FA, Zidani R, Vannetzel JM, Perpoint B, Focan C, Faggiuolo R, et al: Chronomodulated versus fixed-infusion-rate delivery of ambulatory chemotherapy with oxaliplatin, fluorouracil, and folinic acid (leucovorin) in patients with colorectal cancer metastases: a randomized multi-institutional trial. J. Natl.Canc.Inst. 1994; 86 (21): 1608–17.

105. Kamali F, Fry JR, Bell GD: Temporal variations in paracetamol absorption and metabolism in man. Xenobiotica. 1987; 17 (5): 635–41.

106. Halsas M, Hietala J, Veski P, Jurjenson H, Marvola M: Morning versus evening dosing of ibuprofen using conventional and time-controlled release formulations. Int.J.Pharmaceut. 1999; 189 (2): 179–85.

107. Clench J, Reinberg A, Dziewanowska Z, Ghata J, Smolensky M: Circadian changes in the bioavailability and effects of indomethacin in healthy subjects. Eur.J.Clin.Pharmacol. 1981; 20 (5): 359–69.

108. Mustofa M, Suryawati S, Dwiprahasto I, Santoso B: The relative bioavailability of diclofenac with respect to time of administration. Brit.J.Clin.Pharmacol. 1991; 32 (2): 246–7.

109. Ollagnier M, Decousus H, Cherrah Y, Levi F, Mechkouri M, Queneau P, et al: Circadian changes in the pharmacokinetics of oral ketoprofen. Clin. Pharmacokinet. 1987; 12 (5): 367–78.

110. Han PY, Duffull SB, Kirkpatrick CM, Green B: Dosing in obesity: a simple solution to a big problem. Clin. Pharmacol.Ther. 2007; 82 (5): 505–8.

111. Abernethy DR, Greenblatt DJ: Drug disposition in obese humans. An update. Clin.Pharmacokinet. 1986; 11 (3): 199–213.

112. Mulla H, Johnson TN. Dosing dilemmas in obese children. Arch.Dis.Child.Educ.Pract.Ed. 2010; 95 (4): 112–17.

113. Anderson BJ, Holford NH: Getting the dose right for obese children. Arch.Dis.Child. 2017; 102 (1): 54–5.

114. Anderson BJ, Holford NH: What is the best size predictor for dose in the obese child? Pediatr.Anesth. 2017; 27 (12): 1176–84.

115. Chidambaran V, Venkatasubramanian R, Sadhasivam S, Esslinger H, Cox S, Diepstraten J, et al: Population pharmacokinetic-pharmacodynamic modeling and dosing simulation of propofol maintenance anesthesia in severely obese adolescents. Pediatr.Anesth. 2015; 25 (9): 911–23.

116. Cortinez LI, Anderson BJ, Penna A, Olivares L, Munoz HR, Holford NH, et al: Influence of obesity on propofol pharmacokinetics: derivation of a pharmacokinetic model. Brit.J.Anaesth. 2010; 105 (4): 448–56.

117. Diepstraten J, Chidambaran V, Sadhasivam S, Esslinger HR, Cox SL, Inge TH, et al: Propofol clearance in morbidly obese children and adolescents: influence of age and body size. Clin.Pharmacokinet. 2012; 51 (8): 543–51.

118. Holford NHG, Anderson BJ: Allometric size: the scientific theory and extension to normal fat mass. Eur.J.Pharm.Sci. 2017; 109S: S59–S64.

119. Allegaert K, Olkkola KT, Owens KH, Van de Velde M, de Maat MM, Anderson BJ: Covariates of intravenous paracetamol pharmacokinetics in adults. BMC Anesthesiol. 2014; 14: 77.

120. Tham LS, Wang LZ, Soo RA, Lee HS, Lee SC, Goh BC, et al: Does saturable formation of gemcitabine triphosphate occur in patients? Canc.Chemother. Pharmacol. 2008; 63 (1): 55–64.

121. McCune JS, Bemer MJ, Barrett JS, Scott Baker K, Gamis AS, Holford NHG: Busulfan in infant to adult hematopoietic cell transplant recipients: a population pharmacokinetic model for initial and bayesian dose personalization. Clin.Canc.Res. 2014; 20 (3): 754–63.

122. Cortinez LI, Anderson BJ, Holford NH, Puga V, de la Fuente N, Auad H, et al: Dexmedetomidine pharmacokinetics in the obese. Eur.J.Clin.Pharmacol. 2015; 71 (12): 1501–8.

123. Van Boxtel C, Holford N, Danhof M: *In Vivo Study of Drug Action*. Amsterdam: Elsevier, 1992.

124. Schnider TW, Minto CF, Shafer SL, Gambus PL, Andresen C, Goodale DB, et al: The influence of age on propofol pharmacodynamics. Anesthesiology. 1999; 90 (6): 1502–16.

125. Lerman J. Pharmacology of inhalational anaesthetics in infants and children. Paediatr.Anaesth. 1992; 2: 191–203.

126. LeDez KM, Lerman J. The minimum alveolar concentration (MAC) of isoflurane in preterm neonates. Anesthesiology. 1987; 67 (3): 301–7.

127. Warner MA, Kunkel SE, Offord KO, Atchison SR, Dawson B: The effects of age, epinephrine, and operative site on duration of caudal analgesia in pediatric patients. Anesth.Analg. 1987; 66 (10): 995–8.

128. Lerman J, Robinson S, Willis MM, Gregory GA: Anesthetic requirements for halothane in young children 0–1 month and 1–6 months of age. Anesthesiology. 1983; 59 (5): 421–4.

129. Molin JC, Bendhack LM: Clonidine induces rat aorta relaxation by nitric oxide-dependent and -independent mechanisms. Vascul.Pharmacol. 2004; 42 (1): 1–6.

130. Chugani DC, Muzik O, Juhasz C, Janisse JJ, Ager J, Chugani HT: Postnatal maturation of human GABAA receptors measured with positron emission tomography. Ann.Neurol. 2001; 49 (5): 618–26.

131. Herlenius E, Lagercrantz H: Development of neurotransmitter systems during critical periods. Exp. Neurol. 2004; 190 Suppl 1: S8–21.

132. Chugani HT, Kumar A, Muzik O: GABA(A) receptor imaging with positron emission tomography in the human newborn: a unique binding pattern. Pediatr. Neurol. 2013; 48 (6): 459–62.

133. Koch SC, Fitzgerald M, Hathway GJ: Midazolam potentiates nociceptive behavior, sensitizes cutaneous reflexes, and is devoid of sedative action in neonatal rats. Anesthesiology. 2008; 108 (1): 122–9.

134. Choudhuri S, Klaassen CD: Structure, function, expression, genomic organization, and single nucleotide polymorphisms of human ABCB1 (MDR1), ABCC (MRP), and ABCG2 (BCRP) efflux transporters. Int.J.Toxicol. 2006; 25 (4): 231–59.

135. Herd DW, Anderson BJ, Keene NA, Holford NH: Investigating the pharmacodynamics of ketamine in children. Paediatr.Anaesth. 2008; 18 (1): 36–42.

136. Sani O, Shafer SL: MAC Attack? Anesthesiology. 2003; 99 (6): 1249–50.

137. Dilger JP: From individual to population: the minimum alveolar concentration curve. Curr.Opin. Anaesthesiol. 2006; 19 (4): 390–6.

138. de Jong RH, Eger EI: 2nd. MAC expanded: AD50 and AD95 values of common inhalation anesthetics in man. Anesthesiology. 1975; 42 (4): 384–9.

139. Gourlay GK, Kowalski SR, Plummer JL, Cousins MJ, Armstrong PJ: Fentanyl blood concentration-analgesic response relationship in the treatment of postoperative pain. Anesth.Analg. 1988; 67 (4): 329–37.

140. Dutta S, Matsumoto Y, Ebling WF: Is it possible to estimate the parameters of the sigmoid Emax model with truncated data typical of clinical studies? J.Pharm. Sci. 1996; 85 (2): 232–9.

141. Dixon WJ: Staircase bioassay: the up-and-down method. Neurosci.Biobehav.Rev. 1991; 15 (1): 47–50.

142. Gorges M, Zhou G, Brant R, Ansermino JM: Sequential allocation trial design in anesthesia: an introduction to methods, modeling, and clinical applications. Paediatr. Anaesth. 2017; 27 (3): 240–7.

143. Hansen MS, Mathiesen O, Trautner S, Dahl JB: Intranasal fentanyl in the treatment of acute pain – a systematic review. Acta.Anaesthesiol.Scand. 2012; 56 (4): 407–19.

144. Lotsch J, Skarke C, Liefhold J, Geisslinger G: Genetic predictors of the clinical response to opioid analgesics: clinical utility and future perspectives. Clin. Pharmacokinet. 2004; 43 (14): 983–1013.

145. Hannam J, Anderson BJ, Veyckemans F: Tears at breakfast. Pediatr.Anesth. 2012; 22 (4): 419.

146. Jimenez N, Anderson GD, Shen DD, Nielsen SS, Farin FM, Seidel K, et al: Is ethnicity associated with morphine's side effects in children? Morphine pharmacokinetics, analgesic response, and side effects in children having tonsillectomy. Pediatr.Anesth. 2012; 22 (7): 669–75.

147. Myles PS, Buchanan FF, Bain CR: The effect of hair colour on anaesthetic requirements and recovery time after surgery. Anaesth. Intensive Care. 2012; 40 (4): 683–9.

148. Kaitin KI: Deconstructing the drug development process: the new face of innovation. Clin.Pharmacol. Ther. 2010; 87 (3): 356–61.

149. Long LS, Ved S, Koh JL: Intraoperative opioid dosing in children with and without cerebral palsy. Paediatr. Anaesth. 2009; 19 (5): 513–20.

150. Valkenburg AJ, de Leeuw TG, Tibboel D, Weber F: Lower bispectral index values in children who are intellectually disabled. Anesth.Analg. 2009; 109 (5): 1428–33.

151. Hallett BR, Chalkiadis GA: Suspected opioid-induced hyperalgesia in an infant. Br.J.Anaesth. 2012; 108 (1): 116–18.

152. Meibohm B, Beierle I, Derendorf H: How important are gender differences in pharmacokinetics? Clin. Pharmacol. 2002; 41 (5): 329–42.

153. Beierle I, Meibohm B, Derendorf H: Gender differences in pharmacokinetics and pharmacodynamics. Int.J.Clin.Pharm.Ther. 1999; 37 (11): 529–47.

154. Apfelbaum JL, Grasela TH, Hug CC, Jr., McLeskey CH, Nahrwold ML, Roizen MF, et al: The initial clinical experience of 1819 physicians in maintaining anesthesia with propofol: characteristics associated with prolonged time to awakening. Anesth.Analg. 1993; 77 (4 Suppl): S10–14.

155. Hoymork SC, Raeder J, Grimsmo B, Steen PA: Bispectral index, predicted and measured drug levels

of target-controlled infusions of remifentanil and propofol during laparoscopic cholecystectomy and emergence. Acta Anaesth. Scand. 2000; 44 (9): 1138–44.

156. Hoymork SC, Raeder J, Grimsmo B, Steen PA: Bispectral index, serum drug concentrations and emergence associated with individually adjusted target-controlled infusions of remifentanil and propofol for laparoscopic surgery. Br.J.Anaesth. 2003; 91 (6): 773–80.

157. Vuyk J, Oostwouder CJ, Vletter AA, Burm AG, Bovill JG: Gender differences in the pharmacokinetics of propofol in elderly patients during and after continuous infusion. Br.J.Anaesth. 2001; 86 (2): 183–8.

158. Hoymork SC, Raeder J. Why do women wake up faster than men from propofol anaesthesia? Br.J.Anaesth. 2005; 95 (5): 627–33.

159. Niesters M, Dahan A, Kest B, Zacny J, Stijnen T, Aarts L, et al: Do sex differences exist in opioid analgesia? A systematic review and meta-analysis of human experimental and clinical studies. J.Pain. 2010; 151 (1): 61–8.

160. Sarton E, Olofsen E, Romberg R, den Hartigh J, Kest B, Nieuwenhuijs D, et al: Sex differences in morphine analgesia: an experimental study in healthy volunteers. Anesthesiology. 2000; 93 (5): 1245–54; discussion 6A.

161. Dahan A, Kest B, Waxman AR, Sarton E: Sex-specific responses to opiates: animal and human studies. Anesth.Analg. 2008; 107 (1): 83–95.

162. Rabbitts JA, Groenewald CB, Dietz NM, Morales C, Rasanen J: Perioperative opioid requirements are decreased in hypoxic children living at altitude. Pediatr. Anesth. 2010; 20 (12): 1078–83.

163. Sadhasivam S, Chidambaran V, Ngamprasertwong P, Esslinger HR, Prows C, Zhang X, et al: Race and unequal burden of perioperative pain and opioid related adverse effects in children. Pediatrics. 2012; 129 (5): 832–8.

164. Sadhasivam S, Krekels EH, Chidambaran V, Esslinger HR, Ngamprasertwong P, Zhang K, et al: Morphine clearance in children: does race or genetics matter? J. Opioid Manag. 2012; 8 (4): 217–26.

165. Chidambaran V, Ngamprasertwong P, Vinks AA, Sadhasivam S: Pharmacogenetics and anesthetic drugs. Curr.Clin.Pharmacol. 2012; 7 (2): 78–101.

166. Cohen M, Sadhasivam S, Vinks AA: Pharmacogenetics in perioperative medicine. Curr.Opin.Anaesthesiol. 2012; 25 (4): 419–27.

167. Stamer UM, Stuber F: Pharmacogenetics of anesthetic and analgesic agents: CYP2D6 genetic variations. Anesthesiology. 2005; 103 (5): 1099; author reply 101.

168. Williams DG, Patel A, Howard RF: Pharmacogenetics of codeine metabolism in an urban population of children and its implications for analgesic reliability. Brit.J.Anaesth. 2002; 89 (6): 839–45.

169. Anderson BJ. Is it farewell to codeine? Arch.Dis.Child. 2013; 98 (12): 986–8.

170. Rigby-Jones A, Sneyd JR: Cardiovascular changes after achieving constant effect site concentration of propofol. Anaesthesia. 2008; 63 (7): 780.

171. Hutchinson MR, Coats BD, Lewis SS, Zhang Y, Sprunger DB, Rezvani N, et al: Proinflammatory cytokines oppose opioid-induced acute and chronic analgesia. Brain.Behav.Immun. 2008; 22 (8): 1178–89.

172. Candiotti KA, Yang Z, Morris R, Yang J, Crescimone NA, Sanchez GC, et al: Polymorphism in the interleukin-1 receptor antagonist gene is associated with serum interleukin-1 receptor antagonist concentrations and postoperative opioid consumption. Anesthesiology. 2011; 114 (5): 1162–8.

173. Lotsch J, Geisslinger G: Relevance of frequent mu-opioid receptor polymorphisms for opioid activity in healthy volunteers. J. Pharmacogenomics. 2006; 6 (3): 200–10.

174. Walter C, Lotsch J: Meta-analysis of the relevance of the OPRM1 118A> G genetic variant for pain treatment. J. Pain. 2009; 146 (3): 270–5.

175. Ross JR, Rutter D, Welsh K, Joel SP, Goller K, Wells AU, et al: Clinical response to morphine in cancer patients and genetic variation in candidate genes. J. Pharmacogenomics. 2005; 5 (5): 324–36.

176. Liem EB, Joiner TV, Tsueda K, Sessler DI: Increased sensitivity to thermal pain and reduced subcutaneous lidocaine efficacy in redheads. Anesthesiology. 2005; 102 (3): 509–14.

177. Lotsch J, Geisslinger G: Pharmacogenetics of new analgesics. Br.J.Pharmacol. 2011; 163 (3): 447–60.

178. Tournier N, Decleves X, Saubamea B, Scherrmann JM, Cisternino S: Opioid transport by ATP-binding cassette transporters at the blood-brain barrier: implications for neuropsychopharmacology. Curr. Pharm.Des. 2011; 17 (26): 2829–42.

179. Holford NH, Buclin T: Safe and effective variability-a criterion for dose individualization. Ther. Drug Monit. 2012; 34 (5): 565–8.

180. Palomaki GE, Bradley LA, Douglas MP, Kolor K, Dotson WD: Can UGT1A1 genotyping reduce morbidity and mortality in patients with metastatic colorectal cancer treated with irinotecan? An evidence-based review. Genet.Med. 2009; 11 (1): 21–34.

181. Fredriksson A, Archer T, Alm H, Gordh T, Eriksson P: Neurofunctional deficits and potentiated apoptosis by neonatal NMDA antagonist administration. Behav. Brain Res. 2004; 153 (2): 367–76.

182. Wang C, Sadovova N, Fu X, Schmued L, Scallet A, Hanig J, et al: The role of the N-methyl-D-aspartate receptor in ketamine-induced apoptosis in rat forebrain culture. Neuroscience. 2005; 132 (4): 967–77.

61

183. Bates E, Reilly J, Wulfeck B, Dronkers N, Opie M, Fenson J, et al: Differential effects of unilateral lesions on language production in children and adults. Brain. Lang. 2001; 79 (2): 223–65.

184. Ansermino M, Basu R, Vandebeek C, Montgomery C: Nonopioid additives to local anaesthetics for caudal blockade in children: a systematic review. Paediatr. Anaesth. 2003; 13 (7): 561–73.

185. Dodwell ER, Latorre JG, Parisini E, Zwettler E, Chandra D, Mulpuri K, et al: NSAID exposure and risk of nonunion: a meta-analysis of case-control and cohort studies. Calcif.Tissue.Int. 2010; 87 (3): 193–202.

186. Anderson BJ, Ralph CJ, Stewart AW, Barber C, Holford NH: The dose-effect relationship for morphine and vomiting after day-stay tonsillectomy in children. Anaesth.Intens.Care. 2000; 28 (2): 155–60.

187. Weinstein MS, Nicolson SC, Schreiner MS: A single dose of morphine sulfate increases the incidence of vomiting after outpatient inguinal surgery in children. Anesthesiology. 1994; 81 (3): 572–7.

188. Bouillon T, Bruhn J, Radu-Radulescu L, Andresen C, Cohane C, Shafer SL: A model of the ventilatory depressant potency of remifentanil in the non-steady state. Anesthesiology. 2003; 99 (4): 779–87.

189. Standing JF, Hammer GB, Sam WJ, Drover DR. Pharmacokinetic-pharmacodynamic modeling of the hypotensive effect of remifentanil in infants undergoing cranioplasty. Paediatr.Anaesth. 2010; 20 (1): 7–18.

Chapter 5

Signal Analysis and Response Measurement

Umberto Melia, Erik W. Jensen and José F. Valencia

Introduction

Monitoring during anaesthesia is based on the measurement of physiological signals that are recorded during surgical or other procedures requiring anaesthetic drug administration. The methods used to process these signals, calculate derived parameters and develop the different indicators of the physiological status of the patient or depth of anaesthesia are difficult to understand for anaesthesia providers without an engineering background. The present chapter aims to fill this gap by introducing the reader to the main concepts related to signal analysis commonly used to measure the response of human physiological systems under anaesthesia.

The purpose is to describe how biomarkers, signals and responses from the human body can be recorded, collected and mathematically analysed to quantify drug effect. The reader will learn about how a signal of the body is transformed into a parameter that is displayed on the screen and how it correlates with human responses or outcomes. The examples used to introduce these concepts will pertain to the measurement of (components of) 'depth' of anaesthesia that include: (a) the autonomic nervous system (ANS) response to noxious stimuli, such as haemodynamic responses [1], heart rate variability (HRV) [1], plethysmographic responses [2], and pulse wave analysis [2]; and (b) the electroencephalogram (EEG). The EEG is a direct measurement of brain activity from which indices of hypnotic effect and even a measure of pain/nociception have been and are being developed [3, 4, 5, 6, 7].

Signal Analysis: An Overview

A signal is commonly defined as a physical quantity or a source of information that is a function of independent variables such as time and/or space. For example, a signal that varies with time (e.g. the EEG) is represented as a function of the time variable, 't', which is denoted as 'x(t)', with 'x' being the value of the signal at the time 't'.

Signals are classified by different features. A signal can be periodic or non-periodic. A periodic signal contains a sequence of values that is repeated after a fixed time period, 'T'. The reciprocal of the 'T' value is defined as the fundamental frequency, 'f', of the signal. A signal is called deterministic if it can be expressed by a mathematical expression, while a signal is random if it is not predictable.

By using different signal processing techniques, it is possible to calculate several parameters that allow all the information that a signal can provide to be extracted. There are two commonly used methods to extract information from signals: analysis in the time domain and analysis in the frequency domain. The information contained in the time domain expresses the occurrence of some events by signal amplitude variation. This is the simplest and more intuitive way to represent a signal. In contrast, information in the frequency domain is more indirect and can be extracted by several methods. One of the more important methods is Fourier analysis, which is based on the theory that every signal (periodic or non-periodic, random or deterministic) can be decomposed into a sum of infinite periodic signals with different frequencies. The range of these frequency values is defined as the bandwidth of the signal.

The purpose of this section is to list and illustrate the basic concepts that are related to the processing and analysis of physiological signals.

Recording and Representation of Physiological Signals

A physiological signal is a biological electric potential variation which can be recorded from any part of the body. Recording a physiological signal can provide relevant information to assess the underlying physiological system that generates the signal.

Physiological signals are acquired by a device that measures the electrical activity using sensors that are placed in different parts of the body. Because the

63

amplitude of this type of signal is quite weak compared to the electrical activity from other sources, these devices are equipped with amplifiers. Furthermore, an ideal recording system should be able to separate the physiological components of interest from any other unwanted electrical activity, which is considered to be noise. Accordingly, the input signal 'x(t)' of a recording device can be written as the sum of two terms (Equation 1), the physiological signal of interest 's(t)' and a noise term 'n(t)':

$$x(t) = s(t) + n(t) \qquad (1)$$

where 'n(t)' is any kind of electrical activity, physiological or not, that contaminates the signal of interest 's(t)' and might cause misinterpretation of its real features.

Before being processed, the recorded signal must be also converted from analogue to digital. Indeed, biological systems generate signals that are continuous over an interval of time. In order to be able to be processed by software, the analogue signal has to be converted into a digital signal, that is, a sequence of numbers that is discrete in time and amplitude. Thus, the signal x(t) is sampled by taking discrete x values at a fixed time interval Ts. The reciprocal of the period Ts is defined as the sampling frequency of the digital signal, fs. The outcome of the digitalization process is that the fundamental frequencies that can be analysed from the obtained digital signal are only in the range from 0 to half of the fs value, according to the Nyquist theorem. On the other hand, also the signal amplitude is discretized during the recording because the voltage values are converted into digital numbers that are discrete and have a limited range. The number of available discrete values and the range of the analogue values determine the resolution of the recording system (see 'EEG Recording in the Operating Room' in this chapter for more explanation). A low resolution, which occurs when a small number of discrete values are used to represent the whole range of the analogue signal, implies that a range of amplitudes of the analogue signal will have the same discrete value. Therefore, a variation of the analogue signal smaller than the resolution could be undetected after the analogue to digital conversion of the signal. Resolution can be enhanced by both

increasing the number of available discrete values and limiting the analogue input range of the recording system. The former will increase the computational cost of the system and the latter alternative will cause loss of high amplitude signal values. For these reasons, before recording and converting a physiological signal, it is very important to know the bandwidth and the amplitude of the signal of interest in order to design an acquisition system with appropriate sampling frequency, amplitude range and resolution. Fig. 5.1 shows the block diagram of a typical system that records and processes a signal.

Filtering

An important aspect of recording and processing digital signals is the elimination or reduction of 'noise', the unwanted component n(t) that can affect the interpretation of the physiological information, which is contained in s(t). When the bandwidth of the original signal s(t) is different from the bandwidth of noise n(t), it is possible to eliminate the frequency components of noise n(t) by using filters. A filter is a signal processing tool that reduces or removes the energy of a signal in certain frequency bands. There are several types of filters and different criteria to classify them, such as linear or nonlinear, time-invariant or time-variant, causal or not-causal, analogue or digital, discrete-time (sampled) or continuous-time, passive or active, infinite impulse response (IIR) or finite impulse response (FIR) type. An important feature of the filters is the associated frequency response that describes which frequency bands the filter allows to pass (the passband) and which it rejects (the stopband). Table 5.1 shows the list of the most relevant filters with a short description of which frequency band passes and which is reduced.

The transition band of a filter is defined as the band between the passband and the stopband. The cut-off frequency of the filter is the frequency that lies at the division between the passband and the transition band, in which the filtered signal has an attenuation of 3 dB compared to the original signal. That means that a filtered sinusoidal signal with frequency equal to the cut-off frequency will have half of the energy compared with the original signal (signal without filtering).

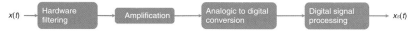

Fig. 5.1 Block diagram of a typical system that records and processes a physiological signal. x(t) = analogue signal; xs(t) = processed digital signal.

Table 5.1. List of the most known filters and their behaviour.

FILTER	PASS	REDUCE
Low-pass	Frequencies lower than a specific frequency	Frequencies higher than a specific frequency
High-pass	Frequencies higher than a specific frequency	Frequencies lower than a specific frequency
Band-pass	Frequencies in a specific frequency band	All the frequencies that are not in a specific frequency band
Band-stop	All the frequencies that are not in a specific frequency band	Frequencies in a specific frequency band
Notch	All the frequencies except one	One specific frequency
Comb	Regularly spaced narrow frequency band	All the frequencies that are not included in the regularly spaced narrow frequency band
All-pass	All frequencies	All frequencies (only modify the phase of the output)

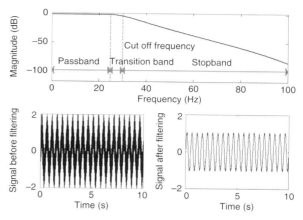

Fig. 5.2 (a) Frequency response of a low-pass filter with cut-off frequency at 30 Hz. (b) A periodic signal sum of two sinusoids at 2 Hz and 50 Hz before and (c) after filtering by the 30 Hz cut-off low-pass filter.

Figure 5.2 shows an example of a frequency response of a low-pass filter with cut-off frequency of 30 Hz and an example of a periodic signal after and before the filtering process.

Time and Frequency Domain Analysis

As mentioned above, a signal can be analysed in time and/or in frequency domains. The following sections provide the basic concepts of the tools most commonly used to represent the signal features in time and frequency domains. First, the parameters that can be extracted from time domain analysis are described. Then, a selection of methods for signal representation in frequency and in both the time and frequency domains are introduced.

Time Domain Analysis

Time domain analysis involves analysing the data over a time period. Periodic signals can be easily characterized by calculating the maximum or minimum amplitude, the mean value and the root mean square (RMS) amplitude with respect to time. The RMS amplitude is defined as the square root of the arithmetic mean of the squares of the signal amplitude. It represents the effective amplitude of a varying signal. In case of a signal with mean value equal to 0, the root mean square amplitude is the same as the standard deviation of the signal amplitude in a defined time frame. A physiological signal that can be easily analysed in the time domain is the electrocardiogram (ECG). Figure 5.3

illustrates an example of maximum, mean, root mean square value and duration of a PQRST segment calculated from an ECG signal, and also an example of the interval between 2 R peaks.

However, most physiological signals have random features that can be approximated by a normal, Gaussian distribution. In this case, signals can be summarized by calculating the mean and standard deviation of the amplitude, assuming that the investigated periods have more or less constant statistical properties. Other statistical methods that are widely applied to characterize a signal in the time domain are kurtosis and the autocorrelation function. Kurtosis is a descriptor of the shape of the probability distribution of a random variable that is used to quantify its 'tailedness'. The autocorrelation function is calculated as the correlation of a signal with a delayed copy of itself as a function of delay. It represents the similarity between observations as a function of the time lag between them. The analysis of autocorrelation is mostly used for finding repeating patterns or identifying the fundamental frequency in a signal.

A particular use of time domain parameters in signal analysis occurs when an evoked potential is studied, which is a cortical response to a specific stimulus. The traditional methods for analysing evoked potentials are based on measurements of the amplitude and duration of the waveform. Since the amplitude of these evoked potentials is smaller than the EEG background activity, epochs that contain evoked responses are often averaged. Evoked potentials are widely used in neuromonitoring during different types of surgeries

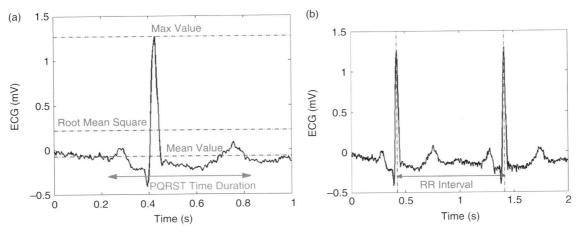

Fig. 5.3 An example of time domain analysis of a PQRST wave from an ECG signal: (a) mean, maximum, root mean square values and PQRST time duration, (b) time interval between two R peaks.

to help minimize iatrogenic trauma. Also, auditory evoked potentials have been used to assess depth of hypnotic effect during anaesthesia.

Frequency Domain Analysis: Fourier Transform

The most important method for signal analysis in the frequency domain is Fourier transformation. The Fourier transform is a mathematical method that decomposes a function of time (a signal) into the frequencies that make it up, allowing the energy or the power of a signal to be computed at each frequency. In signal processing, the energy of a signal is defined as the integral of the square of the amplitude in the time domain, while the power is defined as the energy per time unit. Parseval's theorem demonstrates that the signal energy can be also computed from the sum across all frequencies of the signal spectral energy density that are obtained with the Fourier transform. For example, considering a signal that represents the electric potential (in volts) of a biological phenomenon, the units of measurement for the signal energy would be volt^2 × seconds or volt^2/Hz and the power would be volt^2. The resulting distribution of frequencies that results from Fourier analysis is also called the spectrum or power spectral density (PSD) of the signal if it is calculated per unit of frequency. The sum of the PSD values for all the frequencies gives the total power of the signal. The PSD is often normalized by its maximum value or by the area under the curve so it can be expressed in arbitrary units (AU).

In digital signal processing applications, the Fourier Transform is widely computed by an optimized algorithm that is called the Fast Fourier

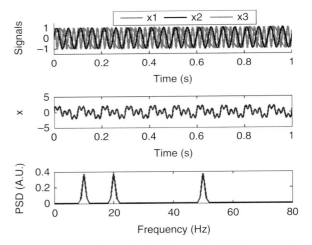

Fig. 5.4 The periodic signal x (middle pane) can be decomposed into three sinusoids x1, x2 and x3 at 10, 20 and 50 Hz, respectively (upper pane). The power spectral density (lower pane) is computed by the Fourier transform, and provides a measure of how much each frequency contributes to the original signal.

Transform (FFT). This algorithm, instead of applying the simple definition of the Fourier Transform, uses mathematical properties that permit the computational costs and the complexity of the algorithm to be reduced yet obtains the same result. Figure 5.4 shows an example of the sum of sinusoidal signals with different frequencies and the corresponding PSD in the frequency domain, obtained with the FFT. It can be noted that the PSD shows peaks at the frequency values corresponding to the fundamental frequencies of the sinusoids that compose the signal, while it tends to be 0 at the other frequencies.

In the case of digital real signals, many limitations can affect the PSD estimation. First of all, the frequency resolution increases with the length of the signal segments of which the PSD is estimated: longer segments provide better frequency resolution. However, too lengthy segments may not be stationary, affecting the estimation of the PSD. Furthermore, the theory of the PSD is based on signals of infinite length, while the real signal has finite length. The effect of this limitation on the PSD estimation is named spectral leakage and consists of the generation of new frequency components (that are not real) around the main frequency component in the spectrum. Also, the limitation provided by the discretization of time can cause noise in the PSD estimation, since for example the frequencies that are not an integer multiple of the sample frequency are not correctly evaluated. For this reason the PSD is often estimated using averaging methods in order to minimize the error in the estimation of the spectral power. Indeed, the EEG is normally divided into segments, with or without overlap, with a fixed length and it is multiplied by window signals of specific shapes that reduce the spectral leakage. The final spectral density is achieved as the average of the spectral densities estimated on all the processed segments. Hence, the goodness of the PSD estimation depends on the choice of the shape of the windows, the length of the windows and how they are adapted with the characteristic of the signal.

One of the parameters that can be extracted from the PSD is the spectral power in specific frequency bands, which can be calculated as the area under the PSD curve in the desired bands. In a digital signal the spectral power is often calculated by summing the power at each frequency in one defined frequency range. Another parameter is the centroid, which is defined as the mean frequency of the PSD curve and can be computed with respect to the entire frequency spectrum or in different frequency bands. The mean frequency is the sum of each PSD value multiplied by the respective frequency value and divided by the sum of all the PSD values (the total power). A parameter that quantifies one aspect of frequency characteristics is the 'spectral edge frequency' or SEF. SEF is defined as the highest frequency at which a significant amount of energy is present in the signal (usually calculated at 50% or between 75% and 95% of total power contents). The SEF50 represents the value of the median frequency of the spectrum and it has been used as a surrogate measure of anaesthetic drug effects. The median frequency is the frequency that divides the spectrum into two parts with equal power.

Spectrogram

The main disadvantage of the Fourier transform is the lack of information about how the energy at each frequency evolves over time. Furthermore, because the theory of the Fourier transform is based on comparing the signal with sinusoids that extend through the whole time domain, it also needs to fulfill the requirement of stationarity, which means that the signal always carries the same information during the entire duration of observation. If the signal is not stationary, an isolated alteration might affect the whole Fourier spectrum. Since the Fourier transform does not include time information, also a short time event might be represented in the frequency domain as part of the signal spectrum and it can be misinterpreted as a signal component that is part of the signal for the entire recording period.

Time–frequency analysis is a tool that permits description of the evolution of the periodicity and frequency components with respect to time. Different time–frequency analysis methods with different properties have been proposed over the last decades [8]. The result of the time–frequency analysis can be visualized in a spectrogram, a 3D representation of the time, frequency and energy of the signal. A common 2D display of the 3D spectrogram represents time on the horizontal axis, frequency on the vertical axis and the amplitude of a particular frequency at a particular time by the colour of each point.

The simplest method to obtain a spectrogram is the short time Fourier transform which consists of dividing the signal into short segments of equal length and then computing the Fourier transform of each segment separately. Figure 5.5 shows an example of two sinusoidal signals, their PSD and the spectrogram. In the signal in Fig. 5.5a the frequency components of the signal evolve with respect to time while the signal in Fig. 5.5b contains the same frequency components for all the time instants. As can be noted, with the spectrogram it is possible to observe the evolution of the frequencies of both signals with respect to time, while with only the PSD computed by Fourier transform, all frequencies are represented without the information of time. Although the two sinusoidal signals are different, it is almost impossible to distinguish them from their respective PSD, because they have the same morphology.

Nonetheless, the main limitation of the short time Fourier transform remains that it is not possible to simultaneously obtain a very good time resolution and a very good frequency resolution. For that reason,

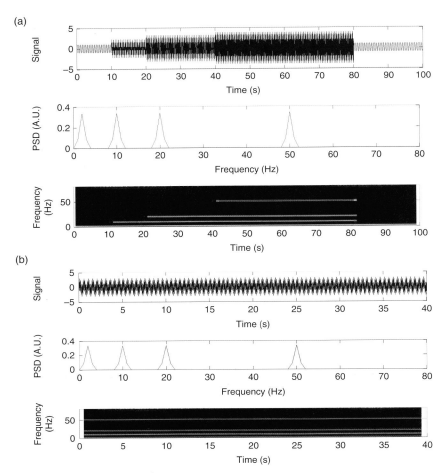

Fig. 5.5 (a) A periodic signal composed of different sinusoids whose frequencies change over time with values: 2, 10, 20 and 50 Hz, the power spectral density and the spectrogram; (b) another periodic signal sum of four sinusoids at 2, 10, 20 and 50 Hz whose frequencies do not change over time, the power spectral density and the spectrogram.

methods based on quadratic transformation and signal windowing, such as the Cohen class distributions, permit improvement of the performance of the time–frequency analysis. A detailed discussion, however, is outside the scope of this chapter.

All the parameters explained in this section that can be computed from the PSD (power, mean frequency or centroid and SEF) can also be calculated by using the time–frequency representation of the signal, obtaining their evolution over time.

Wavelet

A specific class of time–frequency analysis contains the wavelet transform. The main difference with the Fourier transform from the other time–frequency representation techniques is that the signal is not decomposed into sinusoids and cosinusoids. The wavelet transform uses different functions belonging in both the time

and Fourier space in which the concept of frequency is replaced by the concept of time scale. Hence, while traditional spectral analysis is used to represent a signal in the frequency domain, the frequency being the inverse of time, wavelet analysis permits representation of a signal in the time scale domain, the time scale being the time divided by a predefined factor. Instead of using sinusoid waves of infinite time length as Fourier transforms, the wavelet transform performs a mathematical projection of the signal to several wave oscillations with an amplitude that begins at zero, increases, and then decreases back to zero with different time durations. These wave oscillations are called wavelets, and their duration determines the different time scale at which the signal is represented. By using wavelets of different shapes and durations it is possible to recognize or detect specific pattern(s) in a signal. Continuous wavelet transform (CWT) is an implementation of the

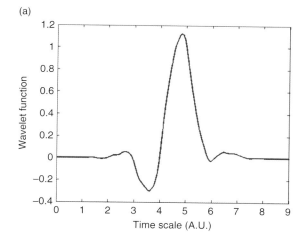

(a)

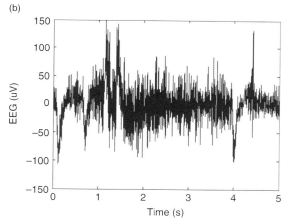

(b)

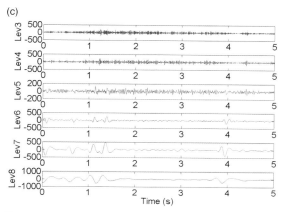

(c)

Fig. 5.6 An example of (a) discrete wavelet transform that is similar to EOG activity, (b) an EEG segment that contains EOG activity and (c) the results of the discrete wavelet decomposition of levels from three to eight. The results of the DWT in (c) is reached by mathematical projection of the signal in (b) to the wavelet in (a) in which the time (x-axis) is scaled by six different factors: Lev3: scale factor is 2^3, Lev4: scale factor is 2^4, Lev5: scale factor is 2^5, Lev6: scale factor is 2^6, Lev7: scale factor is 2^7, Lev8: scale factor is 2^8. It can be observed that at higher time scales, 2^6, 2^7, 2^8, it is possible to observe better the slower oscillations of the signal that are included in (b) and that have a shape that is similar to the wavelet shape in (a).

wavelet transform using arbitrary scales and almost arbitrary wavelets. This transform can be used also for the discrete time series, with the limitation that the smallest wavelet translations must be equal to the sampling frequency. Discrete wavelet transform (DWT) decomposes the signal by progressively dividing the bandwidth by a power of two at each level of decomposition. Hence, the time scale factor is always a power of two and the signal components that are represented at each level contain only the lowest frequencies of the original signal, and therefore this kind of representation can also act as a pass band or a low pass filter.

The choice of the wavelet that is used for signal decomposition is the most important point. Depending on the choice, it might be possible to influence the time and frequency resolution of the result and to steer the focus of the analysis towards specific patterns of the signal. Wavelet techniques are mostly used to detect known waveforms in a noisy background signal. An example of wavelet application is electro-oculogram (EOG) pattern recognition in the EEG signal. Since eye blinking or eye movement can be represented by specific patterns at low frequencies mimicking delta waves, the wavelet decomposition of the EEG at low time scale can help detect the EOG components. In this case the wavelet of choice should be one that is most similar to the EOG waves.

Figure 5.6 shows an example of a DWT decomposition of an EEG segment containing ocular activity. It can be noted that at high decomposition levels (lower frequencies) the EOG components are more visible and separated from the EEG activity, while at low decomposition levels (higher frequencies) the EEG activity is dominant. Another option for EOG detection with wavelet transform can be the design of a specific CWT as a model of experimental EOG recorded data.

Figure 5.7 shows an example of an EOG wavelet generated from real EEG data recording and the CWT of an EEG window containing EOG patterns. As can be seen, the energy of the wavelet representation (colour scale on the right) is higher in the x-axes at the time of blinking and in the y-axes at the time scales that match with duration of blinking.

Nonlinear Analysis

The state of a dynamical system (output) is given by a set of variables (inputs) that describe it at a particular time. The system is classified as linear if the change of the output is proportional to the change of their inputs, acting individually or in combination. Otherwise, the system is defined as nonlinear. Most physiological

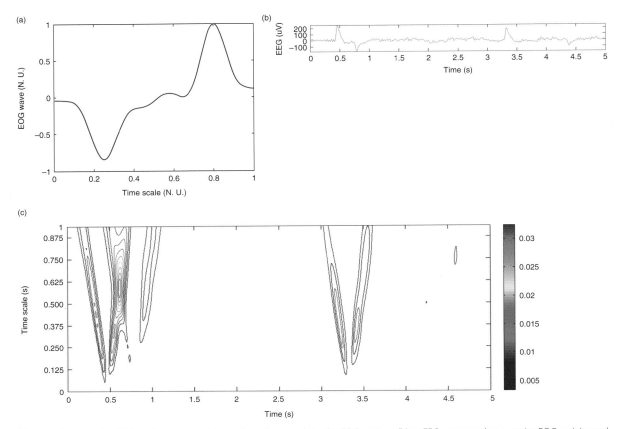

Fig. 5.7 An example of (a) continuous wavelet transform that simulates the EOG pattern, (b) an EEG segment that contains EOG activity and (c) the results of the continuous wavelet decomposition.

systems are inherently nonlinear, showing outputs that may appear chaotic, unpredictable or counterintuitive, contrasting with the much simpler linear systems. Although nonlinear systems can be approximated by linear equations for some range of the input values, this procedure could hide important features of the system.

Physiological signals can be adequately described also with methods derived from chaos theory including nonlinear dynamics analysis. Most of these methods are usually based on the concepts of entropy, fractals, symbolic dynamics and Poincare plots. They all are mathematical methods that are used to quantify nonlinear dynamics and system complexity. They can be correlated with physiological conditions.

The fundamental assumption of nonlinear techniques is that the physiological signals are generated by nonlinear deterministic systems with nonlinear coupling interactions, for example between neuronal populations in case of the EEG. Every neuron can be represented as a signal source and the EEG is the signal that is the result of the nonlinear interactions between the signals of all sources. Hence, the neuronal populations can be represented as a nonlinear deterministic system with nonlinear coupling interactions whose output is the EEG signal. The analysis of the EEG signal by nonlinear techniques permits one to assess the features and the state of the nonlinear system that has generated it, and thus may be used to assess the physiological state of the neurological system. In a complex dynamic system, a large number of interrelated variables are involved. The state of the system at a particular moment in time can be represented by a point in a space (the state space or phase space) with as many dimensions as there are variables. Nonlinear analysis is used to convert data from one dimension (the signal) into a multidimensional phase space that expresses each state of the system by a point, with as many coordinates as the values of the governing variables that are used to describe this specific state. When the system is observed for a long period of time, the sequence of those points in the phase space allows one to obtain a subspace called the attractor of the system. The nonlinear measures are the methods that are used to quantify the geometric and dynamical properties of the attractor.

In general, nonlinear approaches that have mostly been applied to various physiological data are based on attractor feature computation [9, 10, 11, 12, 13]. Table 5.2 shows a list of the parameters that are involved in the most frequently used nonlinear approaches. With these approaches it is possible to evaluate the nonlinearity and complexity of the physiological signals and then to classify their behaviour as deterministic, chaotic or random.

Signal Measurement and Processing during Anaesthesia and Surgical Procedures

The purpose of the following sections is to illustrate basic concepts related to measurement, storage and processing of signals during general anaesthesia. Special attention will be given to electroencephalographic and heart signals by providing clinical examples.

Table 5.2. List of the parameters that are involved in the most used nonlinear approaches.

Nonlinear Dynamics Approach	Estimation Parameter	Scope
Attractor dimension	Correlation dimension Katz dimension Higuchi dimension Petrosian dimension	This approach quantifies the complexity of a dynamical system by analysing the topological dimension of its attractor
Attractor stability	Lyapunov exponent	The trajectories of a chaotic attractor can diverge exponentially fast from similar initial conditions (expansion) or fold back into it as time evolves. The Lyapunov exponent measures the average rate of expansion and folding that occurs within an attractor
Attractor entropy	Kolmogorov entropy Approximate entropy Shannon entropy Renyi entropy Sample entropy Multiscale entropy	This approach quantifies the rate of information loss of the attractor dynamics

The Electroencephalographic Signal

The effect of several anaesthetic agents (i.e. hypnotic drugs) on the brain can be detected by analysing the changes in EEG signal that can be related to drug-induced biochemical changes in different structures of the brain. During induction of anaesthesia, EEG changes and depth of anaesthesia in terms of clinical signs are correlated with the administration of different drugs or drug combinations such as propofol and remifentanil. In order to extract information from the EEG, appropriate EEG recording and processing techniques should be applied.

Electroencephalography Recording in the Operating Room

EEG recording is generally done on the scalp. Electrodes are placed at specific locations according to the International 10–20 System. In the operating room, however, only two to four electrodes are placed on the forehead for practical reasons. It is important that electrode impedance is low (less than 10 kΩ) and equal for all electrodes. Because proper skin preparation can reduce the impedance, it is common practice to scrub and clean the areas where the electrodes are to be placed. Electrode impedance can increase if electrode paste and conductive gel dry out. Most EEG recording devices contain a system for electrode impedance checks. Electrode leads should be as short as practically feasible to avoid electrical interference.

The EEG is measured as the difference of potential between two electrodes that are referred to a third electrode (ground electrode), which is connected to the ground of the amplifier; this is performed by using a differential amplifier (Fig. 5.8). The EEG recording amplifier must be able to suppress noise and other interfering signals that are synchronized at different electrode positions, for example the power line noise. As specified above, the EEG is widely recorded by using differential amplifiers that, in theory, measure two values of voltage (one positive and one negative) from two electrodes and give an output voltage as the difference between the two voltages multiplied by a factor that is called the differential gain. However, in real differential amplifiers, electrical phenomena cause the output to contain another term which is a function of the sum of the two measured voltages multiplied by a factor that is called the 'common-mode gain'. Because this term represents undesired noise in the amplifier output, the differential gain in an ideal recording device should exceed common-mode gain as much as

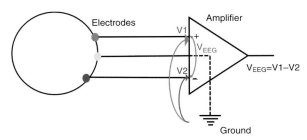

Fig. 5.8 EEG recording system with a differential amplifier. See text for details.

possible. The so called 'common mode rejection ratio' is defined as the ratio of the power of the differential gain over the common-mode gain, measured in decibels. It is an important specification of the amplifiers that has to be taken into account during the design of an EEG recording device. If the impedances of the electrodes are not balanced, the common-mode rejection could be altered and some interferences could affect the recording.

Another important specification is the sampling frequency which, according to the Nyquist theorem, should be above the double of the band of interest (see 'Recording and Representation of Physiological Signals', this chapter). The other important feature is the input range of the amplifier, which must be sufficient to record the normal amplitude range of the EEG with good resolution. It is often recommended to sample the EEG with a frequency higher than 100 Hz, and to use at least 16-bit precision in a range of ±500 µV. A sample frequency of 100 Hz means that the amplifier acquires one EEG sample every 0.1 seconds and, according to the Nyquist theorem, will result in an EEG bandwidth of 50 Hz that can be analysed by Fourier transform.

The amplifier also acquires voltage values between −500 µV and +500 µV that are converted into digital samples with a value between zero and $2^{16} - 1$ (using 16-bit precision). In this way, the value zero is associated with an input voltage of −500 µV and the value $2^{16} - 1$ (65535), is associated with an input voltage of +500 µV. With this configuration, a change in the voltage input of 0.015 µV (1000 µV / 65535) is the minimum change of voltage that can be detected since it corresponds to a change in the digital value of one. By using more bits in the digital conversion or a smaller input voltage range, it is possible to detect smaller changes in the input voltage. On the other hand, a voltage value that is out of the ±500 µV range

is either converted to zero if it is lower than −500 µV or to 65535 if it is above +500 µV; this phenomenon is called amplifier saturation. By changing the voltage range and the bit precision of the amplifier, it is possible to design devices with different capabilities to detect small or big changes in the input voltage.

Artefact Rejection

The EEG signal can be affected by several artefacts such as power line noise, biological noise or electrode noise. These artefacts can confound signal analysis because they can be wrongly interpreted as brain cortex activity. The impact of artefacts on signal processing can be minimized by different means. First, artefacts can be prevented during the recording phase by following the recommendations listed in the section 'Electroencelphalogram Recording in the Operating Room' above. Proper annotation should be made of any external causes that might generate an artefact so it can be taken into account during further EEG signal processing. Furthermore, there are other kinds of artefact such as power line noise or the electrocautery unit that must be removed after the recording process by signal processing techniques that permit detection of a period of EEG signal that is affected by noise. Finally, it is possible to have to deal with artefacts that resemble EEG activity and thus are more difficult to eliminate. The most common example is electromyogram (EMG) activity. EMG activity refers to muscle contractions that may be clinically evident or not, but generate an electric potential in a frequency band where cortical activity can also be observed and as such have the potential to cause confusion about whether or not they are related to anaesthetic drug effects. If neuromuscular blocking agents are used, the EMG is flat. But because nowadays several procedures under general anaesthesia are performed without neuromuscular blocking agents, electric activity generated by muscles can contaminate the EEG signal, thereby potentially altering the correct computation of indicators of anaesthetic drug effects.

Several methods are being used to detect and reject artefacts during EEG processing. First, a proper digital filter must be used to eliminate noise that is out of the EEG bandwidth. In general, a low pass filter with a cutoff frequency of 30 or 45 Hz is suggested; such a filter would remove all signal components beyond that given frequency (as explained in the section 'Filtering'). Other techniques are available to reject or correct the contaminated EEG segments. Algorithms that compare the amplitude or derivative of the signal with a

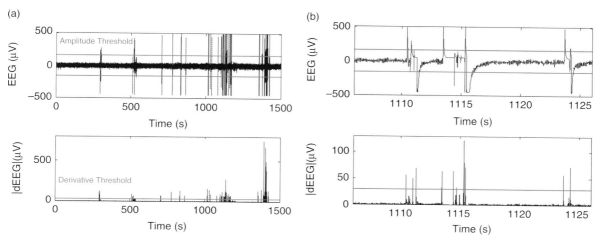

Fig. 5.9 (a) An example of an EEG trace affected by electrocautery interference as well as examples of thresholds that can be applied to the amplitude or the absolute value of the derivative (dEEG) to detect the artefacts. Those EEG samples and absolute derivatives that are out of the threshold ranges should be rejected. (b) Detail of an electrocautery unit artefact.

fixed or adaptive threshold can be applied to EEG in the time domain. Fig. 5.9 shows an example of EEG segments that have some epochs affected by electro-surgical interference. By applying a threshold on the amplitude and on the absolute value of the derivative, it is possible to detect the parts of the EEG that are corrupted and thus should be removed before further signal processing.

Because the number of available EEG channels that are recording during surgical procedure is often limited, it is difficult to apply other techniques that require a large number of channels, such as regression-based techniques or independent component analysis.

Cardiac, Haemodynamic and Respiratory Signals

The following sections provide an overview about signal analysis related to cardiac function and ventilation.

The value of haemodynamic and ventilatory parameters [such as heart rate, noninvasive mean arterial pressure (MAP), noninvasive blood pressure (NIBP), oxygen saturation and capnography] to assess 'depth of anaesthesia' is controversial [14, 15, 16] because some authors do not consider them to define anaesthesia in a narrow sense per se. For example, MAP is more likely to predict increasing and decreasing concentrations of propofol and remifentanil rather than any particular stage of depth of anaesthesia. MAP can thus – at best – only be an indirect parameter to estimate the hypnotic effects.

Heart Rate Variability

ECG monitoring is a standard of care and thus mandatory during anaesthesia. From the ECG signal it is possible to extract clinically relevant information about the function of the heart such as the rhythm, heart rate or its myocardial oxygen balance (myocardial ischaemia might show up as an altered ST segment).

Processing the signal from the heart allows heart rate variability (HRV) to be calculated, the variability of the interval period between two consecutive R peaks. Several parameters computed from the HRV signal in the time and frequency domain are related to the tone of the sympathetic and parasympathetic components of the autonomic central nervous system and to respiration and may therefore provide clinical information on how these systems are influenced by anaesthesia (also see Chapter 8). For example, during isoflurane anaesthesia the decreasing high-frequency and mid-frequency components of HRV are indicative of a reduction of total autonomic nervous system activity [16]. HRV is influenced by changes in levels of drug concentrations and/or intensity of stimulation and thus may be able to act as an indicator of inadequate analgesia [1, 17, 18]. Induction of anaesthesia decreases heart rate; if the patient has received sufficient 'analgesia', HRV does not change if an ensuing noxious stimulus is applied [14, 19].

Respiratory Rate

A well-established technique for respiratory rate monitoring is electrical impedance changes picked up by an ECG electrode. During inspiration, the distance between the ECG electrode on the thoracic wall and the heart increases, increasing impedance. It is important to realize that it will not detect airway obstruction because the chest wall continues to move, which under these conditions will be misinterpreted as breathing.

Another frequently monitored parameter is the CO_2 partial pressure in the respiratory gases, via capnometry. The capnogram displays ins- and expiratory CO_2 over time, and provides quantitative and qualitative measures of ventilation and information about patient homeostasis and proper functioning of the anaesthesia ventilator. It prevents patient injury by helping the clinician to detect adverse respiratory events such as hypoventilation, decreased cardiac output, oesophageal intubation and circuit disconnection or inadvertent extubation.

By multiplying expired CO_2 and expired volume over time it is possible to calculate the volume (amount) of CO_2 in the exhaled breath (volumetric capnography). CO_2 elimination is a measure of metabolism and of the elimination of any exogenous CO_2 (used when applying a CO_2 pneumoperitoneum), and can be used to detect important changes in cardiorespiratory function.

Pulse Oximetry Signal

Pulse oximetry devices record the pulsatile signal in the arterial blood generated by the heart, and measure the absorption of red and infra-red light to calculate oxygen saturation. The combination of the two (differentiating the diastolic and systolic phase and light absorption at two different wavelengths) allows the pulse oximeter to calculate saturation. By analysing the absorption spectra, oxyhaemoglobin (O_2Hb) can be differentiated from reduced haemoglobin (HHb) and functional haemoglobin saturation can be calculated [20]. The most commonly used oximeters in the operating room use two light-emitting diodes (LEDs) that emit light at the 660 nm (red) and the 940 nm (infrared) wavelengths. In the red region, O_2Hb absorbs less light than HHb, while in the infra-red region O_2Hb absorbs more light than HHb. The ratio of absorbencies at these two wavelengths is calibrated empirically against direct (co-oximeter) measurements of arterial blood oxygen saturation (i.e. fractional haemoglobin saturation). While there is no doubt that pulse oximetry monitoring helps detect hypoxaemia, it is unlikely this will ever be 'proven' because not using a pulse oximeter would not be considered ethical. Newer technologies use more wavelengths and thus also allow measurement of fractional saturation of haemoglobin (i.e. they also measure methaemoglobin and carboxyhaemoglobin).

Anaesthetic Drug Effects Quantitation: From the Raw Electroencephalogram to a Consciousness Index

The following sections apply the concepts described earlier to an EEG database owned by the authors to derive a value (index) that quantifies drug effects in real-time during sedation or anaesthesia. Generally speaking, the development of EEG indices is based on the extraction of parameters from the EEG signal whose values are statistically correlated with anaesthetic agent concentrations and different clinical responses related to hypnotic effect. These parameters are used as inputs of mathematical algorithms whose output is usually a normalized, dimensionless value ranging from zero to 100, or a character, letter or score indicating some level of hypnotic effect.

Once the definitive model relating EEG features to drug concentrations and clinical end-points has been generated, it must be prospectively validated against a reference or 'gold standard'. The 'gold standard' is designed to provide observations of hypnotic responses such as sedation, loss of consciousness or consciousness recovery, awareness or observations of nociceptive responses (such as movement after applying a specific stimulus). The 'gold standard' can also include information related to the estimated effect site concentration of the drugs. The resulting scale may consist only of patient 'response' versus 'no response' probability display, or it may have multiple or graded levels (a range of stimuli of a different intensity that are used to define different 'consciousness levels' [21]). The most frequently used gold standards are the Observer's Assessment of Alertness and Sedation (OAAS), the Ramsay Sedation Scale (RSS) and the effect site concentration of the drug. For example, the RSS is a score ranging from one to six, with the two-to-six range describing the clinical response after a nociceptive stimulus: low values correspond to a patient that is conscious and calm, while RSS=6 corresponds to absence of any response to noxious stimulation. Fig. 5.10 shows a typical block diagram of the development process of an anaesthesia index.

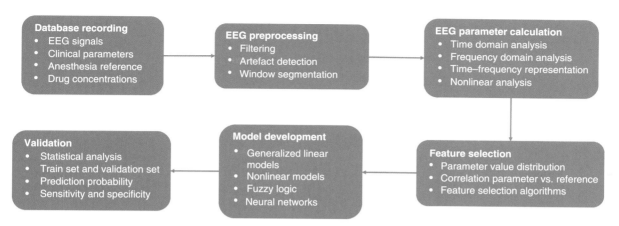

Fig. 5.10 A typical block diagram that illustrates the development process of an EEG-based anaesthesia index.

Electroencephalography for the Assessment of Hypnotic Drug Effect during General Anaesthesia

EEG characteristics during general anaesthesia have been extensively studied over the last decades. In general, many studies concur that increased depth of anaesthesia level is associated with higher frontal α (8–16 Hz) power [22, 23, 24, 25], and that the effects of hypnotic drugs and opioids shift cortical activity from a high-frequency, low-amplitude signal to a low-frequency, high-amplitude signal with a decrease of β activity (16–30 Hz) and increase of α and δ (0.1–4 Hz) activities [25]. However, the increase in δ band can be observed only when the awake state is not perturbed by EOG activity, such as blinking or eye movements. For these reasons, EEG parameters based on the PSD in α and β bands might be good candidates to monitor features related to depth of anaesthesia. The δ band can be used for this purpose too, provided it is associated with an accurate EOG detector.

Figure 5.11 shows an example of three EEG segments recorded in the same patient in three different states: relaxed and awake, awake with frequent blinking and eye movements, and anaesthetized (with a propofol and remifentanil effect-site concentration of 3 μg/mL and 3 ng/mL, respectively). The second EEG segment shows more EOG activity than the first segment, implying higher δ energy in the frequency domain. The PSD of the anaesthesia segment shows a higher peak in the α band and δ band, while the awake segment shows higher power at frequencies above 20 Hz, the β and EMG band. EMG is generally considered to produce an increasing part of the electrical power spectrum above a frequency of

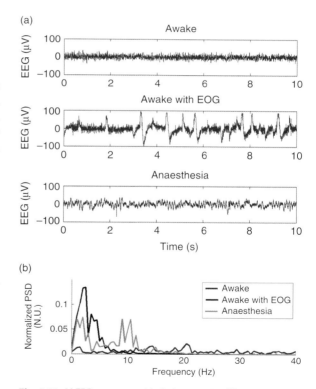

Fig. 5.11 (a) EEG segments with their respective (b) power spectral density (normalized with respect to the total energy) in awake (blue and black) and anaesthetized state (red). In the awake EEG with EOG the PSD can be seen to differ from the awake without EOG activity.

about 30 Hz (also see next paragraph). Fig. 5.12 shows an example of an EEG recording during a surgical procedure under general anaesthesia, along with its relative spectrogram: when the effect-site concentrations of propofol and

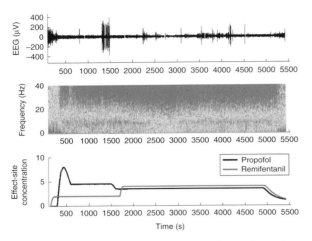

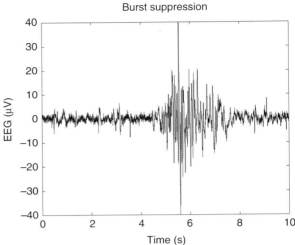

Burst suppression

Fig. 5.12 EEG recording during an entire surgical procedure and the corresponding spectrogram and the effect-site concentration of propofol and remifentanil in μg/mL and ng/mL, respectively. Data obtained from a female 58-year-old patient, 155 cm tall, and weighing 70 kg.

Fig. 5.13 An example of EEG signal during burst suppression period.

remifentanil increase, the energy decreases at high frequency bands, but increases in the low frequency α band.

During anaesthesia, the EEG is recorded from electrodes placed near the centre of the forehead and on the right or left temple because that is where α band changes are mostly detected. Furthermore, this is the most convenient and fastest location to place electrodes. It also avoids hairs becoming entangled between electrodes and skin. Although the recorded voltage predominantly consists of EEG, potentials from facial muscle contraction may contribute to the measured signal. The frequency composition of EEG and EMG artefact overlap in the 30–50 Hz range, and thus simple filtering will not completely remove EMG artefact from single-channel EEG recordings. It is a challenge trying to determine whether the electrical activity detected was generated by the brain or by the frontal muscle. An estimation of the EMG level by computing spectral power in the EMG frequency band is a useful tool that should be taken into account in the interpretation of any EEG-based consciousness index.

At very deep anaesthetic levels, the EEG may develop a peculiar pattern of activity known as 'burst suppression', during which alternating periods of normal to high activity, bursts, and very low voltage (or even electrical silence or 'isoelectricity') are observed (Fig. 5.13). These patterns should be detected using time domain analysis of EEG because they might affect the spectral analysis of the signal, mainly in the period of transitions between burst and suppression where the EEG becomes non-stationary. A parameter that is

widely used to quantify these patterns is called 'burst-suppression ratio' (BSR). After an EEG signal sample of finite length is selected (for example a 30 s window), the amplitude threshold for the EEG is fixed at a specific value, for example 5 μV. The BSR is then computed as the ratio (expressed in percentage) of the seconds during which the EEG is below the amplitude threshold and the total observation period. From a technical point of view, the importance of burst suppression is that the EEG signal has different spectral characteristics during these periods when compared with those of an EEG obtained in other depth stages of anaesthesia: the abrupt changes between the burst and suppression periods can increase the energy in the high frequency of the EEG spectrum and (in the frequency domain) be misinterpreted as the EEG spectrum of an awake subject. A common method to avoid this risk is to correct the value of the index during burst suppression by giving less weight to the parameters obtained from spectral analysis and give more weight to the BSR value.

Several studies also describe how nonlinear dynamics analysis of EEG can be useful for the assessment of depth of anaesthesia features. The main conclusion of these studies is that when a subject becomes unconscious, the EEG signal becomes more regular and less complex. One study [11] showed that changes in various measures of entropy/complexity, such as Shannon entropy, spectral entropy, approximate entropy, Lempel–Ziv complexity and Higuchi fractal dimension, are associated with different levels of sedation. More recent studies show that auto-mutual information measures [26] and refined multi-scale entropy [27] were able to predict the nociceptive responses using the RSS after painful stimulation as a gold standard.

Data Analysis and Feature Selection

The first step in the development of an anaesthesia index consists of finding those EEG parameters in the available database that best correlate with the anaesthetic state. The pre-processing of the EEG and the artefact rejection permit computation of parameters that reflect as well as possible the physiological changes in the signal induced by the hypnotic and analgesic drugs. An important issue is the definition of the length of the segment (window) for which the parameters are to be calculated. Increasing the length of the analysed window permits one to obtain high resolution in the frequency domain, but it requires more computation, which increases the cost and reduces the speed with which the index is updated. A good compromise is to choose a length of one or two seconds and to have a frequency resolution of at least 1 Hz. Next, the correlation should be analysed between the time and frequency domain parameters that have been computed on the windows of interest and the selected gold standard (see above – OAAS, RSS or the effect-site concentration). After this process, that subset of parameters that best correlate with the gold standard are chosen to develop the model. In order to reduce the random noise that in some cases affects data computation, a smoothing technique is often applied on the time evolution of the calculated parameters.

Several approaches can be applied to obtain an appropriate set of parameters, ranging from descriptive statistical analysis to a more complex algorithm of feature selection. Sometimes the analysis of the distribution and the correlation against the gold standard of single parameters might not give the optimal subset to build the model. The most relevant issue is to select only those parameters that are useful to build a good predictive index – any redundant variables should be excluded (so-called Occam's Razor principle or parsimony). By selecting a subset of variables that are well correlated with the gold standard, when they are taken together, it is possible to obtain better results than just by ranking the parameters according to their individual predictive power. Indeed, a variable that seems completely useless in and by itself can still significantly improve performance when combined with others [28].

The feature selection algorithms are divided into three classes: filter methods, wrapper methods and embedded methods. Filter feature selection methods such as the chi-squared test, information gain and correlation coefficient assign a score to each parameter in order to generate a ranking that is used to keep or remove a feature from the dataset. The wrapper methods, such as recursive feature elimination algorithms or genetic algorithms, evaluate different combinations of parameters by using a predictive model and assign a score based on model accuracy. The embedded methods try to learn which parameters best contribute to the performance of the model during the model's creation. The most common type of embedded feature selection methods are regularization methods such as LASSO, Elastic Net and Ridge Regression.

Multi-parameter Model Development

After feature selection procedures (Fig. 5.10), data are ready to be fitted to regression models that characterize the relationship between the parameter subset and the (clinical) gold standard (OAAS, RSS or the effect-site concentration). From a mathematical point of view, the objective is to find a function 'f', the output 'y' of which is the model closest to the gold standard:

$$y = f(x_1, x_2, x_3, \ldots x_N) \tag{2}$$

with 'x_i' being the selected parameters and 'N' the total number of parameters. The process that is used to search for the optimum function 'f' is called 'training'. The training process includes the computation of the best initial model fit. After the training process, a validating process should be performed with data different from the data that were used in the training model, in order to prospectively test the derived model.

Several algorithms can be used to calculate 'y' and then classify the anaesthetic state. The simplest method is the weighted sum of all the parameters. Another approach is to use a classification function, which derives the state of anaesthesia from the extracted features. A fuzzy logic set of rules can also be applied to the selected features to calculate the model output. Other methods that can be used to develop the decision algorithm are: group method of data handling, Naive Bayes, k-nearest neighbour algorithm, Majority classifier, Support vector machines, Random forests, Boosted trees, Classification and Regression Trees, Neural Networks, Ordinary Least Squares, Generalized Linear Models (GLM) and Adaptive Neuro Fuzzy Inference System (ANFIS). The choice of the method depends on the performance of the derived model but also on the complexity of the algorithm. The performance of the derived model is calculated by testing the correlation between the output of the model in the dataset and the clinical gold standard (OAAS, RSS or the effect-site concentration). The best model is the one with the optimal compromise between predictive performances and computational cost. One also needs to consider the fact that the complexity of the algorithm influences the time delay or the response time of the index to an abrupt change in anaesthesia state.

Statistical Analysis and Validation

Validation (Fig. 5.10) is one of the most important steps in the development of a depth of anaesthesia index. It consists of testing the accuracy of the predictions of the developed model in a different population or group of individuals. Firstly, it is suggested to perform the training and the validation in two different sets of data. It is possible to use two different databases or to divide the same database into two subsets of data. The validating process permits one to better prove the index performance with new data that are different from the ones that were used in the training process. In this way, the statistical results of the validation set are independent from those of the training set and they are not biased by the fact that the training data were used for building the model. A good model is the one that is well correlated with the gold standard in both the training and validation sets, while an example of a biased model is one of which the output is very well correlated with the gold standard in the training set but not in the validation set. Analyses to evaluate and validate the performance of a model are numerous and can be numerical, statistic or graphical. Many methods are based on the analysis of the residuals. The residuals are defined as the differences between the responses observed at each value of gold standard and the corresponding model output.

The main performance measures to assess how well model output and clinical gold standard match are (Table 5.3): the familiar parametric t and F statistics and the non-parametric Mann–Whitney statistic; classification measures, such as sensitivity, specificity and percent correct; receiver operating characteristic (ROC) measures, such as parametric and nonparametric ROC area; response curve measures, such as the likelihood value and the slope parameter; and parametric and nonparametric correlation measures, such as the Pearson product–moment correlation, the biserial and the Spearman correlation coefficients, and a variety of measures of association.

In order to determine how well the model output describes the data points according to the gold standard, a threshold can be selected, and index values less than or greater than the threshold are used to predict the value of the gold standard. For example, if we consider a clinical index to describe responsiveness to nociceptive stimulation that ranges between zero and 100, a threshold of 50 can be selected to differentiate a responsive from a no-response state: all the periods when the index is above 50 are classified as samples associated with patients that respond to nociceptive stimulation, while all the periods when the index is lower than 50 are classified as periods associated with patients that do not respond to nociceptive stimulation. When comparing the model predictions to the gold standard, the samples are divided in four groups: (1) the index samples that are above 50 when the gold standard also indicates a responsive state are true positives; (2) the index samples that are above 50 when the gold standard indicates a non-responsive state are false positives; (3) the index samples that are under 50 when also the gold standard indicates a non-responsive state are considered are true negatives; (4) the index samples that are under 50 when the gold standard indicates a responsive state are considered false negatives. Sensitivity is defined as the ratio of true positives over the sum of true positives and false negatives; specificity is defined as the ratio of true negatives over the sum of true negatives and false positives; and percent correct is the ratio of true positives and true negatives over the total number of samples.

Sometimes graphical methods might be preferable over numerical methods because they better illustrate different complex aspects of the relationship between the output and the fitted data, while numerical methods tend to be biased on a particular aspect of the relationship between the model and the data because they try to compress that information into a single descriptive number.

The performance of anaesthesia indexes are often described with the prediction probability (Pk), a rescaled variant of Kim's measure of association [21] that has a value of one when the observed anaesthetic depth is perfectly predicted, and a value of 0.5 when the prediction is no better than a 50:50 chance. Similarly, a Pk value of zero represents a perfect prediction but indicates that the two indicators are correlated reversely. Prediction probability expresses the correlation between the index value and the observed (component of) anaesthetic depth, taking into account both desired performances and the limitations of the data. It is independent of scale units and does not require knowledge of underlying distributions or efforts to

Table 5.3. Main performance measures of difference or separation between model output and clinical gold standard.

Type of Measure	Statistical Method	Scope
Parametric tests	t test	Tests the hypothesis that two sets of data are significantly different from each other. Data should follow normal distribution.
	F test	Tests the hypothesis that the means of a set of normally distributed populations with the same variance are equal or that a regression model fits the data well.
Non-parametric tests	Mann–Whitney test	Tests the hypothesis that two independent samples are selected from populations that have the same distribution.
	Wilcoxon test	Tests the hypothesis that two dependent samples are selected from populations that have the same distribution.
Classification measures	Sensitivity and specificity	Sensitivity: percentage of positives that are correctly identified as such (for example the percentage of people that respond to nociceptive stimulation that are correctly detected).
		Specificity: percentage of negatives that are correctly identified as such (for example the percentage of people that do not respond to nociceptive stimulation that are correctly detected).
	Percent correct	The percent of samples that are correctly classified in their respective state.
	Receiver operating characteristic (ROC) curve	Curve that shows the performance of a binary classifier system as its discrimination threshold is varied. The ROC curve is the plot of the true positive rate (sensitivity) against the false positive rate (1 – specificity) at various threshold settings.
Response curve measures	Likelihood value	The likelihood of a parameter value is a function that describes the probability density for the observed model outputs given that parameter value.
	Slope parameter	The slope of the response curve of a model is a parameter that assesses the performance of the model. The curve slope of the ideal model is vertical: the higher the slope the better the model fits with the clinical gold standard.
Correlation measures	Pearson product–moment correlation	Pearson product–moment correlation quantifies the linear correlation between two variables. It has a value between +1 and −1: 1 is total positive linear correlation, 0 is no linear correlation, and −1 is total negative linear correlation.
	Biserial	The point biserial correlation coefficient is used when one variable is dichotomous. It is mathematically equivalent to the Pearson product moment correlation.
	Spearman correlation	The Spearman correlation coefficient quantifies the statistical dependence between the rankings of two variables, assessing how well the relationship between two variables can be described using a monotonic function. The Spearman correlation between two variables is equivalent to the Pearson correlation between the rank values of those two variables. If there are no repeated data values and each of the variables is a perfect monotone function of the other the Spearman correlation will be +1 or −1.
Association Measures	Chi-square based measures	Chi-square based measures are used to determine whether there is a statistical relationship between two variables after obtaining a cross classification table and calculating whether or not there is a statistical relationship between the variables in the cross classification table.
	Reduction in error	This method predicts the values of one variable in two different ways: the values for one variable without knowing the values of a second variable, and after taking into account the values of the second variable. The reduction in error is based on the range to which the prediction error for values of one variable can be reduced by knowing the value of the second variable.

linearize or to transform scales. Furthermore, its expected value is asymptotically independent of the number of experimental data points.

Another useful validation test is the comparison of the performance of the output model with other anaesthetic depth indices. Pk can be used to perform both grouped and paired data statistical comparisons of the performance of the two indices under the hypothesis that data are recorded with the same response-to-stimulus test procedure and over the same distribution of anaesthetic depths. The test statistic is based on the difference between the two sample values of Pk, divided by an estimated standard deviation of this difference. Usually a t test is performed in order to assess whether the Pk of the two indices are statistically different.

Categorical Responses

When the variables that describe a response are associated with a particular group or nominal category based on a qualitative property, they are called categorical variables. Examples of categorical responses are the OAAS and RSS sedation scores mentioned above, in which each category represents a different level of sedation. If the response only takes on two values, it is called binary or dichotomous, otherwise it is called polytomous.

A robust predictive method that is widely used to model the relationship between predictors and categorical response is the logistic regression model in which a link function is associated with the categorical variables. The use of a logistic regression model allows prediction of the probability, which is continuous, as a function of a variable, e.g. the probability of being at a determined sedation score as a function of propofol concentration.

Response Curve

In some cases the observed anaesthetic depth indicator that is used as the gold standard might be dichotomous having values N1 and N2 that are associated, for example, with response or no response to a stimulus. Those indicators can be represented with the response curve, which permits one to show directly how to achieve a particular probability of no response to stimulus. Having y as the gold standard and x the anaesthesia index, the response curve can be constructed by using a two-parameter function, such as the logistic curve, to fit y versus x in a set of sample data. The obtained curve shows the percent probability of response to a stimulus with respect to the value of x. Common response curve parameters are the value of the index at the 50% probability of no patient response (x50), and the slope of the curve, related to the derivative of the curve. Fig. 5.14 shows an example of the typical morphology of a response curve calculated from an anaesthesia index.

Response curves can be used also to compare the performance of two anaesthetic depth indices with a common scale. The better of the two indices has the response curve with the steeper slope.

Conclusions

The methods and concepts that are used in signal processing and that are commonly used in response measurements and index development for anaesthetic

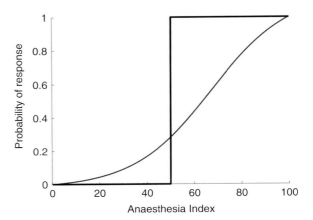

Fig. 5.14 A typical response curve of a generic anaesthesia index (in blue) and the ideal monitor (in black).

depth assessment have been concisely summarized and described. The purpose was to provide an overview of the basics of signal processing techniques that are commonly applied to obtain a parameter displayed on the screen of an anaesthesia monitor that correlates with responses and outcomes relevant to the anaesthetic state. The references in this chapter offer more information to the reader seeking more detailed and specific information on the complex and extended theory that is applied in the search of the ideal anaesthesia response index, an area that is always in progress.

References

1. Win NN, Fukayama H, Kohase H, Umino M: The different effects of intravenous propofol and midazolam sedation on hemodynamic and heart rate variability. Anaesth.Analges. 2005; 101: 97–102.

2. Rantanen M: Novel multiparameter approach for measurement of nociception at skin incision during general anaesthesia. Br.J.Anaesth. 2006; 96: 367–76.

3. Miller RD: *Miller's Anesthesia: 1.* Amsterdam: Elsevier, 2010.

4. Jensen EW, Valencia JF, López A, Anglada T, Agustí M, Ramos Y, Serra R, Jospin M, Pineda P, Gambus P: Monitoring hypnotic effect and nociception with two EEG-derived indices, qCON and qNOX, during general anaesthesia. Acta Anaesthesiol.Scand. 2014; 58: 933–41.

5. Viertiö-Oja H, Maja V, Särkelä M, Talja P, Tenkanen N, Tolvanen-Laakso H, Paloheimo M, Vakkuri A, Yli-Hankala A, Meriläinen P: Description of the Entropy algorithm as applied in the Datex-Ohmeda S/5 Entropy Module. Acta.Anaesthesiol.Scand. 2004; 48: 154–61.

6. Bouillon TW: Pharmacodynamic interaction between propofol and remifentanil regarding hypnosis, tolerance of laryngoscopy, bispectral index, and electroencephalographic approximate entropy. Anesthesiology. 2004; 100: 1353–72.

7. Jensen EW, Lindholm P, Henneberg S: Auto regressive modeling with exogenous input of auditory evoked potentials to produce an on-line depth of anaesthesia index. Methods.Inf.Med. 1996; 35: 256–260.

8. Cohen L: *Time-Frequency Analysis*. New Jersey: Prentice Hall, 1995.

9. Walling PT, Kenneth NH: Nonlinear changes in brain dynamics during emergence from sevoflurane anaesthesia: preliminary exploration using new software. Anesthesiology 2006; 105: 927–35.

10. Lalitha V, Eswaran C: Automated detection of anesthetic depth levels using chaotic features with artificial neural networks. J.Med.Syst. 2007; 31: 445–52.

11. Natarajan K, Acharya R, Alias F, Tiboleng T, Puthusserypady SK: Nonlinear analysis of EEG signals at different mental states. Biomed.Eng.OnLine. 2004; 3: 7–18.

12. Ferenets R, Lipping T, Anier A, Jantti V, Melto S, Hovilehto S: Comparison of entropy and complexity measures for the assessment of depth of sedation. IEEE Trans.Biomed.Eng. 2006; 53: 1067–77.

13. Hornero R, Abásolo D, Escudero J, Gómez C: Nonlinear analysis of electroencephalogram and magnetoencephalogram recordings in patients with Alzheimer's disease. Philos.Trans.Royal.Soc. A. 2009; 367: 317–36.

14. Struys MM, Jensen EW, Smith W, Smith NT, Rampil I, Dumortier FJ, Mestach C, Mortier EP. Performance of the ARX-derived auditory evoked potential index as an indicator of anesthetic depth: a comparison with bispectral index and hemodynamic measures during propofol administration. Anesthesiology. 2002; 96: 803–16.

15. Leslie K, Sessler DI, Smith WD, Larson MD, Ozaki M, Blanchard D, Crankshaw DP: Prediction of movement during propofol/nitrous oxide anaesthesia: performance of concentration, electroencephalographic, pupillary, and hemodynamic indicators. Anesthesiology. 1996; 84: 52–63.

16. Kato M, Komatsu T, Kimura T, Sugiyama F, Nakashima K, Shimada Y: Spectral analysis of heart rate variability during isoflurane anaesthesia. Anesthesiology. 1992; 77: 669–74.

17. Sato A, Sato Y, Shimada F, Torigata Y: Varying changes in heart rate produced by nociceptive stimulation of the skin in rats at different temperatures. Brain.Res. 1976; 110: 301–11.

18. Jeanne M, Logier R, De Jonckheere J, Tavernier B: Heart rate variability during total intravenous anaesthesia: effects of nociception and analgesia. Auton.Neurosci. 2009; 147: 91–6.

19. Jeanne M, Clément C, De Jonckheere J, Logier R, Tavernier B: Variations of the analgesia nociception index during general anaesthesia for laparoscopic abdominal surgery. J.Clin.Monit.Comput. 2012; 26: 289–94.

20. Jubran A: Pulse oximetry. Crit.Care. 2015; 19: 1–7.

21. Smith WD, Dutton RC, Smith NT: Measuring the performance of anesthetic depth indicators. Anesthesiology. 1996; 84: 38–51.

22. Gugino LD, Chabot RJ, Prichep LS, John ER, Formanek V: Quantitative EEG changes associated with loss and return of consciousness in healthy adult volunteers anaesthetized with propofol or sevoflurane. Brit.J.Anaesth. 2001; 87: 421–8.

23. Feshchenko VA, Veselis RA, Reinsel RA: Propofol-induced alpha rhythm. Neuropsychobiology. 2004; 50: 257–66.

24. Hindriks R, van Putten MJ: Meanfield modeling of propofol-induced changes in spontaneous EEG rhythms. Neuroimage. 2002; 60: 2323–34.

25 Ching S, Cimenser A, Purdon PL, Brown EN, Kopell NJ: Thalamocortical model for a propofol-induced alpha-rhythm associated with loss of consciousness. Proc.Natl. Acad.Sci.USA. 2010; 107: 22665–70.

26. Melia U, Vallverdú M, Borrat X, Valencia JF, Jospin M, Jensen EW, Gambus P, Caminal P: Prediction of nociceptive responses during sedation by linear and non-linear measures of EEG signals in high frequencies. PloS.One. 2015; 10: e0123464.

27. Valencia JF, Melia U, Vallverdú M, Borrat X, Jospin M, Jensen EW, Gambus P, Caminal P. Assessment of nociceptive responsiveness levels during sedation-analgesia by entropy analysis of EEG. Entropy. 2016; 18: 103–14.

28. Guyon I: An introduction to variable and feature selection. J.Mach.Learn.Res. 2003; 3: 1157–82.

Application of Pharmacokinetics and Pharmacodynamics and Signal Analysis to Drug Administration in Anaesthesia

R. Ross Kennedy

In the not too distant future the anaesthesiologist, surgeon and patient may arrive at the hospital in self-driving cars. It is hard to imagine they will be content to interact in the operating room with largely manually operated medical equipment (Kuck and Johnson, 2017) [1]

Introduction

In a recent review of the performance of closed-loop systems in anaesthesia, Brogi et al [2] defined a closed-loop system as an automated control system designed to maintain a given variable around a desired set point. The key components of these systems, sensors, controllers and actuators, are outlined in Table 6.1.

To this list we can add a 'supervisor' component. The supervisor (clinician) determines the set point for the various parameters being controlled. These set points include physiological and pharmacological targets. During anaesthesia the 'inputs' for the supervisor include the progress of the procedure, the response of the patient to interventions thus far, and a concept of the way in which the patient and the controller/actuator system will respond to a change in set point. The output of the supervisor is updated set points for one or several controllers. This supervision, or integration, is part of the function of the anaesthesia provider.

Brogi et al reviewed the performance of automated control of a single variable [2]. This general classification can be extended to fully automated anaesthesia with an algorithmic supervisor overseeing a wide range of inputs (sensors and monitors) and controlling multiple outputs (drug delivery systems). The anaesthesia provider now moves outside the system to gain a general oversight (supervision) of the proper functioning of the system in a similar manner to the pilot of a modern airliner monitoring the function of the autopilot.

While the schema in Table 6.1 was developed to describe fully automated systems, the same terminology can be used to describe most methods that maintain a particular drug concentration or component of anaesthesia. In many parts of the world, and within the working lifetime of many practising anaesthetists in the most developed economies, the anaesthesia provider, perhaps aided by some basic monitoring, fills all four roles, i.e. acting as sensor, supervisor, controller and actuator. Clinical signs (feeling the pulse, sweating, pupil size, breath sounds etc.), possibly aided by very basic monitors, make up the 'sensors'. The 'actuator' directly injects drugs and adjusts the vaporizer The supervisor and controller functions might appear similar in this model, but it is useful to think of them as separate, with, for instance, the controller focussing on maintaining a given vapour concentration while the supervisor is thinking about the overall progress of the procedure.

As available technology improves, various tasks are handed off from the provider to various devices. Devices such as automated blood pressure measurement and pulse oximetry are generally more reliable because the measurement is not dependent on the user physically taking the measurement. In addition, these devices can be particularly useful at times of high workload. Finally, they can give information that is not otherwise available such as S_pO_2, respiratory gas composition and the degree of neuromuscular blockade.

Target controlled infusion (TCI) is specifically discussed below. A concept underlying this chapter is that every anaesthetic represents some form of target control with the anaesthesia provider performing

Table 6.1. Components of a closed-loop system (after Brogi et al [2]).

	Input	Function	Output
Sensor	Appropriate monitors and sensors	Measures the target parameter	Produces a feedback signal
Controller	Set point Feedback signal	Compares feedback signal and desired set point	Instructions to delivery device
Actuator	(Digital) signal for controller	Controls physical device (e.g. syringe driver)	

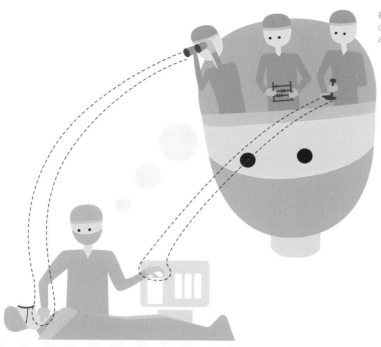

Fig. 6.1 The anaesthetist as an integrated closed-loop system acting as supervisor, and also as sensor, controller and actuator.

a variable number of the roles described above. There is always a desired set point (or target) for each component of the anaesthetic mix. These targets may be clinical end-points, such as keeping the blood pressure within a range, or intermediate targets relating to anaesthesia delivery, such as vapour or O_2 partial pressure. Different providers and providers in different settings use a variety of approaches to achieve and maintain similar targets.

The aim of this chapter is to briefly discuss emerging tools available to the clinical anaesthetist and how they can help optimize delivery of anaesthesia to the individual patient using the concept of a closed-loop system as a framework. While recognizing and touching on the importance and increasing role of an increasing number of sensors, the primary focus of this chapter is on tools that aid delivery of drugs to achieve desired set points and on the improved understanding of the concepts underlying these tools. The emphasis is on commercially available devices with occasional reference to research systems and those available to the enthusiast to illustrate various concepts. The examples chosen are representative of the various concepts and technologies rather than representing a comprehensive review.

The following abbreviations will be used: end-expired partial pressure = F_A; inspired partial pressure = F_I; fresh gas flow = FGF; effect site partial pressure (inhaled agents) or effect site concentration (IV drugs) = C_e. When discussing the kinetics of inhaled anaesthetics, the term 'partial pressure' rather than concentration is used because it is the partial pressure gradient that drives transport (concentration = partial pressure × solubility according to Henry's Law).

The Problem of Achieving a Desired Set Point

Although most anaesthesia providers would think of the set point for these control systems as a given drug concentration in a particular compartment, in fact the objective of the supervisor is a given anaesthetic state.

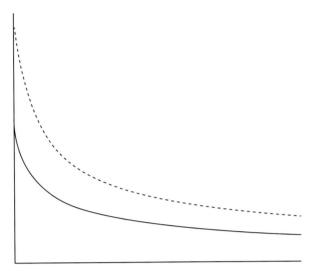

Fig. 6.2 A stylized isobologram. The concentration of hypnotic is on the y-axis and the opioid concentration on the x-axis. The solid curve represents the combination at which 50% of a population will (or will not) respond to a standard noxious stimulus. The dashed line is the 90th centile where 90% will not respond (but 10% will). The y-intercept, with no opioid, represents the effect of hypnotic alone and is the MAC fraction for the given effect. The early part of the curve is relatively steep and, in a standard 70 kg person, 100 μg of fentanyl will reduce volatile requirement by 50% for five to ten minutes. Note that the curve does not intercept the x-axis. Early studies used the interaction between single hypnotic opioid pairs. Data on the relative potencies of the volatile agents (MAC equivalents) and synthetic opioids allow different combinations and mixtures to be plotted on the same set of axes.

Glass provides a useful definition of the objectives of anaesthesia [3]. In addition to providing optimal operating conditions and minimizing physiological trespass, the anaesthesia 'state' is (1) absence of recall and (2) absence of both motor and sympathetic response to noxious stimulus [3]. These effects are primarily mediated by hypnotics in the brain and opioids in the spinal cord, respectively. While volatile anaesthetics are frequently used primarily for their role as hypnotics, they also have direct effects in the spinal cord [4, 5] allowing them to be used to provide single agent anaesthesia. There is considerable synergy between these drug groups on these effects [6, 7] as illustrated in Fig. 6.2 (also see Chapter 3).

During surgery the degree of stimulus and hence anaesthetic requirement changes frequently. Once surgery is completed, we want minimal residual effect of our drugs beyond a suitable level of analgesia. This requirement to continually adjust and titrate anaesthesia is made more complex because most drugs used in anaesthesia do not reach equilibrium during the course of a typical procedure, which implies that maintaining a constant plasma (or effect-site) concentration requires a continually decreasing delivery rate (the exponential decreasing transfer component of bolus–elimination–transfer, or BET, scheme) [8]. Increasing the effect of a given drug is relatively straightforward, although as will be discussed below, simply increasing an infusion rate or vaporizer setting does not produce an immediate change in effect.

Anticipating the rate of decrease in drug effect is more complex and in particular has very little to do with conventional pharmacokinetics (PK) based on elimination half-times and equilibrium volumes of distribution. A good illustration of this disconnect is the concept of context sensitive half-time, the time for a drug concentration to decrease by 50%, which is influenced by the duration of infusion ('context' refers to the duration of administration) [9, 10].

Many drugs used in anaesthesia that we consider rapidly acting, including volatile anaesthetics [10] and opioids such as fentanyl, alfentanil and sufentanil, continue to redistribute for many hours [11]. Although the rate of elimination of inhaled agents via the lungs can be manipulated, redistribution still plays a role and is the basis for the influence of duration of delivery [10] and differing physico-chemical characteristics of different agents on the rate of elimination [12].

The combination of changing stimulus intensity, hysteresis, context sensitive half-times and drug interactions makes drug delivery in anaesthesia surprisingly complex and makes the conventional approach to drug dosing and delivery which considers just amount and timing of drug delivered to the patient less useful. In anaesthesia we have a target that is changing and are working with drug kinetics that change over time. Measuring or modelling drug levels that are more closely related to drug effect considerably simplifies this control task.

The Volatile Cascade

To illustrate the issues with drug delivery during anaesthesia, consider the 'cascade' in volatile anaesthetic partial pressure from the vaporizer of a conventional anaesthetic machine to the effect site. In some ways, this is analogous to the oxygen cascade with a partial pressure gradient from outside the body to the final site of action.

The major steps to consider are: (1) fresh gas mix and FGF; (2) the breathing circuit; (3) the lung (including FRC); (4) arterial blood; (5) brain (or effect site). These are illustrated in Fig. 6.3.

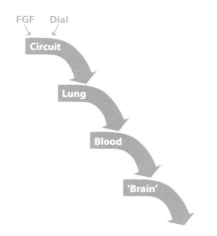

Fig. 6.3 The 'volatile cascade'. Each compartment has an effective volume. Transfer between compartments is determined by the partial pressure gradient and the rate of mixing between compartments (ventilation or blood flow).

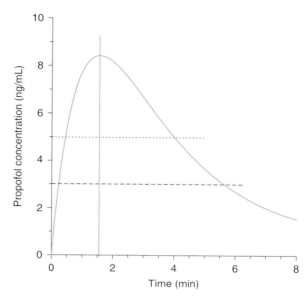

Fig. 6.4 The time course of the effect-site concentration (C_e) of propofol following a 150 mg bolus in a 70 kg 40-year-old male using Schnider's parameters [17]. For this discussion assume the patient will stay unarousable until they return to the C_e at which they became unconscious. The dashed horizontal line is at a propofol concentration of 3 ng/mL and the dotted line is at 5 ng/mL. If loss of consciousness occurs at 3 ng/mL (dashed horizontal line) this will be about 20 seconds after injection with recovery occurring at 5.5 min. If 5 ng/mL is required for loss of consciousness (dotted horizontal line), this will occur at 35 seconds and last for 3.5 min. Peak hypnotic effect of propofol in this model is 8 ng/mL and occurs at 1.6 min (vertical solid line), well after the time of loss of conscious for the 3 and 5 ng/mL scenarios.

The effective volume of each compartment is determined by the physical volume of the compartment and (for the blood and brain) the solubility of that drug in the compartment.

Although we cannot physically observe the individual steps, each causes an additional delay in reaching a new target (effect site) partial pressure after making a change in the vaporizer setting, with the total delay being a composite of these steps. The anaesthesia provider can influence some of these steps (e.g. by manipulating FGF, ventilation, and theoretically cardiac output), but much of the process is determined by the physical characteristics of the system.

Monitoring F_A provides information from part-way along the cascade and approximates the partial pressure in blood [13] but is still several steps removed from the effect site. Even with less soluble agents, there is a delay (hysteresis) at each step, which is discussed in detail in the next section. The half-time for transfer from end-tidal to effect site for the halogenated volatile anaesthetics is two to three minutes [14, 15]. The blood to effect-site transfer half-time for propofol is 1.5–2.5 minutes [16].

To overcome the effect of these compounding delays, we tend to overdose our patients: the initial bolus dose of intravenous hypnotic is usually chosen for speed of onset and duration rather than peak effect. Consequently, the desired change in effect may occur before the maximum C_e change has occurred. Thus we risk overshooting the target. For example, after an induction bolus of propofol, the majority of patients will become unarousable long before the peak drug levels are reached, which may contribute to post-induction hypotension (see Fig. 6.4). Similarly an initial bolus dose of NMB is usually chosen for speed of onset and duration rather than peak effect.

Equilibrium versus Dynamic Changes

With volatile anaesthetic agents, studies of minimum alveolar concentration, or 'MAC' studies, give us some idea of the C_e required for a given effect [18, 19, 20]. These studies are performed using step changes of F_A, and following each step, F_A is kept constant for 10–20 minutes to allow time for equilibrium to occur between compartments. While these studies give us an estimate of partial pressure required to block the response to the given stimulus, use of MAC derivatives is much less useful during periods of change if hysteresis is not taken into account, that is unless C_e is considered. Anaesthesia providers need to recognize that F_A and C_e can differ significantly during periods of rapid change [21]. This is illustrated in Fig. 6.5. This

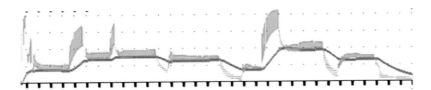

Fig. 6.5 A plot of inspired and expired sevoflurane (yellow band) and calculated effect-site ('brain', grey line) sevoflurane partial pressures using an equilibrium half-time for the effect site $(_{t1/2}k_{eo})$ of 3.2 min [14]. Cross-hatching of the sevoflurane band signifies inspired < expired, or wash-out. This record covers 160 min with solid blocks on the x-axis occuring every five minutes. The lag, or hysteresis, between F_A and C_e is clear in this example.

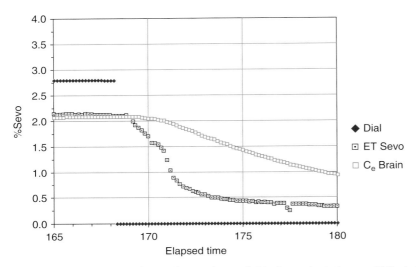

Fig. 6.6 The decline in F_A and C_e sevoflurane after nearly 3 h of anaesthesia. At around 168 min the sevoflurane vaporizer (blue line) is changed from 2.8 to 0. At this time, measured F_A and calculated effect-site (C_e) sevoflurane are similar. Once the vaporizer is turned off F_A falls rapidly towards 0.5% but the decline in C_e is much slower. In this (clinical) example F_A sevoflurane falls below MAC-awake (0.6 vol%) 4 min after the vaporizer is turned off. This delay between FA and C_e is called 'hysteresis'. Eight minutes later, at the right edge of the graph, C_e is still almost 1%. This gives the impression the MAC-awake concept 'does not work' – but it does, provided C_e rather than F_A is considered.

difference between F_A and C_e is particularly relevant at the conclusion of anaesthesia, where 50% of the patients are responsive by the time C_e falls to MAC-awake (around 0.3MAC), but the F_A at the same time will be significantly lower and is thus a much less useful guide to expected recovery time than C_e (Fig. 6.6).

Similar concepts apply with IV agents. The classic Roberts 10/8/6 regime for propofol [22] rapidly achieves and maintains a plasma concentration of around 3 ng/mL but does not guide us if the target needs changing. A common clinical approach is to make a step change in the infusion rate, but it can take a surprisingly long time to approach a new equilibrium. This delay in plasma concentrations after a change in agent delivery, with C_e lagging behind even more, is illustrated in Fig. 6.7. The figure also demonstrates how the effect of a step change in the rate of delivery of a drug continues long after the desired change in effect has been achieved. A similar pattern is seen after a step change in vaporizer dial setting, even at moderately high FGFs.

Is All of Anaesthesia about the Control of Targets?

This chapter has, thus far, developed a number of broad concepts.

Firstly, we can think of all anaesthesia drug delivery in terms of a closed-loop controller, with the anaesthesia provider (or *wetware*[1]) performing more or fewer of the functions of the controller, especially in the supervisor/controller/actuator domains.

---

1   The human nervous system, as opposed to computer hardware or software. www.hacker-dictionary.com/terms/wetware [last accessed 8 June 2019]. See also www.merriam-webster.com/dictionary/wetware) [last accessed 8 June 2019].

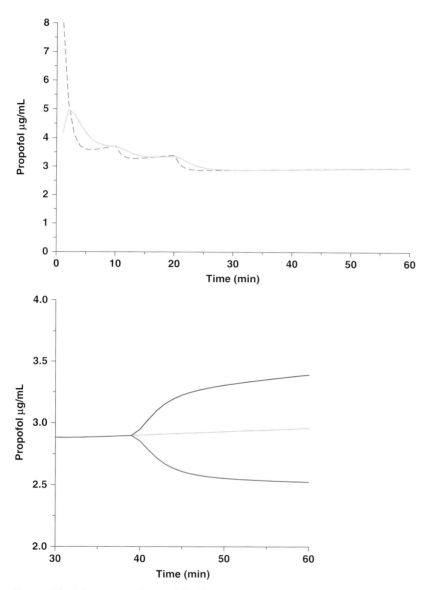

Fig. 6.7 The Roberts regime [22] modelled for a 70 kg 44-year-old 174 cm male using the Schnider model parameters [17]. A 1 mg/kg bolus is followed by an infusion run at 10 mL/kg/h for 10 min, then 8 mL/h for a further 10 min, then 6 mL/h. The upper panel shows calculated plasma (dashed line) and effect-site (solid line) concentrations. The lower panel is the same simulation, but at 40 min from the start of the infusion the rate is increased (blue) or decreased (green) by 20%. After 5 min, C_e has changed by 10% and a further 5% change from baseline has occurred by 20 min. This graph illustrates the way in which the effect of a step change continues for some time. We also see that maintaining a constant infusion (6 mL/kg/h) results in a gradual increase in C_e of about 5%/h.

Secondly, for any drug there are several steps between changing the setting on the delivery device, and a change in effect occurring and reaching equilibrium at the effect site. *Any of these steps can be the 'target' for the control systems.*

Together these concepts suggest that all of anaesthesia is 'target controlled': the anaesthesia provider

always has some idea of the target they are aiming to achieve. The target could be a specific drug level in a given compartment or a given clinical state (unconsciousness, loss of response to a noxious stimulus, control of a physiological parameter ...).

Finally, adjusting drug delivery to match changing patient requirements can be complex, even with drugs considered relatively short acting. Given these issues, we appear to do surprisingly well at matching delivery to need in everyday clinical practice.

There is a place for tools that allow more precise control of the various anaesthetic end-points. In the remainder of this chapter we consider a range of approaches to control 'anaesthesia' in the context of these issues.

Controlling Anaesthetic Drug Delivery

Recipes

A typical basic recipe is a mg/kg dosing regime, such as 'induce with 2 mg/kg of propofol'. A more sophisticated example is the Roberts propofol regime [22] which rapidly achieves and then maintains a predetermined target.

Similar regimes have been described for volatile anaesthetics. In 1972 Cowles et al [23] used computer modelling to develop a series of step changes in dial concentration to achieve and maintain a brain concentration of around 1.3%. For halothane this sequence is 3% for 12 min, 2% for 3 min, 1.5% for 100 min and 1.25% thereafter. Mapleson [24] refined this approach to incorporate changes in flow rates and include all modern halogenated agents. The ultimate in recipe-based low-flow volatile anaesthetic delivery is described in 'The Qualitative Practice of Anesthesia: Use of Closed Circuit' by Lowe and Ernst [25]. This describes in detail the injection of fixed amounts of liquid agent into a closed circuit at increasing intervals following a square root of time rule. All of these approaches require considerable diligence and attention to detail while managing other aspects of induction of anaesthesia and the start of surgery.

Da Silva et al [26] analysed the performance of the 'square root of time model' and found the rate of uptake declined more slowly than predicted with isoflurane and especially with enflurane. This finding was duplicated by Bangaari et al in 2013 [27]. These groups concluded that this approach was not sufficiently accurate for use when agent monitoring is not available, such as in less developed economies [26, 27].

In addition to the intrinsic inaccuracies, these recipes for volatile anaesthetic delivery share the basic weakness of the Roberts propofol regime: they do not allow for a smooth change in effect either because of inter-individual variability in requirement or with a changing surgical stimulus.

These fixed recipe examples are not strictly closed-loop control because there is no feedback (or modification) of the (predetermined) drug dosing. Conversely, the 'control system' is working to control the delivery. These approaches are based on average requirements and do not incorporate any acknowledgement of the considerable inter-patient variability.

More recently Hendrickx et al [28–30] have described simple one or two step sequences to rapidly achieve an approximate end-tidal target and low total FGFs. The vaporizer setting can then be modified based on measured end-tidal concentration and adapted to individual requirements. The important difference between these and earlier regimes is the assumption that the recipe is approximate and will be modified by measurement (or feedback).

Monitoring, Sensors and User Controlled Targets

The preceding paragraph introduces a monitor of drug levels (expired agent partial pressure) as a control variable. Various monitors of the patient state, to be considered in this section, extend this concept.

The simplest form of patient monitoring is observation of vital signs such as palpation of pulses, observation of respiratory rate and pattern, pupillary responses and looking for sweating. These are the basis of the classic signs of anaesthetic depth. Beyond that are simple monitors of pulse, ECG and blood pressure, supplemented by pulse oximetry [31]. Another layer of monitoring is provided by respiratory gas monitoring including O_2, and CO_2. These parameters are general indicators of the patient's physiology rather than specifically related to anaesthesia.

Monitoring anaesthetic agent partial pressures (both volatile and N_2O) in respiratory gases starts to allow more detailed mapping of drug delivery to patient response since it gives some idea of drug levels beyond the rate of delivery. With this technology, the user can adjust the delivered vapour partial pressure and FGF rates to achieve a given F_A and also adjust the target F_A to meet individual patient requirements. Anaesthetic gas monitoring also facilitates different approaches to delivery such as low-flow and closed-circuit.

Despite some initial debate about the value and safety of gas monitoring [32], the place of the monitors listed above is well established. Physiological monitors give an indication of the general well-being of the patient. More recently attention has focussed on developing monitors of the specific components of the anaesthetic state.

An increasing number of monitors use an EEG signal to give an indication of the degree of hypnosis. These include bispectral index (BIS), qCON, Spectral Entropy, Narcotrend, Patient State Analyser and many others [33]. BIS is the most widely studied of these, but most studies suggest equivalence between devices. These devices can be used to guide anaesthesia, with a BIS in the range of 40–60 a commonly reported target.

A number of devices attempt to quantify the degree of response to noxious stimulus with varying success. Monitors include SPI (surgical plethysmographic index), CVI (composite variability index, based on the BIS signal), qNOX, the analgesic nociception index (ANI) and pupillometry. This is an evolving area with many of these approaches showing promise [34, 35]. An alternative approach based on drug levels alone also predicts response to noxious stimulus as well as several monitors [36].

Target Controlled Infusion

With a target controlled infusion (TCI) system, the user enters a target drug concentration and the computer system delivers drug at a rate to achieve and maintain the specified target. Infusion rates are based on combined PKPD models which incorporate patient characteristics ('covariates') such as gender, age, height and weight (see Chapter 4). Although some systems and models target plasma concentrations, increasingly the target used is the effect site.

The unique advantage of TCI is the ability to change the target concentration, not just the delivery rate. A recipe based approach can achieve and approximately maintain a predetermined concentration for a period of time, but changing to a new target is difficult as discussed above. A TCI system will achieve this change rapidly. For example, to decrease the target, a TCI system will stop the infusion for a period of time and then restart it at an appropriate rate, producing a step change as rapidly as drug kinetics allow. TCI systems will maintain a given level (F_A, C_p, or C_e) over a long period of time by gradually decreasing the infusion rate as compartments fill up.

Although several hypnotics and opioids were investigated as prototype TCI systems developed from 1979 onwards [37], the first commercial TCI system, the Diprifusor [38], was introduced in 1996 and specifically designed for propofol. 'Open TCI' systems became available from 2002 allowing the use of a range of drugs including generic brands of propofol, remifentanil, alfentanil and sufentanil [39]. Fentanyl and midazolam are also modelled in some devices. The performance of models used in TCI systems is often described using Varvel's criteria: median performance error (MDPE, a measure of accuracy) or 'togetherness', median absolute percentage error (MDAPE, a measure of bias or 'offset'), divergence (drift over time) and wobble (a measure for stability/oscillations) [40].

The theory, history and development and the contrasting place of TCI systems in the USA and the rest of the world has been reviewed in detail recently [37, 39, 41, 42]. The software for many systems is available for download from the OpenTCI Initiative (www.opentci.org). Several systems, including STANPUMP[2] and RUGLOOP11,[3] continue to be maintained and used in studies where TCI administration is advantageous.

Automated Vapour Control

As with the development of TCI, the components of the control loop including the technology (microprocessors) and the understanding of the underlying kinetics were developed long before these systems became commercially available. Automated feedback control of anaesthetic vapour was first described by a UK group in 1983 for halothane [43] and isoflurane [44]. The key to this system was the availability of an accurate rapid-response monitor of the agent's partial pressure. This system used a computer controlled syringe driver to inject liquid agent into a conventional closed-circle system. This group was able to accurately maintain F_A and quantify the uptake rate of these agents [43, 44]. They found that although the overall rate of uptake followed an exponential washing pattern, there was poor correlation with various anthropometric measurements and there was considerable inter-patient variability [44]. These results support the need for drug delivery to be based on measurements from the individual rather than a population based recipe.

In 1986 Westenskow et al [45] described a custom made closed-loop system for vapour which maintained the halothane F_A and also adjusted O_2 delivery to keep the circuit volume constant, thus allowing vapour and

---

2. Available at www.opentci.org/code/stanpump [last accessed 8 June 2019].
3. Available at www.demed.be/rugloopII.htm [last accessed 8 June 2019].

oxygen uptake to be measured [46]. This controller incorporated aspects of modelling as well as information from the sensor. This group demonstrated more accurate and stable control of vapour partial pressure with the controller than with manual control.

The first commercial anaesthesia delivery system incorporating target controlled vapour delivery was the Physioflex™ (Dräger) introduced in the late 1990s, and followed by the Zeus™ (Dräger) in 2003. More recently existing anaesthetic delivery systems have been enhanced to include automated vapour control. End-tidal control was added to the GE-Aisys in 2010 and more recently a modified Maquet ICU ventilator, the FLOW-i, was released. These devices all allow the user to directly set a target F_A. These machines adjust both the FGF and rate of delivery of vapour to the system to achieve and maintain the desired target. The maintenance, or minimum, FGF can also be set by the user, with the lowest FGF being 0.3 L/min, 0.1 L/min and closed circuit with the Aisys, FLOW-i and Zeus, respectively; all are likely to evolve to (near) closed-circuit conditions in the very near future.

By targeting F_A, automated vapour control systems offer several features in addition to the ability to achieve and maintain the target F_A. These systems minimize FGF and consequently reduce the amount of volatile agent used [47, 48, 49]. With modern inhalational agents, this leads to considerable cost savings and decreases the potential environmental impact of these agents [50, 51]. The control point is moved further down the 'volatile cascade', closer to the end-point of the cascade, the theoretical C_e, which reduces the delay between a change in delivery initiated by the user and a change in effect, improving the ability to match drug delivery and effect.

Unlike systems for IV drugs which rely on models only, end-tidal agent controllers are able to directly measure the end-point being targeted. This allows the system to compensate for physiological changes affecting the uptake and distribution of volatile anaesthetics. For instance, changes in cardiac output (and hence blood flow through the lungs) affect the rate of removal from the gas phase into the blood and thence to the rest of the body. If cardiac output falls, the partial pressure in the lungs rises (and so will that in the blood leaving the lungs). These changes and the adaptation of the controller can be clearly seen and are illustrated in Fig. 6.8 and Fig. 6.9. Zbinden et al [46] were able to demonstrate this interaction using a closed-loop control system in sheep in 1986. Although some argue that true manual control of agent delivery requires a detailed understanding of agent kinetics, we have suggested that observing and understanding how such a controller reacts to these changes can provide much better insights into the underlying process [52].

Most TCI and automated vapour controllers manipulate drug delivery to achieve the new target *as*

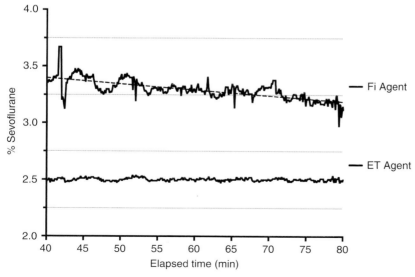

Fig. 6.8 This figure illustrates the decrease in uptake of sevoflurane over a 40-min period as an example of how automated control of anaesthetic agent can illustrate the underlying kinetics. In this sample, an F_A of 2.5% sevoflurane (ET Agent) was set on a GE-Aysis machine. The lower solid line is the measured F_A sevoflurane which remains relatively constant. The inspired sevoflurane partial pressure (Fi Agent, with measured = upper solid line, linear best fit = dashed) decreases from around 3.4% to 3.2%, or approximately 3%/h. (Reproduced with permission from [52]).

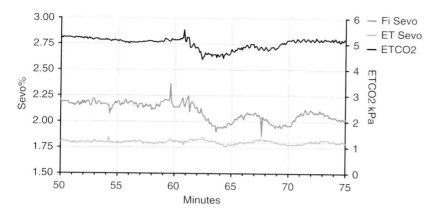

Fig. 6.9 A demonstration of how the response of the end-tidal controller to physiological perturbation can in and by itself illustrate the kinetics of inhalation anaesthetics. During off-pump CABG, the end-tidal target was set at 1.8% on a GE-Aisys machine. The top trace is F_ACO_2 (ETCO$_2$ on right Y-axis), middle and lower traces are inspired and expired sevoflurane partial pressures (left Y-axis), respectively. At 61 min, the surgeon manipulates the heart, resulting in a fall in cardiac output and pulmonary blood flow. As a result, at about 61.5 min, F_ACO_2 starts to fall and $F_A$sevo (ETsevo) rises slightly. This is followed by a large fall in F_I sevo as the controller works to maintain the target F_A sevo. This example again shows the utility of automated control; if F_I sevo had not changed, F_A sevo would have increased by about 0.25% (equivalent to the fall in F_I sevo). Furthermore, the change in F_I sevo illustrates the changes in uptake because uptake is proportional to the inspired – expired gradient and F_A remains nearly constant. (Reproduced with permission from [52]).

quickly as possible within the physical limits of the delivery system and the kinetics of the drug. Although the electronic delivery systems have the potential to achieve any vapour concentration up to saturated vapour pressure, current systems limit the rate of delivery to that achievable with an out of circuit vaporizer with high flows. The Maquet FLOW-i has the ability to set a rate of change that is slower than the maximum, which allows changes in F_A to occur gradually [53]. This may be useful for instance in anticipation of the start of surgery or to allow F_A to gradually fall towards the end of surgery.

These automated systems also allow the user to target the control O_2 partial pressure. For the Zeus and FLOW-i the target is the *inspired* O_2 partial pressure, for Aisys it is the end-expired partial pressure. The FGF rates of O_2 and either air or N_2O are continually adjusted to ensure delivery of adequate amounts of O_2, facilitate changes in vapour partial pressure, and to minimize FGF and thus agent usage, all while ensuring the desired O_2 target partial pressure is maintained.

These systems have been used to provide anaesthesia in millions of patients over the past decade [1]. They have been shown to reduce vapour consumption and more accurately achieve and maintain the chosen target when compared to manual control [54]. The number of actions required by the anaesthetist is significantly reduced [49]. This can be especially advantageous at the start of a complex case since the user is freed from the task of controlling drug delivery [55] and the risk of unintended overshoot is reduced. The versatility of

these systems is demonstrated by a report of an automated targeted vapour control using an adaptive algorithm based on direct injection of liquid isoflurane into a closed circuit used in horses of up to 630 kg [56].

Guided Targeting

Guided targeting is a step back from automated target control (both for IV drug infusion and vapour delivery). In these systems, a computer assembles information on drug delivery and, using the same models used in automated systems, displays current, past and future drug levels. The anaesthesia provider can use this information and adjust the rate of drug delivery to maintain a constant concentration or to have the concentration change over time or to see the effect of various dose regimes over time. Shafer and Egan describe this as 'passive TCI' [41].

Many TCI infusion pumps can be operated in this mode. This approach can be useful during induction with propofol. Stopping or reducing a fixed rate infusion when the patient becomes unarousable minimizes (and optimizes) the dose delivered, gives some idea of the concentration required to reach a certain clinical end-point in the individual patient and potentially reduces side effects. This technique avoids the overshoot commonly seen with bolus induction given manually or after setting a high initial target.

Commercial interaction displays (see below) provide real-time C_p and C_e information for a wide range of drugs, including many hypnotics, synthetic opioids and

91

neuromuscular blocking agents. These systems allow 'manual targeting' of many drugs not included in TCI systems.

Manually targeting a drug towards a clear measure of effect, such as neuromuscular blocking drugs, illustrates many of the principles discussed in the opening section of this chapter. Furthermore, combining the time course of C_e of a drug with a measure of effect allows the drug amount to be titrated in such a manner that the effect (and by definition C_e) is kept constant, or that the effect can be adjusted in a predictable way, for instance by giving a small additional dose of an NMB agent a minute or two before the start of closure of an abdomen.

Manual targeting also demonstrates the time course of the effect of a bolus. In the abdominal closure example, it becomes clear that a dose of neuromuscular blocking agents given when the surgeon complains 1/4 of the way along the muscle closure will be having its maximal effect about the time the wound is closed (Fig. 6.10). In the same way, the relationship between propofol C_e and loss of consciousness becomes explicit by having it displayed and gives an indication of the likely duration of effect of the induction propofol bolus as illustrated in Fig. 6.4 above.

Guided targeting is also possible with inhaled agents. We developed a model-based system which provided the user with forward projections of both end-tidal and effect-site agent partial pressure as shown in Fig. 6.11 (and also Fig. 6.5 above) [57, 58]. A similar display is included in the Dräger Perseus machine.

While manual targeting may require more input from the anaesthesia provider than automated target control delivery, it does make the relationship between dosing and effect explicit to the user and also clearly illustrates the variability in patient response. This approach also offers many of the advantages of TCI in areas where TCI technology is not available [41] and for drugs not included in TCI systems.

Interaction Modelling

Many drug control systems, including early closed-loop feedback systems, use a single effect such as blood pressure as the feedback signal to modulate delivery of a single drug such as isoflurane. Anaesthesia is not this simple.

Anaesthesia involves two main classes of drugs (hypnotics and opioids) and two main effects (lack of recall and lack of response to noxious stimulus) [3]. However, there is considerable synergy between these drug groups, especially for the effect of response to noxious stimulus (immobility and cardiovascular responses in particular). The synergistic effect of opioids on explicit recall on the other hand is much less profound, with moderately high opioid concentrations, of up to 4 ng/mL fentanyl C_e equivalent [59] or moderate morphine doses [60], having no significant effect. The nature of these interactions which we 'empirically' incorporate into anaesthesia practice (i.e. without necessarily fully understanding them) has been studied in detail over the past 20 years and is discussed in detail in Chapter 3.

These principles have been now incorporated into commercial devices [61, 62], the SmartPilot View (Dräger, Lubeck, Germany) and the Navigator (GE Healthcare, Madison, WI, USA) [63]. These devices are illustrated in Fig. 6.12 and Fig. 6.13. Van den Berg et al have recently reviewed the science and theory behind these devices [64].

While the primary function of these systems is to display interactions [65], there are a number of useful 'by-products' of these displays, many of which are

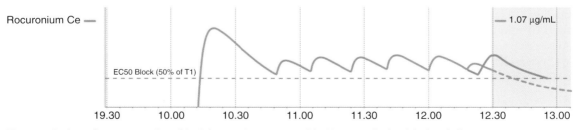

Fig. 6.10 Redrawn from a screen shot of the 'relaxation' component of the Navigator display. Calculated effect-site rocuronium concentration is plotted over time. After an initial 40 mg bolus of rocuronium at 10:45, five incremental 10 mg doses are given when the response to a train-of-four reaches one or two twitches. In any individual, this return occurs at a relatively consistent rocuronium concentration. Towards the end of surgery one can take proactive (blue line) or reactive (green line) approach. In the proactive scenario, at approximately 12:20, a 5 mg bolus of rocuronium is administered in anticipation of abdominal closure. This allows reasonable surgical conditions but does not delay reversal of residual blockade. In the reactive scenario, an additional 10 mg of rocuronium is administered at about 12:25 in response to surgical request. Although closure will be rapidly completed (say by 12:30) it will be 12:40 before 1–2 twitches of the train-of-four return.

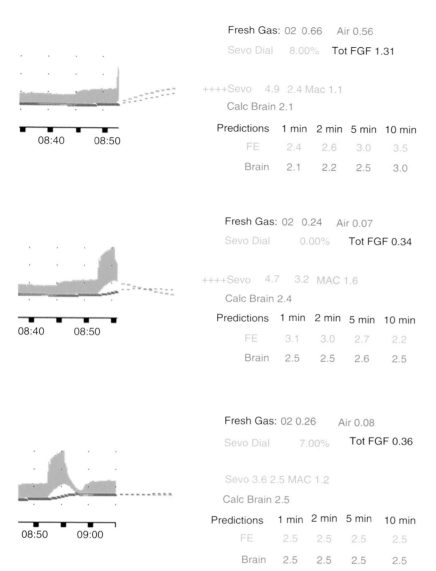

Fresh Gas: 02 0.66   Air 0.56
Sevo Dial   8.00%   Tot FGF 1.31

++++Sevo   4.9 2.4 Mac 1.1
Calc Brain 2.1

Predictions	1 min	2 min	5 min	10 min
FE	2.4	2.6	3.0	3.5
Brain	2.1	2.2	2.5	3.0

08:40   08:50

Fresh Gas: 02 0.24   Air 0.07
Sevo Dial   0.00%   Tot FGF 0.34

++++Sevo   4.7 3.2 MAC 1.6
Calc Brain 2.4

Predictions	1 min	2 min	5 min	10 min
FE	3.1	3.0	2.7	2.2
Brain	2.5	2.5	2.6	2.5

08:40   08:50

Fresh Gas: 02 0.26   Air 0.08
Sevo Dial   7.00%   Tot FGF 0.36

Sevo 3.6 2.5 MAC 1.2
Calc Brain 2.5

Predictions	1 min	2 min	5 min	10 min
FE	2.5	2.5	2.5	2.5
Brain	2.5	2.5	2.5	2.5

08:50   09:00

Fig. 6.11 A sequence from the 'Christchurch Predictor' System [57, 58] which used data from Datex-Ohmeda ADU and AS/3 and S/5 series monitors to display and predict vapour partial pressures. The plot shows the history of inspired and expired inhaled agent partial pressure as a solid block, in this case yellow signifying sevoflurane. The grey line that in Frame A is rising to meet then following F_A sevoflurane is the calculated C_p. The dotted lines at the right of the plot are the 10 min predictions of F_A and C_e for the current FGF and vapour dial settings. On the right of the images are, from the top, current values for fresh gas and vapour dial settings; current measured F_I and F_A sevoflurane; current C_e (shown as 'calc brain'); and the forward predictions of expired ('FE') and effect-site ('brain') partial pressures. In Frame A, shortly after 8:50 h, the vaporizer dial has been set to 8% and the total FGF increased to 1.31 L/min with the objective of increasing C_e sevo from 2.0% to around 2.5vol%. In Frame B, C_e is approaching the target, the vaporizer has been set to '0' and the flow reduced to 340 mL/min. The F_A will drift down to meet C_e. Frame C shows the situation about 5 min later with steady (and matched) sevoflurane F_A and C_e which are predicted to remain constant over the next 10 min. At about 8:57 when the falling F_A met the C_e, the user would gradually increase the vaporizer dial setting, watching the forward predictions and choosing the setting (7%) that gave a constant forward prediction. Modified from a figure originally published in *Anaesthesia and Intensive Care* [58] and reproduced with the kind permission of the Australian Society of Anaesthetists.

relevant to this chapter. These features have recently been discussed in detail [96] and fall into two broad groups: information that results from displaying the past and predicted (future) time course of the C_e of individual drugs and information that can be derived from the interaction display itself. These are elaborated below.

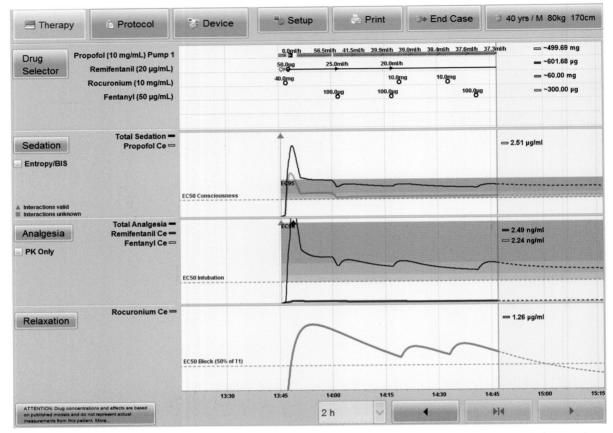

Fig.6.12 The GE Navigator Display. In this simulation, TCI propofol is being administered along with a non-TCI remifentanil infusion and boluses of fentanyl and rocuronium. Drug dosing is shown in the top pane. The middle pane shows C_e for propofol (yellow) while the black line is the combined effect of propofol and the opioids on the likelihood of response to command. The third pane shows the combined effect on response to noxious stimulus (intubation) while the lowest pane displays calculated C_e for neuromuscular blocking drugs, in this case rocuronium. The response probabilities, or isoboles, are represented by the shaded grey bands, with the lower border representing 50% and the upper border 95% probability of no response. Individual drug levels are presented as effect-site concentrations. C_e at the present time are shown in the yellow area to the right of each band. The dotted lines in the yellow zone are forward predictions. In this example, the propofol alone is having an effect on lack of response command at just above the 50% isobole. However, the opioid concentrations alone will have minimal effect on the response to noxious stimulation. We also see that the fentanyl boluses have a greater effect on response to noxious stimulation than on response to command.

Advantages of Displaying the Kinetics of Individual Drugs

The display of individual drug concentrations helps move from thinking about drug doses to drug concentrations and makes the use of effect-site concentrations the norm. While it is rare to talk about the total amount of vapour or of remifentanil used (except for financial reasons), we still commonly discuss total fentanyl dose, irrespective of the duration of the case. Once we think in terms of effect sites and concentrations and have a predictive display, moving between bolus and infusion dosing becomes straightforward.

Guided targeting, or manual target control (as discussed in the previous section), becomes possible (and easy) for a wide range of hypnotics, opioids and neuromuscular blocking agents once the history and predictions of drug concentrations are displayed. The ability to see forward predictions of a drug concentration from a delivery system being automatically logged can help detect errors such as failing to restart a pump after changing a syringe or altering a setting.

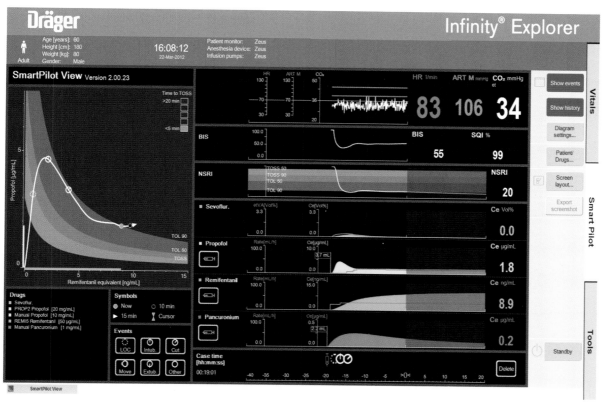

Fig. 6.13 Drager SmartPilot View. The two dimensional plot on the left illustrates the interaction between opioids (in this case remifentanil) and hypnotics (sevoflurane and propofol). The white line shows the patient's 'progress' across the diagram over time and projected into the future. Individual drug effect-site concentrations are shown on the right along with the NSRI, an index of responsiveness to noxious stimulus. Forward predictions of drug concentrations and NSRI are plotted in the shaded area. (Image copyright Dräger, Lubeck, Germany reproduced with permission.)

With the display of drug concentrations, switching between drugs of the same class becomes straightforward. For example, it is possible to move between different opioids while keeping an equivalent effect as long as the relative potencies are known. The differences in kinetics, including context sensitive half-times, are displayed by the models and allow suitable adjustment of doses to maintain a given combined effect appropriate for the degree of surgical stimulation and anticipating postoperative analgesic requirements.

Using Interaction Displays

Thus far we have discussed exploring the relationship between drug dosing, C_e and measured effect for a single drug and a specific effect. However, the interaction display component of Navigator and SmartPilot View also demonstrate the combined effect (predominantly synergy) between opioids and hypnotics, for two different clinical end-points: response to command (as an indicator of the likelihood of recall) and response to intubation (indicating response to noxious stimulus). This allows more sophisticated titration of drug delivery to effect than just considering a single drug.

Both systems describe the likelihood of response as population-based probabilities. This can be confusing when first meeting these devices because there is no way of predicting in advance where an individual sits within the population distribution. Conceptually, targeting a given response (non-)probability is no different from targeting a drug level such as a MAC-fraction, except that it is making the uncertainty and variability in patient response explicit by displaying it as such.

The effects 'response to command' and 'response to intubation' are much closer to the actual end-points of anaesthesia than considering drug–effect pairs in isolation. Similarly, the inclusion of interaction effects simplifies titration to the desired effect in an individual. For example, while 1.3MAC of a volatile agent alone will block the response to a specified noxious stimulus in 95% of patients, addition of 100 µg of fentanyl will, for a brief period, allow the same effect to be achieved with half the volatile partial pressure [59]. This synergistic effect is clearly illustrated by interaction displays, as is the waning influence of a fentanyl bolus over time.

A question commonly asked by new users of TCI systems is: 'What number should I aim for?' Writing about propofol and TCI infusion systems, Coppens et al [66] stated:

> The major strength of effect-site controlled TCI lies not in predicting the resulting hypnotic effect in the individual patient but rather in its ability to maintain the pharmacological condition once a predetermined clinical effect has been reached

In other words, rather than targeting a predetermined propofol concentration, which is similar to a recipe-based 1.3 MAC vaporizer setting, **the user first has to determine the propofol concentration that meets the needs of the individual patient**, and then the TCI system will maintain that patient's level in the face of the complexity of the pharmacokinetics of the drug. In contrast, a constant infusion state will lead to a gradual increase in propofol levels.

This same approach can be applied with interaction displays when the new user asks: 'What number [on the isoboles] should I aim for?' The user should first establish the requirements of the individual patient, and then the advisory drug display will advise the user how drugs can be delivered at the appropriate rate to maintain that 'state'. Hence the name 'advisory display system'.

These concepts do not, however, directly answer the new user's question. We are accustomed to thinking about individual drug levels and, although $1 \times$ MAC actually represents a population probability, we generally think of MAC values as a surrogate for volatile anaesthetic partial pressures. Thinking about where an individual patient, or opioid–hypnotic drug combination, is located within a population distribution is not a familiar approach for many users.

Most anaesthetists appreciate that responses are binary, i.e. a patient either responds or doesn't respond, or putting it yet another way: a patient on the 80%

isobole is not 20% awake. Similarly, being on the 80% isobole does not mean there is a 20% likelihood this patient will respond; the 80% isobole represents the combination of drugs at which 80% of patients will not respond, or conversely one in five patients will respond, it does not tell us anything about the response of an individual patient.

The width of the bands of isoboles on the displays of SmartPilot View and Navigator (see Fig. 6.12 and Fig. 6.13) gives some indication of the variability between patients. Consider two patients undergoing similar surgical stress, one is satisfactorily anaesthetized on the 33% isobole while the other requires to be on the 80% isobole. Administering drug doses to both patients to achieve the 80% (or 90%) isobole represents a dramatic overdose for the first patient which may result in cardiovascular depression and a delayed recovery. Placing both patients on the 50% isobole will still overdose the first patient but will now be insufficient for the second. These are not abstract concepts: one in three patients will require no more than the patient on the 33% isobole while one in five will need more than the 80% patient. Determining the anaesthetic requirements of each individual patient is the underlying concept of this book. As outlined above, the value of interaction displays lies in making it easier to determine individual requirements and then to maintain that level.

Used in this way, interaction displays can improve drug titration, supported by the finding that use of these systems is associated with decreased vapour use [67]. Interaction displays also facilitate the use of a wide range of drug combinations to achieve the same effect. For instance, by altering the hypnotic/opioid mix, the same level of unresponsiveness can be achieved across a wide range of responses to noxious stimulus. Whilst the need for lack of recall is consistent across many types of surgery, the need for antinociception varies greatly between cases. This ability to see the effect of different combinations gives the anaesthetist improved flexibility in choosing the appropriate recipe for the individual patient and procedure. The increased understanding of drug interactions that these devices give the clinician may help us understand some of the drug choices fully automated systems may make.

Some of the functionality and underlying principles of these displays is incorporated into a number of standalone 'apps' such as FentaSim[4] and AnestAssisit.[5] These apps can provide useful information, such as the

---

4. pkpdtools.com/iphone/fentasim/ [last accessed 9 June 2019].
5. palmahealthcare.com [last accessed 9 June 2019].

C_e-time profile of fentanyl after a series of boluses and at least one includes interaction probabilities. However, the user needs to enter all data and drug doses. A particular advantage of SmartPilot View and Navigator is that they are integrated into the anaesthesia workstation so that vapour and infusion dosing is continuously imported and updated in real time.

Short et al [68] have developed a system which incorporates interaction models into a multi-drug TCI system in which the user sets a BIS value as the target BIS. This work opens the way for a whole new class of models and control systems utilizing models derived from clinical end-points rather than modelled drug levels or measures of effect that are not familiar to the clinical anaesthetist. As examples of unfamiliar end-points, spectral edge frequency was the effect-site measure used to develop the Minto remifentanil model [17].

Feedback Control

Much of the discussion thus far in this chapter has considered a model of feedback control where the anaesthesia provider is very much part of the control loop. With the various approaches considered above, the anaesthesia provider can fill several roles within the control loop. For instance, when manually targeting a drug level, the user has the supervisor role (determining the desired level) and also performs the sensor (what is the current level?) and actuator (setting the pump rate) functions. Even with modern TCI or end-tidal targeting systems, the user is still setting the desired end-point.

In this final section, we briefly explore fully automated delivery of some or all of the components of anaesthesia. This is a rapidly developing area. We can consider this control at three levels of complexity:

a) control of delivery of a **single drug level** at a specified (measured) level such as occurs with automated end-tidal control where the system targets a predetermined end-tidal vapour concentration. This has been discussed above;

b) control of delivery of a **single** drug guided by some measure of the **effect** of the drug. This can be extended to multiple systems each controlling a single drug;

c) integrated control of **multiple effects**.

Feedback control of anaesthesia is thought of as a relatively recent development facilitated by the development and availability of digital microprocessors [69]. However in 1950 Bickford developed a system which administered small increments of ether or thiopentone at a rate determined by an integrator of the power of the EEG [70]. This system was used to keep animals anaesthetized for several days, and was also used in at least 50 patients undergoing surgery. This system was able to adapt to changes in surgical stimulus.

In anaesthesia, neuromuscular blockade is the prototypical example of using a specific measure of effect to control delivery of a drug. Neuromuscular blocking drugs have the advantage of a distinct, easily quantifiable effect and formed the basis of early work on the concept of the effect site [71, 72]. An automated feedback system controlling delivery of a number of neuromuscular blocking drugs was described by Cass in 1976 [73, 74]. At around the same time systems to control blood pressure using vasoactive drugs were described [75, 76]. These systems were found to be at least as accurate as expert human control, echoing an earlier assertion that these systems would free up the time taken by these tasks allowing better patient care [77].

In 1987 Schwilden et al [78] used the median frequency of the EEG as the sensor for closed-loop control of methohexitone delivery and then adapted this for propofol [79]. BIS was used as the signal by Mortier et al [80] while Kenny used auditory evoked potentials (AEP) as the signal for controlling propofol delivery in the presence of alfentanil at a target plasma concentration of 15 ng/mL [81]. Morley et al used BIS to control either isoflurane in N_2O or a mixture of propofol and alfentanil [82]. This principle of a relatively fixed analgesic component while a controller varied the hypnotic component based on BIS was explored further by Struys et al using remifentanil at 0.25 µg/kg/min (equivalent to an effect-site contraction of 6 ng/mL) [83, 84]. Locher et al demonstrated that a closed-loop system maintained BIS more accurately than manual control with both propofol- and isoflurane-based anaesthesia [85].

Recognizing the need to specifically target the response to noxious stimulus, Luginbuhl et al used alfentanil to control blood pressure [86] using a dual-input single-output controller to maintain a given MAP while minimizing alfentanil. Other groups have used changes in BIS (and other similar measures such as spectral entropy and WaveSense™ [87]) to drive separate control loops for propofol and remifentanil [55, 88, 89]. These systems have been used in a large number of patients in a wide variety of procedures including cardiac bypass surgery and to guide sedation.

Several approaches to quantifying the balance between noxious stimulus and analgesia balance during anaesthesia have been described and several are available as commercial products. Hemmerling et al have used the Analgoscore, derived from blood pressure and pulse rate, as a specific input to their triple-loop anaesthesia 'robot' [90, 91].

In their recent meta-analysis, Pasin et al [92] concluded that BIS guided closed-loop propofol delivery compared to manual BIS guided delivery reduced the induction dose, maintained better control of BIS and reduced recovery time. Interestingly, there was little improvement when moving from TCI to closed-loop systems. What is missing from this review is workload as an end-point. It is well established that a trained, attentive operator can match the performance of a closed-loop controller. Moving to TCI (or perhaps even a model-based advisory system) gives the human controller the same tool set as the automated controller. Data with both intravenous [55] and vapour [48, 49] delivery clearly show a reduction in workload with automated systems.

Brogi et al showed that for systems with a wide range of targets (including depth of anaesthesia, insulin administration and ventilation) automated systems consistently provided more accurate control with less over- or undershoot of the consent variable [2].

Again, this is a rapidly expanding area. Fully automated anaesthetic drug delivery is being reported for increasingly complex surgical procedures such as adult [93] and paediatric [94] cardiac surgery and sedation for TAVI [95]. Despite the complexity of the patients and the rapidly changing anaesthetic demands in these settings, the automated systems require minimal intervention. Where these approaches lead in clinical practice remains to be seen.

A Summary and Some Thoughts on the Near Future

While anaesthetic drug delivery can be controlled in a variety of ways, and although we may not recognize them as such, all delivery methods use or actually 'are' some type of feedback control. An increasing number of systems are available to help optimize drug delivery and titrate the anaesthetic state to individual patient needs.

Patients differ in their requirements and responses to anaesthetic drugs and to surgical insults. We are increasingly able to quantify these responses and adjust

therapy to match the changing needs **of the individual**. It is no longer sufficient to administer drugs based only on targets defined on a population basis and give everyone 1.3MAC of inhalation anaesthetic.

Currently available commercial systems allow automated or guided delivery, targeting concentrations at the effect site, and give the user much better control over the actual levels of individual drugs, regardless of the complexity of the drug kinetics. Many drugs used in anaesthesia are not given as a single bolus, and because steady state is seldom reached during an anaesthetic, the change in C_e will follow a different time course after every dose.

A number of studies suggest drug levels are better controlled with both advisory displays and automated systems when compared to manual control and this improved control requires less intervention by the user [55] and less vapour [48, 49]. Systems under development with improved monitors and sensors will automate the anaesthesia drug delivery further. Interestingly, as sensors and algorithms become more sophisticated, drug kinetics models may lose importance as systems learn to match drug delivery and effects in the same way that early neuromuscular blocking agents and isoflurane control systems were model independent [45, 73].

There is a considerable amount of work being done on developing better measures of the response to noxious stimulus, but no commercial device has yet reached widespread clinical acceptance. Models to describe individual drug kinetics and dynamics and of interactions are also being further developed. Innovative approaches to modelling interactions are emerging, such as the recent work of Short et al [68] which has the potential to completely change the 'targets' of many anaesthesia systems from drug levels to measured patient variables.

Newer systems will allow more precise titration of drugs towards a range of clinical end-points and will match changes in patient requirements with less direct user input. This will allow the anaesthesia provider to take on the role of really supervising the case rather than having to concentrate on the technical aspects of manipulating the delivery rate of individual drugs [1]. Loeb and Cannesson [96] suggest that '... there will be a continued need for anaesthesia professionals ... but it (increasing automation) will change their role.' Although some might see these changes as a threat, it is part of the natural development of anaesthesia that goes hand-in-hand with rapid and ever expanding technological innovations. It will allow us to safely anaesthetize increasingly complex patients for new procedures while continuing to improve our safety record. They will become an essential element of and help define what constitutes 'Personalized Anaesthesia'.

A recent article on the rapid evolution of medical technology summed up what I believe should be our approach to tools that help optimize drug dosing:

> Don't use the force, Luke, use the targeting computer.[6]

References

1. Kuck K, Johnson KB: The three laws of autonomous and closed-loop systems in anesthesia. Anesth.Analg. 2017; 124 (2): 377–80.

2. Brogi E, Cyr S, Kazan R, Giunta F, Hemmerling TM: Clinical performance and safety of closed-loop systems: a systematic review and meta-analysis of randomized controlled trials. Anesth.Analg. 2016; 124 (2): 446–55.

3. Glass PS: Anesthetic drug interactions: an insight into general anesthesia – its mechanism and dosing strategies. Anesthesiology. 1998; 88 (1): 5–6.

4. Rampil IJ, King BS: Volatile anesthetics depress spinal motor neurons. Anesthesiology. 1996; 85 (1): 129–34.

5. Sonner JM, Antognini JF, Dutton RC, Flood P, Gray AT, Harris RA, et al: Inhaled anesthetics and immobility: mechanisms, mysteries, and minimum alveolar anesthetic concentration. Anesth.Analg. 2003; 97 (3): 718–40.

6. Vuyk J, Engbers FH, Burm AGL, Vletter AA, Griever GE, Olofsen E, et al: Pharmacodynamic interaction between propofol and alfentanil when given for induction of anesthesia. Anesthesiology. 1996; 84 (2): 288–99.

7. Hendrickx JFA, Eger EI, Sonner JM, Shafer SL: Is synergy the rule? A review of anesthetic interactions producing hypnosis and immobility. Anesth.Analg. 2008; 107 (2): 494–506.

8. Krüger-Thiemer E: Continuous intravenous infusion and multicompartment accumulation. Eur.J.Pharmacol. 1968; 4 (3): 317–24.

9. Hughes MA, Glass PS, Jacobs JR: Context-sensitive half-time in multicompartment pharmacokinetic models for intravenous anesthetic drugs. Anesthesiology. 1992; 76 (3): 334–41.

10. Bailey JM: Context-sensitive half-times and other decrement times of inhaled anesthetics. Anesth.Analg. 1997; 85 (3): 681–6.

11. Youngs EJ, Shafer SL: Pharmacokinetic parameters relevant to recovery from opioids. Anesthesiology. 1994; 81 (4): 833–42.

12. Eger EI, Shafer SL: Tutorial: context-sensitive decrement times for inhaled anesthetics. Anesth. Analg. 2005; 101 (3): 688–96.

13. Frei FJ, Zbinden AM, Thomson DA, Rieder HU: Is the end-tidal partial pressure of isoflurane a good predictor of its arterial partial pressure? Br.J.Anaesth. 1991; 66 (3): 331–9.

14. Kennedy RR, Minto C, Seethepalli A: Effect-site half-time for burst suppression is longer than for hypnosis during anaesthesia with sevoflurane. Br.J.Anaesth. 2008; 100 (1): 72–7.

15. Lerou JGC, Mourisse J: Applying a physiological model to quantify the delay between changes in end-expired concentrations of sevoflurane and bispectral index. Br.J.Anaesth. 2007; 99 (2): 226–36.

16. Absalom AR, Mani V, De Smet T, Struys MM: Pharmacokinetic models for propofol – defining and illuminating the devil in the detail. Br.J.Anaesth. 2009; 103 (1): 26–37.

17. Schnider TW, Minto CF, Gambus PL, Andresen C, Goodale DB, Shafer SL, et al: The influence of method of administration and covariates on the pharmacokinetics of propofol in adult volunteers. Anesthesiology. 1998; 88 (5): 1170–82.

18. Quasha AL, Eger EI, Tinker JH: Determination and applications of MAC. Anesthesiology. 1980; 53 (4): 315–34.

19. Gaumann DM, Mustaki JP, Tassonyi E: MAC-awake of isoflurane, enflurane and halothane evaluated by slow and fast alveolar washout. Br.J.Anaesth. 1992; 68 (1): 81–4.

20. Kimura T, Watanabe S, Asakura N, Inomata S, Okada M, Taguchi M: Determination of end-tidal sevoflurane concentration for tracheal intubation and minimum alveolar anesthetic concentration in adults. Anesth. Analg. 1994; 79 (2): 378–81.

21. Kennedy RR: Effect-site estimation of volatile anaesthetic agents: Beyond MAC fractions as a target for anaesthesia delivery. Trends in Anaesthesia and Critical Care 2013; 3 (4): 211–15.

22. Roberts FL, Dixon J, Lewis GT, Tackley RM, Prys-Roberts C: Induction and maintenance of propofol anaesthesia. A manual infusion scheme. Anaesthesia. 1988; 43 Suppl: 14–17.

23. Cowles AL, Borgstedt HH, Gillies AJ: Digital computer prediction of the optimal anaesthetic inspired concentration. Br.J.Anaesth. 1972; 44: 420–5.

24. Mapleson WW: The theoretical ideal fresh-gas flow sequence at the start of low-flow anaesthesia. Anaesthesia. 1998; 53 (3): 264–72.

---

6. https://www.theatlantic.com/technology/archive/2017/04/force-computer-vision/522720/?utm_source=atltw [last accessed 9 June 2019].

25. Lowe HJ, Ernst EA: *The Qualitative Practice of Anaesthesia: Use of Closed Circuit*. Baltimore/London: Williams & Wilkins, 1981.

26. da Silva JM, Mapleson WW, Vickers MD: Quantitative study of Lowe's square-root-of-time method of closed-system anaesthesia. Br.J.Anaesth. 1997; 79 (1): 103–12.

27. Bangaari A, Panda NB, Puri GD: A simple method for evaluation of the uptake of isoflurane and its comparison with the square root of time model. Indian.J.Anaesth. 2013; 57 (3): 230–5.

28. Hendrickx JF, Vandeput DM, De Geyndt AM, De Ridder KP, Haenen JS, Deloof T, et al: Maintaining sevoflurane anesthesia during low-flow anesthesia using a single vaporizer setting change after overpressure induction. J.Clin.Anesth. 2000; 12 (4): 303–7.

29. Hendrickx JFA, Dewulf BBC, De Mey N, Carette R, Deloof T, De Cooman S, et al: Development and performance of a two-step desflurane-O(2)/N(2)O fresh gas flow sequence. J.Clin.Anesth. 2008; 20 (7): 501–7.

30. Van Zundert T, Brebels A, Hendrickx J, Carette R, De Cooman S, Gatt S, et al: Derivation and prospective testing of a two-step sevoflurane-O_2-N_2O low fresh gas flow sequence. Anaesth.Intens.Care. 2009; 37 (6): 911–17.

31. Albert V, Mndolo S, Harrison EM, O'Sullivan E, Wilson IH, Walker IA: Lifebox pulse oximeter implementation in Malawi: evaluation of educational outcomes and impact on oxygen desaturation episodes during anaesthesia. Anaesthesia. 2017; 72 (6): 686–93.

32. Sykes MK: Continuous monitoring of alveolar and inspiratory concentrations of anesthetic and respiratory gases is difficult and potentially unsafe. J. Clin.Monit. 1987; 3 (2): 116–22.

33. Fahy BG, Chau DF: The technology of processed electroencephalogram monitoring devices for assessment of depth of anesthesia. Anesth.Analg. 2017 3. doi:10.1213/ANE.0000000000002331. [Epub ahead of print]

34. Absalom AR, De Keyser R, Struys MMRF: Closed loop anesthesia: are we getting close to finding the holy grail? Anesth.Analg. 2011; 112 (3): 516–18.

35. Upton HD, Ludbrook GL, Wing A, Sleigh JW: Intraoperative analgesia nociception index guided fentanyl administration during sevoflurane anesthesia in lumbar discectomy and laminectomy. Anesth.Analg. 2017; 125 (1): 81–90.

36. Hannivoort LN, Vereecke HEM, Proost JH, Heyse BEK, Eleveld DJ, Bouillon TW, et al: Probability to tolerate laryngoscopy and noxious stimulation response index as general indicators of the anaesthetic potency of sevoflurane, propofol, and remifentanil. Br.J.Anaesth. 2016; 116 (5): 624–31.

37. Struys MMRF, De Smet T, Glen JIB, Vereecke HEM, Absalom AR, Schnider TW: The history of target-controlled infusion. Anesth.Analg. 2016; 122 (1): 56–69.

38. Glen JB: The development of "Diprifusor": a TCI system for propofol. Anaesthesia. 1998; 53 Suppl 1: 13–21.

39. Absalom AR, Glen JIB, Zwart GJC, Schnider TW, Struys MMRF: Target-controlled infusion. Anesth. Analg. 2016; 122 (1): 70–8.

40. Varvel J, Donoho D, Shafer S: Measuring the predictive performance of computer-controlled infusion pumps. J.Pharmacokinet.Biopharm. 1992; 20 (1): 63–94.

41. Shafer SL, Egan T: Target-controlled infusions. Anesth. Analg. 2016; 122 (1): 1–3.

42. Schnider TW, Minto CF, Struys MMRF, Absalom AR: The safety of target-controlled infusions. Anesth. Analg. 2016; 122 (1): 79–85.

43. Ross JA, Wloch RT, White DC, Hawes DW: Servo-controlled closed-circuit anaesthesia. A method for the automatic control of anaesthesia produced by a volatile agent in oxygen. Br.J.Anaesth. 1983; 55 (11): 1053–60.

44. O'Callaghan AC, Hawes DW, Ross JA, White DC, Wloch RT: Uptake of isoflurane during clinical anaesthesia. Servo-control of liquid anaesthetic injection into a closed-circuit breathing system. Br.J.Anaesth. 1983; 55 (11): 1061–4.

45. Westenskow DR, Zbinden AM, Thomson DA, Kohler B: Control of end-tidal halothane concentration. Part A: anaesthesia breathing system and feedback control of gas delivery. Br.J.Anaesth. 1986; 58 (5): 555–62.

46. Zbinden AM, Frei F, Westenskow DR, Thomson DA: Control of end-tidal halothane concentration. Part B: verification in dogs. Br.J.Anaesth. 1986; 58 (5): 563–71.

47. Lortat-Jacob B, Billard V, Buschke W, Servin F: Assessing the clinical or pharmaco-economical benefit of target controlled desflurane delivery in surgical patients using the Zeus® anaesthesia machine. Anaesthesia. 2009; 64 (11): 1229–35.

48. Tay S, Weinberg L, Peyton P, Story D, Briedis J: Financial and environmental costs of manual versus automated control of end-tidal gas concentrations. Anaesth.Intens.Care. 2013; 41 (1): 95–101.

49. Lucangelo U, Garufi G, Marras E, Ferluga M, Turchet F, Bernabè F, et al: End-tidal versus manually-controlled low-flow anaesthesia. J.Clin.Monit.Comput. 2014; 28 (2): 117–21.

50. Ryan SM, Nielsen CJ: Global warming potential of inhaled anesthetics: application to clinical use. Anesth. Analg. 2010; 111 (1): 92–8.

51. Sulbaek Andersen MP, Sander SP, Nielsen OJ, Wagner DS, Sanford TJ, Wallington TJ: Inhalation anaesthetics and climate change. Br.J.Anaesth. 2010; 105 (6): 760–6.

52. Kennedy RR: New technology in anaesthesia: friend or foe? J.Clin.Monit.Comput. 2014; 28 (2): 113–16.

53. Carette R, De Wolf AM, Hendrickx JFA: Automated gas control with the Maquet FLOW-i. J.Clin.Monit. Comput. 2016; 30 (3): 341–6.

54. Sieber TJ, Frei CW, Derighetti M, Feigenwinter P, Leibundgut D, Zbinden AM: Model-based automatic feedback control versus human control of end-tidal isoflurane concentration using low-flow anaesthesia. Br.J.Anaesth. 2000; 85 (6): 818–25.

55. Dussaussoy C, Peres M, Jaoul V, Liu N, Chazot T, Picquet J, et al: Automated titration of propofol and remifentanil decreases the anesthesiologist's workload during vascular or thoracic surgery: a randomized prospective study. J.Clin.Monit.Comput. 2014; 28 (1): 35–40.

56. Franci P, Bertamini A, Bertamini O, Pilla T, Busetto R: Clinical evaluation of an end-tidal target-controlled infusion closed-loop system for isoflurane administration in horses undergoing surgical procedures. Vet.J. 2012; 192 (2): 206–11.

57. Kennedy RR, McKellow MA, French RA: The effect of predictive display on the control of step changes in effect site sevoflurane levels. Anaesthesia. 2010; 65 (8): 826–30.

58. Kennedy RR, French RA: The development of a system to guide volatile anaesthetic administration. Anaesth. Intens.Care. 2011; 39 (2): 182–90.

59. Katoh T, Uchiyama T, Ikeda K: Effect of fentanyl on awakening concentration of sevoflurane. Br.J.Anaesth. 1994; 73 (3): 322–5.

60. Katoh T, Suguro Y, Kimura T, Ikeda K: Morphine does not affect the awakening concentration of sevoflurane. Can.J.Anaesth. 1993; 40 (9): 825–8.

61. Gin T: Clinical pharmacology on display. Anesth. Analg. 2010; 111 (2): 256–8.

62. Struys MMRF, Sahinovic M, Lichtenbelt BJ, Vereecke HEM, Absalom AR: Optimizing intravenous drug administration by applying pharmacokinetic/pharmacodynamic concepts. Br.J.Anaesth. 2011; 107 (1): 38–47.

63. Kennedy RR: Seeing the future of anesthesia drug dosing: moving the art of anesthesia from impressionism to realism. Anesth.Analg. 2010; 111 (2): 252–5.

64. van den Berg JP, Vereecke HEM, Proost JH, Eleveld DJ, Wietasch JKG, Absalom AR, et al: Pharmacokinetic and pharmacodynamic interactions in anaesthesia. A review of current knowledge and how it can be used to optimize anaesthetic drug administration. Br.J.Anaesth. 2017; 118 (1): 44–57.

65. DeCou J, Johnson K: An introduction to predictive modelling of drug concentration in anaesthesia monitors. Anaesthesia. 2017; 2;72: 58–69.

66. Coppens M, Van Limmen JGM, Schnider T, Wyler B, Bonte S, Dewaele F, et al: Study of the time course of the clinical effect of propofol compared with the time course of the predicted effect-site concentration: Performance of three pharmacokinetic-dynamic models. Br.J.Anaesth. 2010; 104 (4): 452–8.

67. Cirillo V, Zito Marinosci G, De Robertis E, Iacono C, Romano GM, Desantis O, et al: Navigator® and SmartPilot® View are helpful in guiding anesthesia and reducing anesthetic drug dosing. Minerva.Anestesiol. 2015 19; 81 (11): 1163–9.

68. Short TG, Hannam JA, Laurent S, Campbell D, Misur M, Merry AF, et al: Refining target-controlled infusion. Anesth.Analg. 2016; 122 (1): 90–7.

69. O'Hara DA, Bogen DK, Noordergraaf A: The use of computers for controlling the delivery of anesthesia. Anesthesiology. 1992; 77 (3): 563–81.

70. Mayo CW, Bickford RG, Faulconer A: Electroencephalographically controlled anesthesia in abdominal surgery. J.Am.Med.Assoc. 1950 25; 144 (13): 1081–3.

71. Hull CJ, Van Beem HB, McLeod K, Sibbald A, Watson MJ: A pharmacodynamic model for pancuronium. Br.J.Anaesth. 1978; 50 (11): 1113–23.

72. Stanski DR, Ham J, Miller RD, Sheiner LB: Pharmacokinetics and pharmacodynamics of d-tubocurarine during nitrous oxide-narcotic and halothane anesthesia in man. Anesthesiology. 1979; 51 (3): 235–41.

73. Cass NM, Lampard DG, Brown WA, Coles JR: Computer controlled muscle relaxation: a comparison of four muscle relaxants in the sheep. Anaesth.Intens. Care. 1976; 4 (1): 16–22.

74. Lampard DG, Brown WA, Cass NM, Ng KC: Computer-controlled muscle paralysis with atracurium in the sheep. Anaesth.Intens.Care. 1986 Feb; 14 (1): 7–11.

75. Murchie CJ, Kenny GN: Comparison among manual, computer-assisted, and closed-loop control of blood pressure after cardiac surgery. J.Cardiothorac.Anesth. 1989; 3 (1): 16–19.

76. Monk CR, Millard RK, Hutton P, Prys-Roberts C: Automatic arterial pressure regulation using isoflurane: comparison with manual control. Br.J.Anaesth. 1989; 63 (1): 22–30.

77. Mitchell RR: The need for closed-loop therapy. Crit. Care.Med. 1982; 10 (12): 831–4.

78. Schwilden H, Schuttler J, Stoeckel H: Closed-loop feedback control of methohexital anesthesia by quantitative EEG analysis in humans. Anesthesiology. 1987; 67 (3): 341–7.

79. Schwilden H, Stoeckel H, Schuttler J. Closed-loop feedback control of propofol anaesthesia by

quantitative EEG analysis in humans. Br.J.Anaesth. 1989; 62 (3): 290–6.

80. Mortier E, Struys M, De Smet T, Versichelen L, Rolly G: Closed-loop controlled administration of propofol using bispectral analysis. Anaesthesia. 1998; 53 (8): 749–54.

81. Kenny GN, Mantzaridis H: Closed-loop control of propofol anaesthesia. Br.J.Anaesth. 1999; 83 (2): 223–8.

82. Morley A, Derrick J, Mainland P, Lee BB, Short TG: Closed loop control of anaesthesia: an assessment of the bispectral index as the target of control. Anaesthesia. 2000; 55 (10): 953–9.

83. Struys MM, De Smet T, Versichelen LF, Van De Velde S, Van den Broecke R, Mortier EP: Comparison of closed-loop controlled administration of propofol using bispectral index as the controlled variable versus "standard practice" controlled administration. Anesthesiology. 2001; 95 (1): 6–17.

84. Struys MMRF, De Smet T, Greenwald S, Absalom AR, Bingé S, Mortier EP: Performance evaluation of two published closed-loop control systems using bispectral index monitoring: a simulation study. Anesthesiology. 2004; 100 (3): 640–7.

85. Locher S, Stadler KS, Boehlen T, Bouillon T, Leibundgut D, Schumacher PM, et al: A new closed-loop control system for isoflurane using bispectral index outperforms manual control. Anesthesiology. 2004; 101 (3): 591–602.

86. Luginbühl M, Bieniok C, Leibundgut D, Wymann R, Gentilini A, Schnider TW: Closed-loop control of mean arterial blood pressure during surgery with alfentanil: clinical evaluation of a novel model-based predictive controller. Anesthesiology. 2006; 105 (3): 462–70.

87. West N, Dumont GA, van Heusden K, Petersen CL, Khosravi S, Soltesz K, et al: Robust closed-loop control of induction and maintenance of propofol anaesthesia in children. Paediatr.Anaesth. 2013; 23 (8): 712–19.

88. Liu N, Chazot T, Hamada S, Landais A, Boichut N, Dussaussoy C, et al: Closed-loop coadministration of propofol and remifentanil guided by bispectral index: a randomized multicenter study. Anesth.Analg. 2011; 112 (3): 546–57.

89. Puri GD, Mathew PJ, Biswas I, Dutta A, Sood J, Gombar S, et al: A multicenter evaluation of a closed-loop anesthesia delivery system: a randomized controlled trial. Anesth.Analg. 2016; 122 (1): 106–14.

90. Hemmerling TM, Arbeid E, Wehbe M, Cyr S, Taddei R, Zaouter C: Evaluation of a novel closed-loop total intravenous anaesthesia drug delivery system: a randomized controlled trial. BJA. 2013; 110 (6): 1031–9.

91. Wehbe M, Arbeid E, Cyr S, Mathieu PA, Taddei R, Morse J, et al: A technical description of a novel pharmacological anesthesia robot. J.Clin.Monit. Comput. 2014; 28 (1): 27–34.

92. Pasin L, Nardelli P, Pintaudi M, Greco M, Zambon M, Cabrini L, et al: Closed-loop delivery systems versus manually controlled administration of total IV anesthesia. Anesth.Analg. 2017; 124 (2): 456–64.

93. Zaouter C, Hemmerling TM, Lanchon R, Valoti E, Remy A, Leuillet S, et al: The feasibility of a completely automated total IV anesthesia drug delivery system for cardiac surgery. Anesth.Analg. 2016; 123 (4): 885–93.

94. Biswas I, Mathew PJ, Singh RS, Puri GD: Evaluation of closed-loop anesthesia delivery for propofol anesthesia in pediatric cardiac surgery. Paediatr.Anaesth. 2013; 23 (12): 1145–52.

95. Zaouter C, Hemmerling TM, Mion S, Leroux L, Remy A, Ouattara A: Feasibility of automated propofol sedation for transcatheter aortic valve implantation: a pilot study. Anesth.Analg. 2017 Nov; 125 (5): 1505–12

96. Kennedy RR: Lessons from drug interaction displays. In Absalom AR & Mason KP (eds), *Total Intravenous Anesthesia and Target Controlled Infusions*. Springer 2017.

Chapter

7

Hypnotic Effect: Inducing Unconsciousness and Emergence from Anaesthesia

Sergio Vide, Catarina Nunes and Pedro Amorim

The Hypnotic Effect

General anaesthesia (GA) is a reversible drug-induced state of altered arousal required for more than 60,000 surgical procedures each day in the USA alone, making it one of the most common manipulations of the brain and central nervous system [1]. It comprises several specific behavioural and physiological end-points – unconsciousness, amnesia, analgesia and akinesia – with concomitant stability of the autonomic, cardiovascular, respiratory and thermoregulatory systems [2, 3].

Many years after the first demonstration of anaesthesia in 1846 by William T. Morton in the 'Ether Dome' of the Massachusetts General Hospital in Boston, the mechanisms by which general anaesthetics render an individual unconscious remain incompletely understood [4].

For many decades, only one 'general' anaesthetic drug with a low therapeutic index [5] was used to induce immobility, analgesia, amnesia and unconsciousness. Nowadays, drugs with higher therapeutic indices and of different drug classes are available. Some combinations display synergism (Fig. 7.1, see also

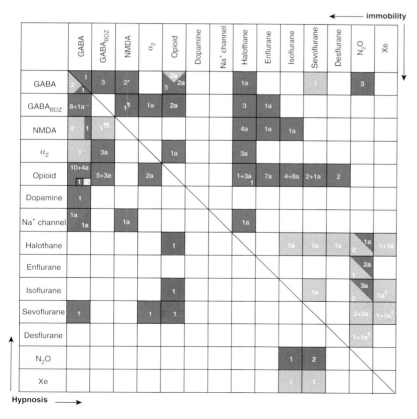

Fig. 7.1 Interaction grid summarizing drug interactions in humans and animals for hypnosis and immobility. Taken from [6], where detailed explanation of these interactions can be sought.

Chapter 3) which may be clinically useful by allowing us to use smaller doses of the individual drug (potentially decreasing side effects). Too much synergy may carry its own risk because there is synergy for side effects as well (e.g. ventilatory depression when benzodiazepines are combined with opioids) [6].

This chapter focuses on the hypnotic component of anaesthesia during induction and maintenance (unconsciousness and amnesia) and during emergence (i.e. regaining consciousness). Unconsciousness and amnesia are defined in Table 7.1.

Except when provided solely and exclusively by inhaled agents, the different components of GA are often provided by a mixture of hypnotic drugs and opioids (see Fig. 7.1). While specific drug classes target specific clinical end-points, i.e. hypnotics for hypnosis and 'analgesics' (opioids) for 'analgesia', opioids also have sedative effects and propofol also has analgesic properties [7]. The sedative effects of propofol result mainly from cortical disruption (discussed in more detail later), whereas those of opioids result from effects on acetylcholine, adenosine and dopamine receptors [3]. With regard to analgesia, propofol decreases the *perception* of pain related to a decreased state of consciousness, while opioids have an antinociceptive mechanism through a pathway-specific reduction of stimulus responses (modulation of afferent noxious stimulation as well) [7].

Several drugs are known to produce hypnosis: γ–aminobutyric acid type A (GABA-A) receptor agonists (propofol, etomidate, methohexital,

thiopental, midazolam and diazepam), N-methyl-d-aspartate (NMDA) receptor antagonists (ketamine), α_2-adrenoceptor agonists (dexmedetomidine, clonidine), μ-opioid receptor agonists (morphine, fentanyl, sufentanil, alfentanil and remifentanil) and dopamine receptor antagonists (droperidol and metoclopramide). Inhaled anaesthetics (halothane, enflurane, isoflurane, sevoflurane, desflurane, nitrous oxide [N_2O] and xenon [Xe]) also induce hypnosis, the mechanisms of which remain enigmatic [6]. Considering this extensive list, it is fascinating to see that so many different drug classes and with such a diverse molecular structure can produce the same effect. Biologically, this phenomenon can be described as degeneracy, which is the ability of structurally different elements to perform the same function or yield the same output. Unlike redundancy, which occurs when the same function is performed by identical elements, degeneracy, which involves structurally different elements, may yield the same or different functions depending on the context in which it is expressed. It is a prominent property of gene networks, neural networks and evolution itself [8].

The mechanisms leading to anaesthetic-induced unconsciousness are complex and constitute a fundamental, unresolved question in both anaesthesiology and neuroscience [4]. Much evidence suggests that both consciousness and anaesthetic-induced unconsciousness depend on higher-order processes of the brain. Some models suggest an impaired capacity of the brain to integrate information across specialized

Table 7.1. Differences between amnesia and unconsciousness. Adapted from [13].

Hypnotic Component	Description
Amnesia	Partial or complete loss of memory. Memory formation occurs at various sites in the brain, including the hippocampus, amygdala, prefrontal cortex and other cortical sensory and motor areas. Patients should be unable to remember what happened during a surgical procedure. In this context, the possibility of both implicit and explicit memory formation is relevant. Explicit memory refers to information that is consciously perceived and retained, and can subsequently be reported. Patients who accidentally awaken from anaesthesia during surgery frequently suffer from an unpleasant experience that is recalled for a long time. Implicit memory refers to information that is unconsciously perceived, and that cannot be reported, but the retained information influences the patient's behaviour without recollection. Anaesthetic-induced amnesia usually affects recall of events that occurred after the onset of anaesthesia (anterograde amnesia).
Unconsciousness	Conscious perception and/or response to environmental stimuli is impaired. Loss of responsiveness is not the same as loss of consciousness, even though sometimes they are used equivalently in the anaesthesia literature. For example, certain anaesthetics may produce behavioural unresponsiveness but not complete unconsciousness [11]. Responsiveness is usually used as a surrogate for consciousness, but it is still an indirect (and incomplete) measure of consciousness [12]. Furthermore, unconsciousness is a dynamic state. Its threshold should be continuously adjusted to the environment (e.g. noxious stimulation). For example, a patient receiving an infusion of propofol titrated to a surrogate measure of unconsciousness is not equivalent to the situation of surgical anaesthesia, because a noxious stimulus such as a scalpel cutting through skin could easily reverse this unconscious state [4].

subsystems as a common denominator. Several studies that investigated the effects of GA on the functional connectivity (FC) in the resting brain [9] illustrate that connectivity networks (cortical and subcortical) change, but the precise mechanisms remain controversial. One hypothesis is the 'bottom-up' paradigm, which argues that anaesthetics suppress consciousness by modulating sleep-wake nuclei and neural circuits in the brainstem and diencephalon that have evolved to control arousal states. The other is the 'top-down' paradigm, which argues that anaesthetics suppress consciousness by modulating the cortical and thalamocortical circuits involved in the integration of neural information [9, 10].

Targeting Optimal Delivery of Hypnotic Drugs

As described in Chapter 2, pharmacokinetic and pharmacodynamic (PK/PD) models allow clinicians to rationally dose and individually titrate anaesthetic drugs [14]. Parameters of several PK/PD models for several drugs are summarized in Table 7.2. The following section considers the clinically relevant parameters for the different anaesthetic drugs.

Propofol

Several PK/PD models exist for propofol. Some have been integrated in commercially available target controlled infusion (TCI) systems, which in and by itself attests to the usefulness of these PK/PD models for propofol: TCI systems facilitate clinical practice and maintenance of intravenous anaesthesia [15].

Commercial TCI devices incorporate the Marsh and the Schnider propofol PK/PD models [15]. For effect-site targeting, the Schnider model should be used, for plasma targeting, the Marsh model.

The use of the lean body mass (LBM) equation in the Schnider model limits its use in obese patients. Different k_{eo} values have been proposed for effect-site targeting, but there is little conclusive evidence to demonstrate the superiority of any particular model or method. Clinicians should use the model and methods with which they are most familiar [15].

Effect-site targeting better maintained drug effect (evaluated with the bispectral index (BIS) as a measure of hypnotic effect) of propofol over time [16]. Out of three compartmental models (Marsh, Schnider, Schütller) and a physiologically based recirculatory PK model, the Schnider model (although not perfect) best predicted propofol plasma concentration with different infusion schemes (including TCI) [17] and is to be recommended, for TCI and advisory drug displays.

Sevoflurane and Isoflurane

Even though the PK of inhalational anaesthetics are most often described with a physiological model, empirical compartmental modelling has been used by Yasuda et al to describe sevoflurane and isoflurane PK [18]. The volume of the central compartment of sevoflurane (2.10±0.62 L) was smaller than that of isoflurane (2.31±0.71 L). The elimination rate constant from the central compartment was greater for sevoflurane than for isoflurane. The pulmonary elimination clearances and the rate constants from the peripheral compartments to the central compartment did not differ between the two drugs. The mammillary time constants were identical for all compartments except for the lung (smaller for sevoflurane). Estimated blood flow to the fat group was larger for sevoflurane. The recovery parameters for sevoflurane and isoflurane did not differ [18].

As part of the development of a model-based closed-loop control system, Gentilini et al built a PK/PD model for isoflurane (combined with alfentanil) and the BIS as measure of hypnotic effect [19]. Yasuda's PK model was combined with a sigmoidal E_{max} model, yielding an EC50 of 0.6 % and a k_{eo}=0.217/min (or $t_{1/2}k_{eo}$ = 3.19 min). Olofsen et al reported the E_{max} models describing the relationship between isoflurane and sevoflurane effect-site concentrations and the BIS and the spectral edge frequency (SEF) of the EEG [20] to only differ with regard to their EC50 values: 0.6% for isoflurane versus 1.14% for sevoflurane using the BIS as end-point.

Others have confirmed k_{eo} values for sevoflurane and isoflurane to be the same [21], indicating that these two inhalational anaesthetic drugs have very similar PD profiles. McKay's PK/PD model parameters describing the sevoflurane response and state entropy relationship ($t_{1/2}k_{eo}$ = 2.65 min and EC50= 1.7%) are similar to those reported by Olofsen above [20, 22]. The PD interaction between propofol and sevoflurane with BIS as the clinical end-point is additive, information that may be helpful to provide a smooth transition between the two anaesthesia techniques and to be used in advisory drug display systems [23].

Ketamine

Ketamine is an unique pharmacological agent with a turbulent history [24]. The racemic mixture R, S(±)-ketamine and its enantiomers S(+)-ketamine and R(−)-ketamine have different effects on the median spectral frequency of the EEG in humans [25]. The maximal decrease (mean ± SD) of the median

Table 7.2. Summary of the main anaesthetic drug models presented in this chapter. Model parameters are expressed as mean population values. PK: Pharmacokinetic; PD: Pharmacodynamic; CI: Confidence Interval; RSE: Relative Standard Error; SE: Standard Error; LBM: Lean Body Mass; TTPE: Time to Peak Effect.

Anaesthetic Drug	Reference	Type of Model	Measure of Effect	Model Parameters
Ketamine	Dahan et al, 2011 [27]	PK/PD	Pain Scores	V1 (L) 53.26 (95% CI 38.71–69.59) V2 (L) 507.28 (95% CI 362.51–717.23) CL1 (L/per 70 kg) 83.34 (95% CI 72.36–95.39) CL2 (L/per 70 kg) 118.32 (95% CI 85.62–162.84) EC50 (ng/mL) 10.5 (95% CI 4.37–21.2) γ 1.89 (95% CI 0.79–3.84) $t\frac{1}{2}k$ (days) 10.9 (95% CI 5.25–20.50)
Ketamine	Schüttler et al, 1987 [25]	PD	Median Frequency of the EEG	E_{max} (Hz) 7.6±1.7 EC50 (μg/mL) 2.0±0.5 γ 3.8 ± 1.5
Dexmedetomidine	Colin et al, 2017 [29]	PD	Bispectral Index of the EEG	k_{eo} (min^{-1}) 0.12 (3.80 RSE %) EC50 (ng/mL) 2.63 (15.9 RSE %) ΔC50 1.71 (18.3 RSE %) K_{in} (min^{-1}) 0.130 (24.6 RSE %)
Etomidate	Kaneda, Yamashita, Woo and Han, 2011 [31]	PK/PD	Bispectral Index of the EEG (also for the OAA/S)	V1 (L) 4.45 (7.4 SE %) V2 (L) 74.9 (41.7 SE %) CL1 (L/min) 0.63 (88.0 SE %) CL2 (L/min) 3.16 (21.4 SE %) k_{eo} (/min) 0.477 (9.9 SE %) $t_{1/2}k_{eo}$ (min) 1.55 EC50 (μg/mL) 0.526 (14.9 SE %)
Propofol	Marsh et al, 1991 [15]	PK		V1 (L/kg) 0.228 V2 (L/kg) 0.463 V3 (L/kg) 2.893 k_{10} (/min) 0.119 k_{12} (/min) 0.112 k_{13} (/min) 0.042 k_{21} (/min) 0.055 k_{31} (/min) 0.0033
Propofol	Schnider et al, 1998 [15]	PK/PD	EEG	V1 (L) 4.27 V2 (L) 18.9–0.391x(age – 53) V3 (L) 238 k_{10} (/min) 0.443+0.0107x(weight – 77) -0.0159x(LBM-59)+0.0062x(height – 177) k_{12} (/min) 0.302–0.0056x(age – 53) k_{13} (/min) 0.196 k_{21} (/min) [1.29–0.024x(age – 53)]/ [18.9–0.391x(age-53)] k_{31} (/min) 0.0035 k_{eo} (/min) 0.456 TTPE (min) 1.69
Sevoflurane	Yasuda et al, 1991 [18]	PK		V1(L) 2.10±0.62 k_{10} (/min) 1.78±0.32 k_{12} (/min) 0.709±0.145 k_{13} (/min) 0.223±0.035 k_{14} (/min) 0.125± 0.056 k_{15} (/min) 0.0310±0.0196 k_{21} (/min) 0.194±0.092 k_{31} (/min) 0.0231± 0.0198 k_{41} (/min) 0.00313±0.00180 k_{51} (/min) 0.000502±0.000117 k_{20} (/min) 0.0094±0.0171

Table 7.2. (cont.)

Anaesthetic Drug	Reference	Type of Model	Measure of Effect	Model Parameters
Sevoflurane	Olofsen and Dahan, 1999 [20]	PD	Bispectral Index of the EEG (also for Spectral Edge Frequency)	$t_{1/2}k_{eo}$ (min) 3.5±2.0 E_{max} 94.5±3.1 EC50 (%) 1.14±0.31 γ 4.5±3.5
Isoflurane	Yasuda et al, 1991 [18]	PK		V1(L) 2.31±0.71 k_{10} (/min) 1.64±0.33 k_{12} (/min) 1.26±0.204 k_{13} (/min) 0.402±0.055 k_{14} (/min) 0.243±0.072 k_{15} (/min) 0.0646±0.0414 k_{21} (/min) 0.210±0.082 k_{31} (/min) 0.0230±0.0156 k_{41} (/min) 0.00304±0.00169 k_{51} (/min) 0.000500±0.000119 k_{20} (/min) 0.0093±0.0137
Isoflurane	Olofsen and Dahan, 1999 [20]	PD	Bispectral Index of the EEG (also for Spectral Edge Frequency)	$t_{1/2}k_{eo}$ (min) 3.2±0.7 E_{max} 95.7±2.2 EC50 (%) 0.60±0.11 γ 5.8±4.6
Midazolam	Koopmans et al, 1988 [33]	PD	α – activity of the EEG	EC50 (ng/mL) 42.0 – 48.1 γ 3.7 ± 1.8

Table 7.3. Components needed to define depth of anaesthesia. Reproduced with permission from [7].

Afferent stimulus

Efferent response

Concentrations of analgesic components

Concentrations of hypnotic components

Concentrations of other relevant drugs (e.g. beta blockers, muscle relaxants, local anaesthetics)

Interaction surface relating the drug concentrations to the probability of the given response to the given stimulus

frequency (E_{max}) for R,S(±), R(–) and S(+) ketamine were 4.4±0.5, 7.6±1.7 and 8.3±1.9 Hz, respectively, and the ketamine serum concentration that caused one-half of the maximal median frequency decrease (IC50) 2.0±0.5, 1.8±0.5 and 0.8±0.4 g/mL, respectively. In sheep, the time to peak effect or $t_{1/2}k_{eo}$ of ketamine is identical to that of propofol [26]. A population PK/PD model for S(+)-ketamine-induced pain relief in humans has been described [27].

Dexmedetomidine

Dexmedetomidine is a selective and potent α_2-adrenoceptor agonist with anxiolytic, sedative and analgesic properties. Existing PK/PD models have focused on healthy volunteers and ICU patients[28]. A PK/PD model for haemodynamic effects and for arousal and (BIS-guided) sedation in volunteers has recently been described [29, 30]. The models still have to be tested in a clinical environment. More studies are bound to have been published by the time this book goes to press.

Etomidate

Etomidate, a carboxylated imidazole ester, is an intravenous anaesthetic for which a PK/PD model with the BIS and the Alertness and Sedation (OAA/S) scale as a measure of effect has been described in healthy volunteers, but for which prospective testing in patients is still lacking [31]. In 20 volunteers receiving 5 mg/min etomidate eyelash reflex was lost after a mean etomidate dose of 24 mg. A two-compartment PK model described the concentration data well, no inter-individual variability was incorporated, the $t_{1/2}k_{eo}$ was 1.55 min, and the E_{max} and EC50 of the sigmoidal E_{max} model were 67 and 0.526 μg/mL, respectively.

Propofol is faster than etomidate to induce loss of eyelash reflex and to lower BIS to 60, and also has a shorter intubating time [32].

Measuring the Effect

Prior to the induction of anaesthesia, consciousness of a subject can be easily assessed by a traditional clinical neurological exploration that includes verbal response, response to commands and brainstem reflexes. However, after induction of anaesthesia, when unconsciousness has been induced, one is forced to rely on surrogates to assess the hypnotic component of anaesthesia, even reflexes can no longer be used if neuromuscular blocking agents are used (the exception being pupillary reflexes). After initial loss of consciousness, unconsciousness has to be maintained and monitored in such a manner that both excessive and insufficient hypnotic effects are avoided. This is usually referred to as assessing depth of anaesthesia although it belongs directly to the hypnotic component of anaesthesia. The full assessment of adequacy of anaesthesia should involve a postoperative interview to exclude explicit recall.

The hypnotic state during anaesthesia can be measured to guide hypnotic drug targets and dosing by several methods and to several end-points, each of them useful in different phases of the procedure. These will be explained in more detail in this section.

Loss of consciousness

Unconsciousness is attained when the required amount of hypnotic drug reaches the presumably multiple required sites in the cerebral cortex, brainstem and thalamus that alter neurotransmission and induce hypnosis [33]. As the hypnotic drug concentration increases at these sites, individuals transition from wakefulness to unconsciousness. This transition process is a continuum that can be clinically observed as an all-or-none effect [34]. By careful assessment of the different stages it is possible to identify surrogates of the hypnotic effect.

Clinical End-points

The clinical end-points usually used as surrogates reflect both cortical, subcortical and/or spinal functions or indirectly measure their activity.

Cortical

In the continuum to unconsciousness we can determine the moment of loss of behavioural responsiveness (LOBR) to stimulation, when different strengths and types of stimuli cease to cause a response in the patient. This is mediated at the level of the cortex and happens because hypnotics render patients unwilling or unable to interact with their external environment [35]. Classifying the adequacy of the hypnotic effect based on cortical function is also possible using the

Observers' Assessment of Anaesthesia and Sedation score (OAAS/S). OAAS/S is a score that ranges from five (alert) to zero (unconsciousness) and includes end-points such as unresponsiveness to verbal commands and loss of response to shaking and shouting.

Subcortical

Hypnotics can have a profound impact on most actions of the nerves originating in the brainstem, actions that disappear during induction and reappear with recovery of consciousness. This supports the use of the brainstem reflexes as clinical end-points [36], namely the eyelash reflex, corneal reflex, oculocephalic reflex, gagging reflex and the pupillary light reflex [37]. These are non-specific indicators of impaired brainstem function due to the actions of the hypnotic agent on the oculomotor, trochlear, abducens, trigeminal, facial and glossopharyngeal nuclei in the midbrain, pons and medulla [34, 36].

The corneal reflex, for example, is elicited by mechanical stimulation of the cornea, resulting in the closure of the eyelid and requires the integrity of all these structures: (1) afferent nerves from the free nerve endings in the cornea; (2) the ocular division of the trigeminal nerve; (3) ganglion, root and spinal trigeminal tracts; (4) the spinal trigeminal nucleus in the pons. Then, some of the axons synapse into the (5) reticular formation interneurons, which send their axons bilaterally to (6) facial motor neurons in the facial nucleus (resulting in a consensual reflex), and subsequently through the (7) facial nerve, to the (8) orbicularis oculi, finally closing the eyelid.

Even though the assessment of different brainstem reflexes can provide useful insight into the actions of hypnotics in the brain and the integrity of the different structures, most anaesthesiologists use only the eyelash reflex, and even then, not consistently.

Spinal

Loss of muscular tone is also a possible clinical indicator to assess the hypnotic effect. It is usually tested by detecting the moment a patient drops an object held by the hand, a method known as 'syringe drop' because a 50 mL filled syringe was used in clinical studies. The rapid atonia that occurs after a bolus administration of most hypnotic agents can be due to their actions along the motor pathway and brainstem, but is most likely due to the actions of the drug in the spinal cord [34]. While muscle tone is also lost during REM sleep, brainstem reflexes are preserved.

Electroencephalography

There is increasing evidence that electroencephalography (EEG) can be used in the assessment of loss of consciousness [38, 39]. In a volunteer study [38] loss of consciousness coincided with an increase in low-frequency EEG power (< 1 Hz), the loss of spatially coherent occipital alpha oscillations (8–12 Hz), and the appearance of spatially coherent frontal alpha oscillations. These changes in the EEG reversed with recovery of consciousness. This study [38] also suggested that alpha amplitudes could predict the transition into and out of unconsciousness and profound unconsciousness.

In another volunteer study [39], the propofol concentration was gradually increased until the subjects were no longer able to interact with their external environment (= LOBR). After reaching LOBR, the amplitude of slow-wave activity (0.5 to 1.5 Hz) increased sharply, attaining saturation even though propofol concentrations continued to rise afterwards. Following discontinuation of the infusion, as drug levels dropped, the slow-wave power began to decrease and returned to baseline levels before recovery of the behavioural response. Therefore, it was proposed that slow-wave activity saturation could potentially be used as an individualized indicator of perception loss and be useful for monitoring the hypnotic component of depth of anaesthesia and studying altered states of consciousness.

Another approach to using EEG to identify the transition between consciousness and unconsciousness [40] combined data from other sources. This multimodal integration was entitled Anaesthesia Multimodal Index of Consciousness (AMIC), and comprised EEG, standard monitoring data (heart rate, arterial blood pressure, oxygen concentrations, end-expiratory carbon dioxide concentration, peak inspiratory pressure), individual patient data and drug information (MAC and/or plasma concentration). The AMIC not only identified the transition between consciousness and unconsciousness but was also able to separate out different levels of anaesthesia (from wakefulness to burst suppression).

Adequacy of Depth of Anaesthesia

Depth of anaesthesia assessment has been sought after since the beginning of anaesthesia itself. John Snow divided the effects of ether into five stages or degrees, which included end-points such as level of consciousness (awake to deep coma), muscle flaccidity and apnoea [41]. Guedel later refined these stages, introducing in 1937 the concept of different stages based on alterations in breathing, muscle tone, pupil diameter, lacrimation and eyelid reflex. Philip Woodbridge subsequently included the newer agents available in 1957 and presented an alternative way of looking at anaesthetic depth [42], which gained increasing interest with the widespread use of muscle relaxants. This spawned concerns regarding unintended intraoperative awareness, which is still a major concern nowadays. The incidence of awareness has been reported to range from 0.13% to 0.16% and can cause post-traumatic stress disorder in as many as 70% of these patients [43].

The impact of awareness on a patient's well-being postoperatively has since long been recognized. Early methods proposed to assess depth of anaesthesia in an attempt to avoid it were based on clinical observations [42]. However, the assessment of adequacy of the depth of anaesthesia is very important not only in preventing intraoperative awareness, but also in tailoring drug delivery to each patient. This can reduce the amount of anaesthetic given, decrease the time to eye opening and extubation, and shorten the duration of postanaesthesia care unit stay [44].

We now know that depth of anaesthesia depends on other factors than those resulting from the action of hypnotics, thus it is important to recognize these other components, as Shafer and Stanski describe [7]:

1. Afferent stimulus
2. Efferent response
3. Concentrations of analgesic components
4. Concentrations of hypnotic components
5. Concentrations of other relevant drugs (e.g., beta blockers, muscle relaxants, local anaesthetics)
6. Interaction surface relating the drug concentrations to the probability of the given response to the given stimulus.

The assessment of the hypnotic effect during maintenance can therefore be combined with information gathered from other sources. For this there are several methods available.

Pharmacokinetic End-points

Minimum Alveolar Concentration – One of the most widely used indicators to guide depth of anaesthesia, the minimum alveolar concentration (MAC), is a composite index of nociception and immobility as it represents the partial pressure of a volatile anaesthetic needed to prevent movement in 50% of the patients in response to a painful stimulus. This in fact shows the suppression of the withdrawal reflex, reflecting the volatile anaesthetic's actions leading to immediate immobility via the spinal cord (Fig. 7.2).

To better assess the hypnotic and amnestic effects that volatile anaesthetics mediate in the brain cortex, the concept of MAC-awake was introduced. MAC-awake represents the volatile anaesthetic partial pressure needed to suppress a voluntary response to verbal command in 50% of patients. Besides producing unconsciousness, MAC-awake also prevents explicit memory from developing in 50% of patients. MAC-awake is considerably lower than MAC (the partial pressure required to prevent movement in response to surgery) [42], but even more interesting was the observation that MAC-awake could differ from MAC-unawake (the concentration at which 50% of the patients regain consciousness) [45]. The difference in volatile partial pressure between these two states indicates that they are not mirror images of one another, suggesting an asymmetry in the role of some arousal nuclei in the process of induction and emergence. This anaesthetic hysteresis [45] implies that the process of 'coming out' of a state is not simply the reverse process of 'going in', with higher partial pressures needed to lose than to regain consciousness, suggesting the existence of a resistance to state transitions, termed neural inertia [4].

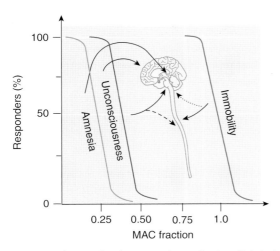

Fig. 7.2 Behavioural end-points and sites of action of inhaled agents. Immobility is mediated in the spinal cord, although supraspinal effects (dotted arrow) are likely to be important for some anaesthetics. Anaesthetic action in the spinal cord blunts ascending impulses arising from noxious stimulation and might indirectly contribute to anaesthetic-induced unconsciousness and amnesia (dashed arrow). (Reproduced with permission from [46].)

Isolated Forearm Technique

The isolated forearm technique (IFT) was described by Tunstall in 1977, and consists of inflating a cuff around the arm after inducing hypnosis, and delaying injection of neuromuscular blocking agents until after full inflation of this cuff. The cuff prevents paralysis of the hand, allowing the patient to communicate to an observer through predefined hand movements, typically following a command such as 'squeeze my hand twice'. Patients can show goal-directed responsiveness (following the requested command), but rarely show spontaneous responsiveness [47]. This technique allows the assessment not only of awareness with recall (AWR), but also of connected consciousness because it is not dependent on memory.

Monitors of Depth of Anaesthesia

Depth of anaesthesia results from the dynamic balance and interaction between effect-site concentrations of hypnotic and analgesic drugs, and the intensity of surgical stimulation [48].

Each drug has to be titrated independently, taking into account the individual patient and procedure and the fact that there are several functional end-points (such as suppression of stress responses and hypnosis) that should ideally be monitored independently and simultaneously to ensure that therapeutic goals of the general anaesthetics are being achieved [41].

Currently, there is no monitor that can measure depth of anaesthesia in its full complexity. However, some of the individual components can be assessed through surrogates of the effects, e.g. monitors to assess the hypnotic effect. There are several monitors for this purpose (see Table 7.4), and they mainly focus on the processing of EEG. Changes in EEG for most of the hypnotics typically follow a similar pattern. Initially, during light sedation, there is an increase in higher (β, 20–30 Hz) frequencies. Next, the dominant frequency shifts towards lower frequencies: β to α (8–13 Hz) to θ (4–8 Hz) to δ (< 4 Hz). If the dose of anaesthetic is further increased, burst suppression activity ensues. During burst suppression, low voltage periods (suppressions) are followed by high amplitude activity (bursts). After burst suppression, the EEG will change to suppression (i.e. iso-electricity). In addition to the changes in the frequency bands, the hypnotic component of anaesthesia also produces topographical changes such as anteriorization of EEG power (the EEG power shifts from posterior to anterior regions of the brain), and a decrease in coherence of homologous regions of the two hemispheres [49].

Table 7.4. Some of the commercially available monitors and indexes of depth of anaesthesia based on processed EEG.

Index	Monitor	Company	Frequency Band (Hz)	Ranges	Recommended Target for GA
Bispectral Index	A2000™/BIS, XP™/BIS, VISTA™	Medtronic-Covidien, Dublin, Ireland	1–47	98 (awake)–0 (isolectric).	40–60
PSI	SedLine	Masimo Corp, California, USA	0.5–50	0–100	25–50
State Entropy (SE) and Response Entropy (RE)	M-Entropy™	GE Healthcare, Helsinki, Finland	SE: 0.8–32 RE: 0.8–47	RE: 0 (no brain activity) to 100 (fully awake) SE: 0 (no brain activity) to 91 (fully awake)	RE: 40–60 SE: values near 40 indicate a low probability of consciousness
qCON	CONOX	Quantium Medical, Barcelona, Spain	?	0–99	40–60
Narcotrend™	Narcotrend™	Narcotrend-Gruppe, Hannover, Germany	0.5–45	A (awake) to F (very deep hypnosis) and ranging from 100 (awake) to 0 (very deep hypnosis)	D0–D2 37–57
Cerebral State Index (CSI™)	Cerebral State Monitor™ (CSM)	Danmeter A/S, Odense C, Denmark	6–42.5	0–100	40–60

The EEG signal is the best window we have on cortical brain activity [50] and provides fair PD feedback on the effects of hypnotics [51]. Depth of anaesthesia monitors process the raw EEG, and their algorithms try to present any changes as a simple index that the anaesthesiologist can easily interpret and act on. Each of the monitors has its own algorithm, and BIS is the most validated of all. However, anaesthesiologists using EEG-based depth of anaesthesia monitoring should also have (pretty strong) skills to interpret the raw EEG signal correctly in order to understand the influence of several artefacts and their limitations.

Bispectral Index – The BIS is the most validated depth of anaesthesia monitor [52]. It was approved in 1996, has been the subject of over 1500 studies and been used in more than 34 million patients. The BIS processes the raw EEG signal obtained through a sensor placed on the patient's forehead to a dimensionless value ranging from 99 (fully awake patient) to zero (absence of brain activity). BIS values between 40 and 60 indicate adequate depth of hypnotic effect during general anaesthesia for surgery, and values below 40 indicate a deep hypnotic state. The BIS monitor analyses the EEG frequencies through spectral analysis. Another level of complexity in signal analysis used by this monitor is called bispectral analysis and investigates the phase coupling between different EEG frequencies and

contributes to both the BIS and the naming of the monitor itself [52]. Chapter 5 gives a detailed explanation of the methods used to analyse EEG signals.

Several studies found an association between cumulative duration of low BIS and mortality [53–55]. In addition, it was also shown that the combination of low mean arterial pressure, low BIS and low MAC fraction, also known as the 'triple low', is an important predictor of excessive hospital length of stay and postoperative mortality although recent reports seem to contradict those initial results [56].

The BIS cannot be used to help guide depth when ketamine or nitrous oxide is used [57]. It is also important to note that muscle relaxation could by itself lower BIS to values close to the accepted range of GA [58]: after volunteers had received both suxamethonium and rocuronium without any hypnotic, the BIS was < 60 for several minutes. The study suggests that BIS monitoring requires muscle activity, in addition to an awake EEG, in order to generate values indicating that the subject is awake [58].

Patient State Index – The Patient State Index (PSI) monitor records four EEG channels and calculates the index based on the quantitative EEG analysis of the power within the α, β, δ and θ frequency bands, and also the temporal and spatial gradients occurring among these frequency bands when anaesthetic depth changes [52].

Values between 25 and 50 are recommended to ensure unconsciousness. Even though these values are 10–15 points lower than BIS, they closely and linearly correlate with the BIS values, more so with propofol than with sevoflurane.

Still, agreement between the recommended ranges for PSI (25–50) and BIS (40–60) was poor, so that index values within the recommended range in one monitor were outside the recommended range in the other monitor [52].

Awareness – The lack of a standard intraoperative depth of anaesthesia monitor reflects the complexities in understanding the neural correlates of consciousness and memory. This brings us ultimately to the way to assess, retrospectively, the adequacy of depth of anaesthesia: a postoperative interview. Memory can be subdivided into implicit (unconscious) and explicit (conscious) [59], and intraoperative awareness is defined by both consciousness and explicit memory of surgical events. Although there is no 'gold-standard' psychometric test for awareness and memory available, the modified Brice interview has been consistently used [60].

The interview consists of several questions which are presented in Table 7.5.

Recovery of consciousness

While the effect of neuromuscular blocking agent that mediates immobility can be actively antagonized with reversal agents, recovery of consciousness is usually seen as a passive process, the inverse of induction, and the result of the elimination of anaesthetic drugs from their sites of action in the CNS. However, many neurophysiological studies suggest this might not be the case, with orexinergic neurons playing a critical role [61], because (1) impaired orexinergic signalling leads to narcolepsy and genetic/pharmacological blockade of orexin-mediated signalling impairs arousal; (2) orexin agonists decrease anaesthetic duration,

meaning that modifying orexin-mediated signalling affects the anaesthetic state; and (3) orexin-1 receptor antagonists increase anaesthetic duration [61]. Hypnotic agents such as isoflurane and sevoflurane inhibit orexinergic but not adjacent melanin concentrating hormone neurons, suggesting that wake-active orexinergic neurons are inhibited by these anaesthetics [61]. The fact that selective orexin-1 receptor antagonism affects anaesthetic emergence but not induction opens the intriguing possibility that neural substrates for induction and emergence might differ and helps explain the phenomena of hysteresis and neural inertia.

The possibility of turning the passive emergence process into an active one has been explored. Several drugs promote active emergence after GA with isoflurane or propofol in rats: methylphenidate (an inhibitor of dopamine and Noradrenaline reuptake transporters), dextroamphetamine and a D1 dopamine receptor agonist [62]. Electrical stimulation of the ventral tegmental area (VTA), a major dopamine nucleus in the brain, also corroborated the idea that a dopaminergic arousal pathway projecting from the VTA promotes active emergence from GA [62]. Other potential candidates that might prove useful to speed up emergence are the arousal-promoting cholinergic neurons. Some studies suggested physostigmine could enhance recovery of consciousness because it is a cholinesterase inhibitor that crosses the blood–brain barrier and therefore stimulates central cholinergic neurotransmission. However, in a recent study [62] it did not decrease time to emergence from isoflurane GA. However, it can induce EEG changes during burst suppression that are consistent with neurophysiological antagonism of isoflurane anaesthesia. The authors conclude that 'cholinergic and monoaminergic stimulation produce distinct arousal states during isoflurane general anaesthesia'.

Another study explored the role of flumazenil [63]. When given to healthy unpremedicated patients during propofol/remifentanil anaesthesia, flumazenil increased the BIS and hastened emergence. This indicates that flumazenil could be useful to reverse endogenous or exogenous benzodiazepines that might play a role during anaesthesia.

Taken together, current evidence suggests that recovery of consciousness could be modulated in the hope of obviating the need for having to wait for the passive elimination of induction and maintenance drugs.

Table 7.5. Questions comprising the modified Brice interview.

1. What was the last thing you remember before anaesthesia?
2. What is the first thing you remember after waking up?
3. Do you remember anything between going under anaesthesia and waking up?
4. Did you dream during your procedure?
5. What was the worst thing about your operation?

Personalizing the Effect

Given the availability of PK/PD models and EEG-derived parameters to predict and monitor the hypnotic state, can we provide each patient with the correct hypnotic dose during both induction and maintenance?

This is a question that has not received the attention it deserves. In order to personalize anaesthesia during **maintenance**, be it with intravenous or inhalational anaesthesia, one can rely on currently available depth of anaesthesia monitors, because a good correlation exists between drug concentrations and the value of the processed indexes and the clinical end-goal (hypnosis/amnesia). So can we say we 'nailed it down' pretty well and that we have succeeded in 'personalizing hypnosis' during maintenance?

However, to monitor the hypnotic state during *induction* of anaesthesia, such monitors are not the best choice due to the fact that the processing time delay, even if less than 30 seconds, is excessive. The inter-individual variability in propofol requirements for the induction of loss of consciousness is of the order of magnitude of 300%, and this variability is independent of age, weight, height and gender [64]. Many factors contribute to this variability, both genetic and non-genetic. The level of anxiety, the time of day, medication being taken, heart rate, cardiac output, level of hydration, volaemia, hepatic and liver function, protein level, metabolic rate and probably many others account for such variability [65]. Accepting the existence of this variability it is obvious that administering the rather fixed recommended dose of 2 mg/kg of propofol is not the solution. The choice of an induction method that results in administering what a patient requires for loss of consciousness and not more, should be derived from existing PK/PD models. Maybe the most relevant PK parameter is the time to peak of propofol, which is around 90 seconds. That implies that once the clinician stops administering a propofol dose, the cerebral concentration will keep increasing for several seconds. If anaesthesia is induced with a manual bolus administered in 30 or 40 seconds, the patient will lose consciousness rather quickly, because the rapid bolus results in high cerebral concentrations in a matter of 30 or 40 seconds, but a significant overshoot in the cerebral concentration will occur, resulting in a fall in blood pressure and an excessive drop in the depth of anaesthesia index. The anaesthesiologist tends to believe an adequate amount of propofol was given based upon the fact that loss of consciousness was almost simultaneous with stopping the bolus, but the lack of feedback information from modelling the concentration as the bolus gives results that underestimate the magnitude of the concentration overshoot that is actually occurring. The alternative is to give the induction dose of propofol in a manner that will attenuate this overshoot. The use of TCI anaesthesia allows a 'cerebral' effect-site concentration to be targeted. But still there is no way of knowing beforehand what the concentration for loss of consciousness (LOC) in the individual patient will be. One could progressively increase the target while intermittently assessing consciousness (e.g. every 10 seconds). But this will delay induction by several minutes (except for those patients in which LOC happens to occur at a low cerebral effect-site concentration). The alternative that we employ in our clinical practice is to induce anaesthesia with the TCI device in manual mode while viewing the corresponding modelled concentrations. With this approach, induction is performed by infusing propofol at 20–40 mg/kg/h [65, 66]. As propofol is being infused we assess consciousness every 10 seconds. LOC is acknowledged once the patient fails to open his/her eyes to name calling and tapping on the forehead. At that moment, the propofol infusion is stopped, the effect-site concentration displayed on the TCI device is noted, and the TCI system is switched to effect-site TCI mode, with the effect-site concentration set equal to that at which LOC occurred (or lower than that of LOC if a depth of anaesthesia monitor indicates otherwise). Even though the infusion rate and total dose are much lower that of a manual bolus, overshoot still occurs but less so. This technique results in an average induction time of around three minutes, which we consider quite acceptable when placed into perspective with total anaesthesia time and when considering what is gained by individualizing a patient's need. If one does not have access to a TCI system, this induction method can still be used. In that case, following LOC, the anaesthesiologist should set up a manual infusion, titrating propofol to the depth of anaesthesia index. If induction is to be performed with propofol and maintained with a volatile anaesthetic, a syringe pump can be used for induction, with propofol at an infusion rate of 20–40 mg/kg/h. For frail or hypovolaemic patients, we reduce the infusion rate to as low as 10 mg/kg/h.

The above approaches represent how we integrate known pharmacological concepts [66] into our clinical practice with the available tools and monitors. It should be seen as 'a' possible way to personalize anaesthesia induction, and encourage the reader to do away with the general practice of giving little attention to propofol dose with a one-size-fits-all approach based on a recommended weight and age. Observing the effect site concentration at which LOC occurs in the individual patient allows the clinician to set a reference target which may help to avoid excessive anaesthesia and personalize the hypnotic effect.

Conclusion

The Holy Grail to monitor the hypnotic state remains elusive simply because we still do not know what defines consciousness and how exactly it is mediated. Monitors that use PK- and EEG-based PD models that correlate with the hypnotic component of anaesthesia help guide the anaesthesiologist in their quest to personalize anaesthesia. We do not have the perfect awareness prevention tool yet, and monitoring the hypnotic state and by implication ensuring hypnosis and amnesia during induction and full and lasting return of consciousness in the immediate postinduction period remain challenging.

References

1. Flores FJ et al: Thalamocortical synchronization during induction and emergence from propofol-induced unconsciousness. Proc.Natl.Acad.Sci.USA. 2017; 201700148.

2. Brown EN, Lydic R, Schiff ND: GA, sleep, and coma. N.Engl.J.Med. Dec. 2010; 363 (27): 2638–50.

3. Brown EN, Purdon PL, Van Dort CJ: GA and altered states of arousal: a systems neuroscience analysis. Annu.Rev.Neurosci. 2011; 34: 601–28.

4. Mashour GA: Top-down mechanisms of anesthetic-induced unconsciousness. Front.Syst.Neurosci. 2014 June; 8: 1–10.

5. Garcia PS, Kolesky SE, Jenkins A: General anesthetic actions on GABA A receptors. Curr.Neuropharmacol. 2010; 8: 2–9.

6. Hendrickx JFA, Eger EI, Sonner JM, Shafer SL: Is synergy the rule? A review of anesthetic interactions producing hypnosis and immobility. Anesth.Analg. 2008; 107 (2):494–506.

7. Schüttler J, Schwilden H (eds.). *Modern Anesthetics*, 182. Berlin, Heidelberg: Springer, 2008.

8. Edelman GM, Gally JA: Degeneracy and complexity in biological systems. Proc.Natl.Acad.Sci.USA. 2001; 98 (24): 13763–8.

9. Jordan D, Ilg R, Riedl V, Schorer A, Grimberg S: Simultaneous electroencephalographic and functional magnetic resonance imaging indicate impaired cortical top-down processing in association with anesthetic-induced unconsciousness. Anesthesiology. 2013; 119 (5):1031–42.

10. Mashour GA, Hudetz AG: Bottom-up and top-down mechanisms of general anesthetics modulate different dimensions of consciousness. Front.Neural.Circuits. 201; 11: 44.

11. Alkire MT, Hudetz AG, Tononi G: Consciousness and anesthesia. Science. Nov. 2008; 80 (322):876–80.

12. Barttfeld P, Bekinschtein TA, Salles A, Stamatakis EA, Adapa R, Menon DK, Sigman M: Factoring the brain signatures of anesthesia concentration and level of arousal across individuals. NeuroImage.Clin. 2015; 9: 385–91.

13. Rudolph U, Antkowiak B: Molecular and neuronal substrates for general anaesthetics. Nat.Rev.Neurosci. 2004; 5 (9): 709–20.

14. Gambús PL, Trocóniz IF: Pharmacokinetic-pharmacodynamic modelling in anaesthesia. Br.J.Clin. Pharmacol. 2015; 79 (1):72–84.

15. Engbers FH, Sutcliffe N, Kenny G, Schraag S: Pharmacokinetic models for propofol: defining and illuminating the devil in the detail. Br.J.Anaesth. Feb. 2010; 104 (2):261–4.

16. Struys LFM, Versichelen MM, Mortier EP, D. Sc, Dumortier FJE: Comparison of plasma compartment versus two methods for effect compartment-controlled target-controlled infusion for propofol. Anesthesiology. 2000; 92 (2): 399–406.

17. Masui K, Upton R, Doufas A, Coetzee J, Kazama T: The performance of compartmental and physiologically based recirculatory pharmacokinetic models for propofol: a comparison using bolus, continuous, and target-controlled infusion data. Anesth.Analg. 2010; 111 (2): 368–79.

18. Yasuda N, Lockhart S, Eger E, Weiskopf R, Liu J: Comparison of kinetics of sevoflurane and isoflurane in humans. Anesth.Analg. Mar. 1991; 72 (3):316–24.

19. Gentilini A, Rossoni-Gerosa M, Frei C, Wymann R, Morari M: Modeling and closed-loop control of hypnosis by means of bispectral index (BIS) with isoflurane. IEEE. Trans.Biomed.Eng. 2001; 48 (8): 874–89.

20. Olofsen E, Dahan A: The dynamic relationship between end-tidal sevoflurane and isoflurane concentrations and bispectral index and spectral edge frequency of the electroencephalogram. Anesthesiology. May 1999; 90 (5): 1345–53.

21. Kreuer S, Bruhn J, Wilhelm W, Bouillon T: Pharmacokinetic-pharmacodynamic models for inhaled anaesthetics. Anaesthetist. 2007; 56 (6):538–56.

22. McKay IDH, Voss LJ, Sleigh JW, Barnard JP, Johannsen EK: Pharmacokinetic-pharmacodynamic modeling of the hypnotic effect of sevoflurane using the spectral

entropy of the electroencephalogram. Anesth.Analg. 2006; 102 (1):91–7.

23. Diz JC, Del Río R, Lamas A, Mendoza M, Durán M, Ferreira LM: Analysis of pharmacodynamic interaction of sevoflurane and propofol on bispectral index during general anaesthesia using a response surface model. Br.J.Anaesth. 2010; 104 (6): 733–9.

24. Domino EF: Taming the ketamine tiger. Anesthesiology. 2010; 113 (3): 678–86.

25. Schüttler J, Stanski DR, White PF, Trevor AJ, Horai Y, Verotta D, Sheiner LB: Pharmacodynamic modeling of the EEG effects of ketamine and its enantiomers in man. J.Pharmacokinet.Biopharm. 1987: 15 (3): 241–53.

26. Voss LJ, Ludbrook G, Grant C, Upton R, Sleigh JW: A comparison of pharmacokinetic/pharmacodynamic versus mass-balance measurement of brain concentrations of intravenous anesthetics in sheep. Anesth.Analg. 2007; 104 (6): 1440–6.

27. Dahan A., Olofsen, E., Sigtermans, M., Noppers, I., Niesters, M., Aarts, L., Sarton, E: Population pharmacokinetic-pharmacodynamic modeling of ketamine-induced pain relief of chronic pain. Eur.J.Pain. 2011; 15 (3): 258–67.

28. Weerink MAS, Struys MMRF, Hannivoort LN, Barends CRM, Absalom AR, Colin P: Clinical pharmacokinetics and pharmacodynamics of dexmedetomidine. Clin. Pharmacokinet. 2017; 26 (5):335–46.

29. Colin PJ, Hannivoort LN, Eleveld DJ, Reyntjens KMEM, Absalom AR, Vereecke HEM, Struys MMRF: Dexmedetomidine pharmacokinetic-pharmacodynamic modelling in healthy volunteers: 1. Influence of arousal on bispectral index and sedation. Br.J.Anaesth. Aug. 2017; 119 (2): 200–10.

30. Colin PJ, Hannivoort LN, Eleveld DJ, Reyntjens KMEM, Absalom AR, Vereecke HEM, Struys MMRF: Dexmedetomidine pharmacodynamics in healthy volunteers: 2. Haemodynamic profile. Br.J.Anaesth. Aug. 2017; 119 (2):211–20.

31. Kaneda K, Yamashita S, Woo S, Han TH: Population pharmacokinetics and pharmacodynamics of brief etomidate infusion in healthy volunteers. J.Clin. Pharmacol. 2011; 51 (4): 482–91.

32. Moller Petrun A, Kamenik M: Bispectral index-guided induction of general anaesthesia in patients undergoing major abdominal surgery using propofol or etomidate: a double-blind, randomized, clinical trial. Br.J.Anaesth. 2013; 110 (3): 388–96.

33. Koopmans R, Dingemanse J, Danhof M, Horsten GPM, van Boxtel CJ: Pharmacokinetic-pharmacodynamic modeling of midazolam effects on the human central nervous system. Clin.Pharmacol.Ther. Jul. 1988; 44 (1): 14–22.

34. Brown EN, Lydic R, Schiff ND: GA, sleep, and coma. N. Engl.J.Med. Dec. 2010; 363 (27): 2638–50.

35. Warnaby CE, Seretny M, Ní Mhuircheartaigh R, Rogers R, Jbabdi S, Sleigh J, Tracey I: Anesthesia-induced suppression of human dorsal anterior insula responsivity at loss of volitional behavioral response. Anesthesiology. April 2016; x: 1.

36. Bosch L, Fernández-Candil J, León A, Gambús PL: Influence of general anaesthesia on the brainstem. Rev. Española.Anesesiol.Reanim. (English Ed.). 2017; 64 (3): 157–67.

37. Leslie K, Sessler DI, Smith WD, Larson MD, Ozaki M, Blanchard D, Crankshaw DP: Prediction of movement during propofol/nitrous oxide anesthesia. Performance of concentration, electroencephalographic, pupillary, and hemodynamic indicators. Anesthesiology. 1996: 84 (1): 52–63.

38. Purdon PL, Pierce ET, Mukamel EA, Prerau MJ, Walsh JL, Wong KFK, Brown EN: Electroencephalogram signatures of loss and recovery of consciousness from propofol. Proc.Natl.Acad.Sci.USA. 2013; 110 (12): E1142-51.

39. Ní Mhuircheartaigh R, Warnaby C, Rogers R, Jbabdi S, Tracey I: Slow-wave activity saturation and thalamocortical isolation during propofol anesthesia in humans. Sci.Transl.Med. 2013; 5 (208): 208ra148.

40. Schneider G, Jordan D, Schwarz G, Bischoff P, Kalkman CJ, Kuppe H: Monitoring depth of anesthesia utilizing a combination of electroencephalographic and standard measures. Anesthesiology. 2014; 120 (4): 819–28.

41. Urban BW, Bleckwenn M: Concepts and correlations relevant to general anaesthesia. Br.J.Anaesth. 2002; 89 (1): 3–16.

42. Aranake A, Mashour GA, Avidan MS: Minimum alveolar concentration: ongoing relevance and clinical utility. Anaesthesia. 2013; 68 (5):512–22.

43. Avidan MS, Mashour GA: Prevention of intraoperative awareness with explicit recall: making sense of the evidence. Anesthesiology. 2013; 118 (2):449–56.

44. Punjasawadwong Y, Phongchiewboon A, Bunchungmongkol N: Bispectral index for improving anaesthetic delivery and postoperative recovery. In The Cochrane Database of Systematic Reviews. 6, 6, Y. Punjasawadwong, Ed. Chichester, UK: John Wiley & Sons Ltd, 2014.

45. Friedman EB, Sun Y, Moore JT, Hung HT, Meng QC, Perera P, Kelz MB: A conserved behavioral state barrier impedes transitions between anesthetic-induced unconsciousness and wakefulness: evidence for neural inertia. PLoS.One. 2010; 5 (7):.

46. Miller RD: *Miller's Anesthesia*, 8th ed. Amsterdam: Elsevier, 2015.

47. Sanders RD, Tononi G, Laureys S, Sleigh JW: Unresponsiveness ≠ unconsciousness. Anesthesiology. 2012; 116 (4): 946–59.

48. Whyte SD, Booker PD: Monitoring depth of anaesthesia by EEG. Contin.Educ.Anaesth.Crit.Care Pain. 2003; 3 (4):106–10.

49. Aho AJ, Kamata K, Jäntti V, Kulkas A, Hagihira S, Huhtala H: Comparison of bispectral index and entropy values with electroencephalogram during surgical anaesthesia with sevoflurane. Br.J.Anaesth. 2015; 115:258–66.

50. Constant I, Sabourdin N: The EEG signal: a window on the cortical brain activity. Paediatr.Anaesth. 2012; 22 (6):539–52.

51. Robinson N, Vinod AP, Ang KK, Tee KP, Guan CT: EEG-based classification of fast and slow hand movements using wavelet-CSP algorithm. IEEE.Trans. Biomed.Eng. 2013; 60 (8):2123–32.

52. Soehle M, Kuech M, Grube M, Wirz S, Kreuer S, Hoeft A, Ellerkmann RK: Patient state index vs bispectral index as measures of the electroencephalographic effects of propofol. Br.J.Anaesth. 2010' 105: 172–8.

53. Lindholm ML, Träff S, Granath F, Greenwald SD, Ekbom A, Lennmarken C, Sandin RH: Mortality within 2 years after surgery in relation to low intraoperative bispectral index values and preexisting malignant disease. Anesth.Analg. 2009; 108 (2): 508–12.

54. Monk TG, Saini V, Weldon BC, Sigl JC: Anesthetic management and one-year mortality after noncardiac surgery. Anesth.Analg. 2005; 100 (1): 4–10.

55. Leslie K, Myles PS, Forbes A, Chan MTV: The effect of bispectral index monitoring on long-term survival in the B-aware trial. Anesth.Analg. 2010; 110 (3): 816–22.

56. Sessler D. I., Sigl, J. C., Kelley, S. D., Chamoun, N. G., Manberg, P. J., Saager, L., Greenwald, S: Hospital stay and mortality are increased in patients having a 'triple low' of low blood pressure, low bispectral index, and low minimum alveolar concentration of volatile anesthesia. Anesthesiology. 2012; 116 (6): 1195–1203.

57. Dahaba AA: Different conditions that could result in the bispectral index indicating an incorrect hypnotic state. Anesth.Analg. 2005; 101 (3): 765–73.

58. Schuller PJ, Newell S, Strickland PA, Barry JJ: Response of bispectral index to neuromuscular block in awake volunteers. Br.J.Anaesth., 2015; 115: I95–I103.

59. Mashour GA, Orser BA, Avidan MS: Intraoperative awareness. Anesthesiology. 2011; 114 (5):1218–33.

60. Mashour GA, Avidan MS: Intraoperative awareness: controversies and non-controversies. Br.J.Anaesth. 2015; 115: I20–I26.

61. Kelz MB, Sun Y, Chen J, Cheng Meng Q, Moore JT, Veasey SC, Dixon S, Thornton M, Funato H, Yanagisawa M: An essential role for orexins in emergence from GA. Proc.Natl.Acad.Sci.USA. 2008; 105 (4): 1309–14.

62. Kenny J. D., Chemali, J. J., Cotten, J. F., Van Dort, C. J., Kim, S. E., Ba, D., Solt, K: Physostigmine and methylphenidate induce distinct arousal states during isoflurane GA in rats. Anesth.Analg. 2016; 123 (5): 1210–19.

63 Dahaba AA, Bornemann H, Rehak PH, Wang G, Wu XM, Metzler H: Effect of flumazenil on bispectral index monitoring in unpremedicated patients. Anesthesiology. 2009; 110 (5): 1036–40.

64. Ferreira A, Nunes CS, Castro A, Ferreira AL, Pedrosa S, Amorim P: Propofol requirements for anesthesia induction show wide individual variability, independently of age, gender, weight and height [abstract]. In *The Anesthesiology Annual Meeting*, 2015.

65. Nunes CS, Mendonca T, Bras S, Ferreira DA, Amorim P: Modeling anesthetic drugs' pharmacodynamic interaction on the bispectral index of the EEG: the influence of heart rate. In the *29th Annual International Conference of the IEEE Engineering in Medicine and Biology Society*, 2007, pp. 6479–82.

66. Kazama T, Ikeda K, Morita K, Kikura M, Ikeda T, Kurita T, Sato S: Investigation of effective anesthesia induction doses using a wide range of infusion rates with undiluted and diluted propofol. Anesthesiology. 2000; 92 (4): 1017–28.

Analgesia: Effects on Response to Nociceptive Stimulation

Emmanuel Boselli and Mathieu Jeanne

Introduction

Conscious patients undergoing regional anaesthesia are able to interact with caregivers and indicate when they are feeling pain and/or anxiety during surgery. Unconscious patients on the other hand, not only in the operating room but also in intensive care, need antinociception when a nociceptive stimulus is applied. In these patients, the dose of antinociceptive drugs cannot be adjusted or the effect of locoregional anaesthesia supplementing general anaesthesia cannot be determined by simply asking the patient. Thus, the clinician needs to rely on monitors of the nociception/antinociception (N/AN) balance to be able to provide adequate, that is personalized, antinociception.

Defining Analgesia and Nociception in Non-conscious States

The reader will have noticed that the terms 'nociception' and 'antinociception' rather than 'pain' and 'analgesia' are being used. The term 'analgesia' refers to pain, which has been defined by WHO as 'an unpleasant sensory and emotional experience associated with actual or potential tissue damage, or described in terms of such damage'. In other words, it describes how a conscious being integrates a nociceptive stimulus into a negative emotional experience. Therefore, the term 'analgesia' cannot be used in non-conscious states such as those induced by hypnotic drugs during general anaesthesia, and the term 'antinociception' has to be used instead. But given the state of unconsciousness induced by anaesthetic drugs, how can we quantify nociception after a noxious stimulus has been applied to the mechanical or biochemical sensors in the human body that generate nociceptive signals? And how can we account for inter-individual variability?

Antinociception has traditionally been quantified with non-specific measurements of the clinical response to noxious stimuli such as loss of verbal response, immobility and absence of hypertension and tachycardia, which are indicators of loss of consciousness, loss of motor response or loss of haemodynamic reactivity, respectively. How can antinociception (i.e. absence of verbal response, immobility, and absence of hypertension and tachycardia after a noxious stimulus) be provided?

One way to prevent so-called 'purposeful movement' is to administer a potent inhaled anaesthetic. At 1MAC or 1.3MAC, they ensure 50% or 95% of the patients will not move (see Chapter 6 for more details). The end-expired partial pressure needed to attain the same probability of response suppression is decreased by GABA-acting agents (benzodiazepines, propofol), NMDA antagonists (ketamine), α_2-adrenergic agonists (clonidine or dexmedetomidine) and of course the potent opioids (the drugs most commonly used to provide antinociception during general anaesthesia). All these drugs have in common that they attenuate the autonomic nervous system (ANS) response to nociception that we usually observe as tachycardia and hypertension. Regional analgesia prevents noxious stimuli from reaching the central nervous system, thus also attenuating the ANS response. This chapter will mainly focus on monitoring the effects of the nociception/antinociception balance via the ANS response.

Quantitative and Modelling Information

Administration of Opioids: The Pharmacokinetic/Pharmacodynamic Models

Opioids can be administered as intermittent boluses, by manually adjusting a continuous infusion or by using a target controlled infusion (TCI) device, with the target being either the plasma (Cp) or effect-site concentration (C_e). They are often titrated towards haemodynamic goals such as heart rate and blood pressure. TCI systems are based upon pharmacokinetic/pharmacodynamic (PK/PD) models. Targeting effect-site rather than plasma concentration takes the hysteresis into account. The effect-site concentration is by definition directly correlated with the effect. TCI is intended to improve bias ('offset') and accuracy ('togetherness'), and thus helps ensure more stable and predictable opioid concentrations, but biological variability will continue to place a limit on the accuracy and bias of these devices. The benefits related to the use of these devices are still a matter of debate since, from a PD point of view, the optimal target is not the concentration predicted by PK/PD models but an individual's response that should be measured, or at least estimated, in each patient. Based on the measurement of the effect, the concentration of drugs can be adjusted until it attains the targeted effect.

Administering an opioid dose to an individual patient that is likely to provide a certain concentration and a certain effect based on a population model goes a long way towards achieving personalized, 'optimized' or 'tailored' anaesthesia, but ultimately and optimally we must also measure the clinical effect to ascertain that it has indeed been obtained and use the clinical effect in the individual to help steer further drug administration.

How to Achieve Personalized Analgesia

Personalized *anaesthesia* may be achieved by using monitors that measure any of the several components of anaesthetic depth such as immobility provided by neuromuscular blockers [3, 4] (with a neuromuscular transmission monitor), depth of hypnosis (with monitors like the bispectral index (BIS), state entropy (SE), or any other EEG derived index [5, 6]), and the N/AN balance (with several commonly called 'analgesia monitors'). 'Analgesia monitors' actually is a misnomer, 'antinociception monitors' or 'N/AN balance monitors' would be the more correct terms. Most analgesia monitors are based on quantifying measurable responses directly related to the variations *in tonus* of the ANS (sympathetic and parasympathetic activity) in relation to changes occurring in the N/AN balance [7, 8]. These monitors use various physiological signals: heart rate, heart rate variability, blood pressure, skin conductance, plethysmograph waveform, pupil diameter or sometimes a combination of them (composite indicators). They can also integrate signals coming from EEG activity. These monitors are reviewed in the remainder of this chapter.

How to Measure Antinociception

Monitors that Use Signals from the Cerebral Cortex as an Indication of the Nociception/Antinociception Balance

Several monitors derive an 'analgesia index' from cortical activation after a nociceptive stimulus, assuming this response to reflect 'a state of antinociception'. The indices are dimensionless numbers, and are the results from complex signal analysis and indicator extraction (see Chapter 5 for details). The qNOX index for example results from the analysis of four EEG spectral bands between 0.5 and 44 Hz. Clinical studies have shown that the qNOX was mildly correlated with the effect-site concentration of remifentanil and with the probability of response to nociception [9].

Monitoring Sympathetic and Parasympathetic Activity as a Surrogate for the Nociception/Antinociception Balance

The sympathetic and parasympathetic systems are affected by the N/AN balance and simultaneously affect several organ systems, the responses of which can be used to help quantify this balance.

Analgesia/Nociception Index®

The Analgesia/Nociception Index® (ANI) (MDoloris Medical Systems, Lille, France) is a wavelet transform-based heart rate variability index with values between 0 and 100, and is a measure of the relative parasympathetic tone [8, 10]. The ANI is based on the measurement of the impact of ventilation on the R-R interval of the electrocardiogram, and allows a qualitative and quantitative measurement of heart rate variability (HRV), in particular in the high-frequency power (0.15–0.5 Hz) (see Fig. 8.1) [11]. The ANI was primarily developed to assess the N/AN balance during general anaesthesia [11]. In clinical practice, high ANI values (> 55–60) indicate parasympathetic predominance, i.e. adequate antinociception, whereas low ANI values (< 50) indicate sympathetic predominance, i.e. nociception [8, 10]. Briefly, a low ANI denotes insufficient 'analgesia'.

The performance of ANI has been evaluated in several studies both in children and in adults during general anaesthesia.

In children receiving desflurane titrated to a BIS of 50, a standardized nociceptive stimulus (ulnar tetanic

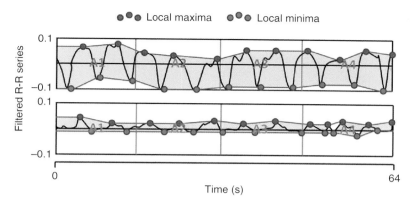

Fig. 8.1 Mean centered, normalized and band pass-filtered R-R series in two different levels of nociception/antinociception balance (upper panel: surgical stimulus in the case of adequate nociception/antinociception balance, lower panel: surgical stimulus in the case of inadequate antinociception (lower panel). Figure reproduced from [8] (with permission).

stimulation) was applied after stepwise reductions of a remifentanil infusion (from 0.2 to 0.04 µg/kg/min). The ANI was always lower after than before stimulation, and lower with lower doses of remifentanil [12]. In another study in children, the ANI was used to predict failure of regional anaesthesia (defined by an increase in heart rate by > 10% within 2 min after skin incision). Area under the receiver-operating curve (ROCAUC) to identify regional anaesthesia failure was 0.747, with a 79% sensitivity and 62% specificity for ANI values <51 [13].

While maintaining the BIS within 30–60 with propofol in adults, a stepwise increase of the remifentanil C_e from 0 to 2 and 4 ng/mL followed by tetanic stimulation of the ulnar nerve resulted in a median ANI of 24, 30 and 13, respectively. Prediction of movement by ANI following stimulation was poor, with a prediction probability (Pk) 0.41; Pk is a statistical measure analogous to ROC AUC, with 0.5 indicating a prediction probability equal to flipping a coin [14]. Similar results were observed in patients under a sevoflurane and fentanyl general anaesthesia: mean ANI decreased from 52 to 33 (p<0.005) after airway manipulation and from 63 to 38 (p<0.001) after skin incision (indicating that the ANI reflected the effect of the noxious stimulus well), but the prediction probability for a 10% increase of heart rate and or systolic blood pressure was low (Pk of 0.61 and 0.59, respectively) [15]. During total knee replacement, the ANI 'early detected' haemodynamic reactivity (defined as a 20% increase in heart rate or systolic blood pressure following intraoperative stimulation) (ROC AUC = 0.92), with 80% sensitivity and 88% specificity at the ANI threshold of 63 [16].

However, if the objective is to optimize analgesic drug titration, it is important to be able to predict whether a decrease in ANI (= poor N/AN balance) will occur after a noxious stimulus rather than merely being able to detect it *post factum*. This has been reported on

in three studies, with various results. During suspension laryngoscopy using propofol/remifentanil or desflurane/remifentanil general anaesthesia, ANI was a good predictor of haemodynamic reactivity (ROC AUC 0.88 and 0.77 with propofol/remifentanil and desflurane/remifentanil, respectively) [17, 18]. The predictive performance of dynamic variations of ANI within 1 min (ΔANI) was even better (ROC AUC = 0.90, with 85% sensitivity and specificity for a variation of –19% in 1 min) [18]. However, when fentanyl rather than remifentanil was used during surgery, the prediction probability of the ANI to predict more than 10% increase in heart rate or systolic blood pressure was poor (P_K 0.61 and 0.59, respectively)[15]. The PK/PD differences in remifentanil (a short-acting opioid with short elimination half-life of < 10 min) and fentanyl (a long-acting opioid with long elimination half-life of > 10 min) may explain these discrepancies [19, 20].

ANI values at the end of surgery and immediately before extubation may help predict immediate postoperative pain [21]. A negative linear relationship was observed between ANI immediately before extubation and NRS [0–10 numerical rating scale (NRS)] on arrival in the PACU. In an observational study performed in 200 patients undergoing ear, nose and throat or lower limb orthopaedic surgery with general anaesthesia using an inhalational agent and remifentanil, the ANI prior to extubation predicted the occurrence of pain (NRS>3) after arrival in PACU well (ROC AUC = 0.89, with 86% sensitivity and specificity for ANI < 50) [21]. In 120 patients undergoing elective laparoscopic cholecystectomy, Szental et al reported that the morphine administration guided by the ANI instead of by clinical signs did not decrease the rate of moderate/severe pain or the use of rescue analgesia in PACU [22]. However, morphine might not have been the optimal choice for ANI guidance considering its slow onset and long acting PK/

PD properties. When fentanyl boluses were titrated to maintain the ANI ≥ 50 instead of using standard clinical administration in 50 patients undergoing lumbar discectomy or laminectomy, postoperative NRS pain scores were lower (1.3 on average), rescue fentanyl administration was less frequent and nausea scores lower [23].

To summarize, the ANI is a continuous 0–100 index of the relative (i.e. parasympathetic/sympathetic) ANS tone. ANI values decrease after insufficiently blunted nociception and its dynamic variations that may help predict haemodynamic reactivity. It intends to optimize intraoperative titration of opioids, but it requires further clinical validation. ANI monitoring cannot be used in patients with cardiac arrhythmia (because the R-R interval is erratic), patients suffering from ANS dysfunction (because this might alter ANI values), and may be impaired in patients receiving inotropic

drugs or β-blockers, although this has to be further evaluated.

Cardiovascular Depth of Analgesia®

The algorithm of the CARdiovascular DEpth of ANalgesia® or CARDEAN index (Alpha-2 Ltd, Lyon, France) predicts hypertension followed by tachycardia based on beat-to-beat analysis of blood pressure and heart rate. The index (0–100%) measures the degree of inhibition of the baroreflex caused by an inadequate N/AN balance [8]. Higher values indicate high levels of baroreflex inhibition, defined as a paradoxical decrease in the R-R interval following an increase in systolic blood pressure and correspond to nociception, whereas an increase in the R-R interval is expected after an increase in systolic blood pressure in the presence of adequate analgesia (see Fig. 8.2). In a

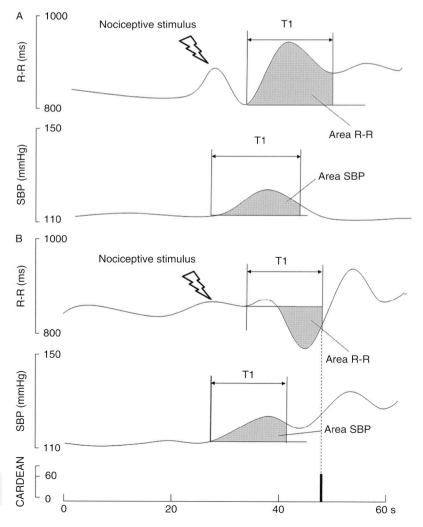

Fig. 8.2 R-R and systolic blood pressure (SBP) series at two different levels of the nociception/antinociception balance; A) surgical stimulus in case of adequate anti-nociception (upper panel), B) surgical stimulus in the case of inadequate antinociception (lower panel). Figure reproduced from [8] (with permission).

retrospective study in 40 ASA 1–2 patients undergoing knee surgery under general anaesthesia without muscle relaxant, the CARDEAN predicted intraoperative movement with high accuracy (ROC AUC = 0.98, with 100% sensitivity and 95% specificity for a CARDEAN index > 60). When propofol was used to maintain the BIS at 40–60 in patients undergoing colonoscopy, titrating alfentanil to the CARDEAN index rather than to conventional signs (e.g. tachycardia, hypertension or movement) decreased the incidence of unexpected movements by 51% [34]. When propofol (titrated to a BIS of 40–60) and remifentanil were used to provide general anaesthesia for spinal disc repair [24], skin incision increased CARDEAN values if C_e remifentanil was 2 ng/mL, but not when it was 4 ng/mL.

Summarized, preliminary data indicate that the CARDEAN index can be related to the N/AN balance; further clinical validation is warranted.

Pupillometry

The pupil diameter results from the balance between the sympathetic dilator tone and the parasympathetic constrictor tone [25]. It can change in many different situations, both in healthy subjects and in several disease states, including brain trauma. During anaesthesia, the pupil diameter changes both after the administration of certain drugs, especially – but not exclusively – after opioid administration and, in a reflex manner, after noxious stimulation. A portable infra-red pupillometry device can be used to measure pupil size and pupillary reflexes, in particular the pupillary dilation reflex (PDR) in response to a homogeneous noxious tetanic stimulation during anaesthesia [8, 25, 26].

In anaesthetized volunteers receiving a constant tetanic electrical stimulus, increasing alfentanil concentrations impaired the PDR but had no effect on the pupillary light reflex (PLR) [27]. The relationship between alfentanil concentrations and the post-stimulus change in pupil size was exponential. The authors concluded that the dilation of the pupil in response to a noxious stimulus was a measure of the A/AN balance in anaesthetized patients.

Several studies attest to the performance of this technique to measure the N/AN balance. During TCI with propofol and increasing concentrations of remifentanil (0 to 5 ng/mL), pupil size after a constant tetanic stimulus decreased from 1.55±0.72 mm to 0.01 ± 0.03 mm with increasing C_e remifentanil; pupil dilation and remifentanil concentration were inversely correlated [28]. The decrease in pupil response to a nociceptive stimulus correlated better with C_e remifentanil than with haemodynamics or BIS measurements.

In children receiving anaesthesia with sevoflurane and alfentanil, pupillary dilation after skin incision was a more sensitive measure of noxious stimulation than haemodynamic variables and BIS values [29]. The pupillary diameter increased by 200 ± 40 % within 1 min after skin incision, with a rapid return to pre-incision values after alfentanil administration.

In 80 female patients undergoing vacuum aspiration while receiving propofol and remifentanil TCI, the PDR amplitude (mean ± SD) was significantly (p<0.001) greater in movers (2.0 ± 1.2 mm) than in non-movers (0.6 ± 0.7 mm) following a homogeneous noxious stimulation (standardized tetanic stimulation) [30]. The performance of PDR amplitude in predicting movement was good, with an AUC ROC of 0.90 (95% CI 0.83–0.96). The PDR amplitude associated with a 50% and 95% probability of non-movement after noxious stimulation was 1.39 mm (95% CI, 0.96–2.20) and 0.29 mm (95% CI, 0.17–0.55). The authors concluded PDR amplitude monitoring could help optimize opioid administration during general anaesthesia.

Pupillometry has been used to assess the effectiveness of regional anaesthesia combined with general anaesthesia in both adults [31] and children [13]. In 24 adult patients undergoing elective foot or ankle surgery under general anaesthesia combined with a popliteal sciatic nerve block, the median [interquartile] PDR response to standardized lower limb tetanic stimulation was blunted to only 2% [1–4] in the blocked leg, whereas a 17% [13–24] increase was observed in the non-blocked leg (p<0.01) [31]. In 58 children undergoing elective surgery with combined general anaesthesia (with sevoflurane) and regional anaesthesia (central or peripheral nerve blocks), the effectiveness of regional anaesthesia was assessed using the pupillary diameter. A PDR cut-off value of > 4.2 mm identified regional anaesthesia failure (defined by a rise in heart rate ≥ 10% from baseline within 2 min after skin incision) with 58% sensitivity and 79% specificity.

Finally, the PDR has been used to assess immediate postoperative analgesia. In 100 patients, postoperative pain intensity was assessed shortly after arrival in the post-anaesthesia care unit using a 0–5 verbal rating scale (VRS) where zero equalled no pain, and five extreme pain. VRS values were linearly correlated with PDR ($\rho = 0.88$, p<0.0001). The threshold value of PDR corresponding to the highest accuracy to have VRS>1 was 23%, with 91% sensitivity and 98% specificity.

In summary, pupillometry seems to be an accurate marker of the N/AN balance, with the pupil diameter increasing with nociception and the PDR decreasing in cases of adequate antinociception. Pupillometry may help assess the efficacy of regional anaesthesia if combined with general anaesthesia, both in adults and in children. In the immediate postoperative period, a PDR value > 23% after noxious stimulation in the awake patient may accurately predict whether (s)he will be suffering from pain. The optimal thresholds to guide intraoperative analgesia need to be determined. The technique has some drawbacks. Pupillometry is not a continuous measurement – intermittent tetanic stimulations are required to measure PDR. In addition, its use may be limited when the eye of the patient is not accessible due to the nature of the surgery (e.g. head and neck or neurosurgery, steep Trendelenburg position) (see Fig. 8.3).

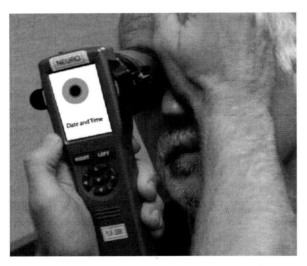

Fig. 8.3 Portable pupillometer in use. Figure reproduced from [25] (with permission).

Skin Conductance

Skin conductance (SC) measures the modulation of electrical conductivity of the skin due to sweat production related to sympathetic activity [7, 8]. Fluctuations in SC in response to noxious stimulation depend on the level of antinociception present. One advantage of SC as compared with HRV or other measures derived from sympathetic nervous system activity is that the neurotransmission to the sweat glands is not adrenergic and thus is not influenced by the administration of β-blockers. The monitor measures SC changes from peak and trough values obtained over time (see Fig. 8.4) via three electrodes placed on palmar or plantar skin, and calculates the number of fluctuations in skin conductance (NFSC) and the corresponding AUC (expressed in µS) [32]. After sympathetic activation, e.g. after intraoperative noxious stimulation, the NFSC increases, which may indicate inadequate analgesia [32].

SC monitoring did not reliably predict changes in stress hormone plasma levels throughout the intraoperative period [33]. In a pilot study in 25 patients admitted to the PACU, a positive linear relationship ($\rho = 0.625$, $p<0.01$) was observed between NRS pain scores and NFSC, with a cutoff value of 0.1 for NFSC to detect NRS > 3 with 89% sensitivity and 74% specificity [34]. This was further confirmed by the same authors in another prospective study with 75 patients, with a prediction probability (P_K) of 0.775 for NFSC > 0.1 to detect NRS > 3, corresponding to 89% sensitivity and 68% specificity [35]. In children aged 1 to 16 years, the ROC AUC for NFSC to detect moderate or severe pain was 0.82 (95% CI, 0.79–0.85), with 90% sensitivity and 64% specificity at a cutoff NFSC of 0.13 [36].

SC was studied for its ability to predict arousal from general anaesthesia. It performed worse than the BIS [37, 38]. SC has also been tested for its ability to predict hypotension after spinal anaesthesia. In 30 elderly

Fig. 8.4 Skin conductance level as a function of time. Figure reproduced from [8] (with permission).

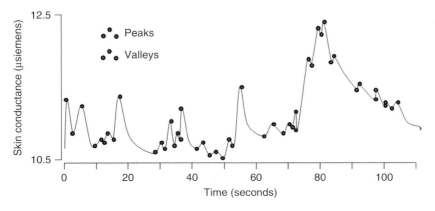

patients older than 60 years receiving spinal anaesthesia for elective urological or orthopaedic surgery [50], SC predicted hypotension (>15% decrease from baseline) with 73% sensitivity and 78% specificity [39]. In 40 pregnant women undergoing caesarean section with spinal anaesthesia, there was no significant relationship between baseline sympathetic tone measured by SC and hypotension [40].

Monitors that Combine Different Signals into One Indicator

Surgical Pleth Index®

The Surgical Pleth Index (SPI) (GE Healthcare, Helsinki, Finland) is a dimensionless number computed from the photoplethysmographic signal of the pulse oximeter. It records the heart beat interval (HBI) and the pulse wave amplitude (PPGA) (see Fig. 8.5). The SPI has been empirically defined as:

$$SPI = 100 - (0.7 * PPGA_{norm} - HBI_{norm}) \quad (1)[8, 41]$$

For clinical use, an SPI value close to 100 indicates a very high stress level, whereas an SPI close to zero indicates a very low stress level. Struys et al studied SPI and heart rate responses to a standard electrical tetanic stimulation under various opioid concentrations. SPI correlated better with opioid concentration than response entropy or heart rate, suggesting that SPI could be a useful

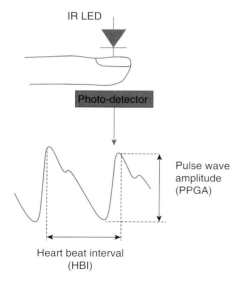

Fig. 8.5 Photoplethysmography and photopletysmographic waveform. An infra-red (IR) LED illuminates the skin and the photodetector measures changes in light absorption due to blood flow. Figure reproduced from [8] (with permission).

measurement of the N/AN balance [42]. Similar results were found in patients undergoing neurosurgery, but hypovolaemia and treated chronic hypertension were identified as factors affecting SPI interpretation [43].

SPI-guided opioid administration lowered intraoperative remifentanil consumption and improved haemodynamic stability compared to standard practice [44] and in another study reduced both opioid and hypnotic drug consumption compared to the use of clinical parameters, which resulted in faster recovery times [45].

The Nociception Level Index

The Nociception Level (NoL) is a multiparameter index that combines the photoplethysmographic waveform amplitude (PPGA), heart rate, heart rate variability (in the 0.15–0.4 Hz power band), skin conductance level (SCL) and the number of skin conductance fluctuations (NSCF) [46]. The estimated multiparameter composite index derived from regression analyses was scaled from 0 to 100 to produce the NoL index. Clinical data at the time of writing are still limited. Skin incision and intubation during propofol and remifentanil anaesthesia increased the mean NoL by eight and 18, respectively, with NoL variations between post- and pre-stimulus values (ΔNoL) being better at differentiating noxious from non-noxious stimuli (ROC AUC = 0.95) than differences in heart rate (0.84) or mean arterial pressure (0.78) [47]. Similar results were observed during general anaesthesia in 58 patients receiving sevoflurane and remifentanil, with good performance (ROC AUC = 0.93) of NoL to discriminate noxious from non-noxious stimuli (tetanic stimulation with and without fentanyl analgesia, intubation, first incision/trocar insertion, and a noxious stimulus free period)[48]. While this suggests the NoL may be a useful index to optimize the intraoperative administration of opioids, this has to be confirmed.

The Noxious Stimulation Response Index

The Noxious Stimulation Response Index (NSRI) is an index based on the analysis of the interaction between hypnotics and opioids. The NSRI has been proposed to predict the likelihood of a response to a noxious stimulus during general anaesthesia [49]. It is incorporated in the Smart Pilot (Dräger, Lübeck, Germany), a drug dosing advisory display.

In 44 patients receiving increasing C_e of propofol and remifentanil, the probability of movement after laryngoscopy was observed. From these data, the prediction probability (P_K) of NSRI different clinical endpoints was calculated using a bootstrap technique [49]. NSRI was then used to predict the response to different noxious stimuli. The median [95% CI] P_K of NSRI for loss of response to tetanic stimulation was 0.87 [0.75–0.96] but only 0.77 [0.68–0.85] for loss of eyelash reflex or sedation score, suggesting that NSRI is an interesting index to predict response to noxious stimulation and to a lesser extent the hypnotic effect. Although promising and despite having been clinically available for many years, this sophisticated index remains poorly studied to date and requires further clinical evaluation.

Closed-loop Anaesthetic Systems

Closed-loop Anaesthesia

The main obstacle to the development of an automatic control closed-loop system to titrate opioids is the lack of a good clinical N/AN end-point that can be translated into a reliable monitor. Currently there is no single or multiple input signal in the human body accurately and specifically reflecting the balance between the response to a nociceptive stimulation during surgery and the effects of antinociceptive drugs and techniques: the ideal N/AN monitor remains elusive at this time. If and when a good surrogate parameter becomes available, it is hoped that closed-loop systems might increase the safety of general anaesthesia in a manner similar to how autopilots increased the safety record of air-travel or to how ABS brake systems improved car driving conditions.

Table 8.1 for example suggests some ranges of parameters of different N/AN monitors that could

be used to titrate remifentanil. Remifentanil could be a particularly useful drug for closed-loop systems because of its time-independent context-sensitive half-time and short hysteresis [20]. The feasibility of using the ANI to guide automated remifentanil administration (Fig. 8.6) has been recently reported [50].

Conclusion

While monitoring the depth of hypnosis or neuromuscular blockade has become routine, N/AN monitoring remains somewhat elusive. Several monitors are currently being developed, and a variety of approaches are being taken. Most of them measure a parameter that is indicative of the balance of the tone of the sympathetic versus the parasympathetic nervous system. All have advantages and limitations, and the clinical potential for basically all still needs to be defined or refined. ANI relies on the analysis of heart rate variability and cardiac rhythm, and can help reduce pain and opioid consumption in PACU. Pupillometry seems a particularly promising technique to help titrate opioids, but

Table 8.1. Monitors and thresholds that could be used for closed-loop antinociception devices.

Index	Threshold for remifentanil overdose (low probability of nociception)	Threshold for remifentanil underdose (high probability of nociception)
ANIm	80–90	45–55
SPI	NA	50–60
PDR	NA	5–10
CARDEAN	NA	50–60

Fig. 8.6 Principle of a remifentanil-ANI/systolic blood pressure-loop.

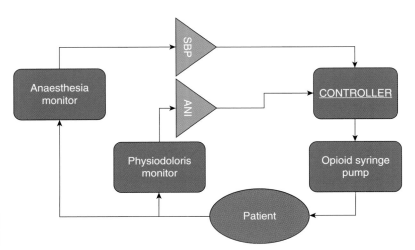

unfortunately can only be used intermittently. The SPI may reduce intraoperative opioid use. Other indexes (CARDEAN, SC, NSRI, NoL) show promising results but require more studies. Closed-loop systems that dose opioids to specific target ranges of N/AN monitors may help personalize analgesia and improve patient safety. The search for the ideal ANC/NC monitor continues to be part of our quest for a 'personalized analgesia'.

References

1. Aranake A, Mashour GA, Avidan MS: Minimum alveolar concentration: ongoing relevance and clinical utility. Anaesthesia. 2013; 68: 512–22.

2. Minto CF, Schnider TW: Contributions of PK/PD modeling to intravenous anesthesia. Clin.Pharmacol. Ther. 2008; 84: 27–38.

3. Checketts MR, Alladi R, Ferguson K, Gemmell L, Handy JM, Klein AA, Love NJ, Misra U, Morris C, Nathanson MH, Rodney GE, Verma R, Pandit JJ: Recommendations for standards of monitoring during anaesthesia and recovery 2015: Association of Anaesthetists of Great Britain and Ireland. Anaesthesia. 2016; 71: 85–93.

4. Lien CA, Kopman AF: Current recommendations for monitoring depth of neuromuscular blockade. Curr. Opin.Anaesthesiol. 2014; 27: 616–22.

5. Punjasawadwong Y, Boonjeungmonkol N, Phongchiewboon A: Bispectral index for improving anaesthetic delivery and postoperative recovery. Cochrane Database Syst. Rev. 2007: CD003843.

6. Chhabra A, Subramaniam R, Srivastava A, Prabhakar H, Kalaivani M, Paranjape S: Spectral entropy monitoring for adults and children undergoing general anaesthesia. Cochrane Database Syst. Rev. 2016; 3: CD010135.

7. Gruenewald M, Ilies C: Monitoring the nociception-anti-nociception balance. Best Pract.Res.Clin. Anaesthesiol. 2013; 27: 235–47.

8. De Jonckheere J, Bonhomme V, Jeanne M, Boselli E, Gruenewald M, Logier R, Richebe P: Physiological signal processing for individualized anti-nociception management during general anesthesia: A review. Yearb.Med.Inform. 2015; 10: 95–101.

9. Jensen EW, Valencia JF, Lopez A, Anglada T, Agusti M, Ramos Y, Serra R, Jospin M, Pineda P, Gambus P: Monitoring hypnotic effect and nociception with two EEG-derived indices, qCON and qNOX, during general anaesthesia. Acta Anaesthesiol. Scand. 2014; 58: 933–41.

10. Boselli E, Bouvet L, Allaouchiche B: Analgesia monitoring using Analgesia/Nociception Index: Results of clinical studies in awake and anesthetized patients. Le Praticien en Anesthésie Réanimation 2015; 19: 78–86.

11. Logier R, Jeanne M, De Jonckheere J, Dassonneville A, Delecroix M, Tavernier B: PhysioDoloris: a monitoring device for analgesia / nociception balance evaluation using heart rate variability analysis. Conf.Proc.IEEE. Eng.Med.Biol.Soc. 2010; 2010: 1194–7.

12. Sabourdin N, Arnaout M, Louvet N, Guye ML, Piana F, Constant I: Pain monitoring in anesthetized children: first assessment of skin conductance and analgesia-nociception index at different infusion rates of remifentanil. Paediatr.Anaesth. 2013; 23: 149–55.

13. Migeon A, Desgranges FP, Chassard D, Blaise BJ, De Queiroz M, Stewart A, Cejka JC, Combet S, Rhondali O: Pupillary reflex dilatation and analgesia nociception index monitoring to assess the effectiveness of regional anesthesia in children anesthetised with sevoflurane. Paediatr.Anaesth. 2013; 23: 1160–5.

14. Jordan D, Steiner M, Kochs EF, Schneider G: A program for computing the prediction probability and the related receiver operating characteristic graph. Anesth.Analg. 2010; 111: 1416–21.

15. Ledowski T, Averhoff L, Tiong WS, Lee C: Analgesia Nociception Index (ANI) to predict intraoperative haemodynamic changes: results of a pilot investigation. Acta.Anaesthesiol.Scand. 2013; 58: 74–9.

16. Jeanne M, Delecroix M, De Jonckheere J, Keribedj A, Logier R, Tavernier B: Variations of the analgesia nociception index during propofol anesthesia for total knee replacement. Clin.J.Pain. 2014; 30: 1084–8.

17. Boselli E, Bouvet L, Bégou G, Torkmani S, Allaouchiche B: Prediction of hemodynamic reactivity during total intravenous anesthesia for suspension laryngoscopy using Analgesia/Nociception Index (ANI): a prospective observational study. Minerva.Anestesiol. 2015; 81: 288–97.

18. Boselli E, Logier R, Bouvet L, Allaouchiche B: Prediction of hemodynamic reactivity using dynamic variations of Analgesia/Nociception Index (ANI). J. Clin.Monit.Comput. 2016; 30: 977–84.

19. Boselli E, Jeanne M: Analgesia/nociception index for the assessment of acute postoperative pain. Br.J.Anaesth. 2014; 112: 936–7.

20. Egan TD: Remifentanil pharmacokinetics and pharmacodynamics. A preliminary appraisal. Clin. Pharmacokinet. 1995; 29: 80–94.

21. Boselli E, Bouvet L, Bégou G, Dabouz R, Davidson J, Deloste JY, Rahali N, Zadam A, Allaouchiche B: Prediction of immediate postoperative pain using the analgesia/nociception index: a prospective observational study. Br.J.Anaesth. 2014; 112: 715–21.

22. Szental JA, Webb A, Weeraratne C, Campbell A, Sivakumar H, Leong S: Postoperative pain after laparoscopic cholecystectomy is not reduced by intraoperative analgesia guided by analgesia nociception index (ANI(R)) monitoring: a randomized clinical trial. Br.J.Anaesth. 2015; 114: 640–5.

23. Upton HD, Ludbrook GL, Wing A, Sleigh JW: Intraoperative "Analgesia Nociception Index"-guided fentanyl administration during sevoflurane anesthesia in lumbar discectomy and laminectomy: a randomized clinical trial. Anesth.Analg. 2017; 125: 81–90.

24. Rossi M, Cividjian A, Fevre MC, Oddoux ME, Carcey J, Halle C, Frost M, Gardellin M, Payen JF, Quintin L: A beat-by-beat, on-line, cardiovascular index, CARDEAN, to assess circulatory responses to surgery: a randomized clinical trial during spine surgery. J.Clin. Monit.Comput. 2012; 26: 441–9.

25. Larson MD, Behrends M: Portable infrared pupillometry: a review. Anesth.Analg. 2015; 120: 1242–53.

26. Guignard B: Monitoring analgesia. Best.Pract.Res.Clin. Anaesthesiol. 2006; 20: 161–80.

27. Larson MD, Kurz A, Sessler DI, Dechert M, Bjorksten AR, Tayefeh F: Alfentanil blocks reflex pupillary dilation in response to noxious stimulation but does not diminish the light reflex. Anesthesiology. 1997; 87: 849–55.

28. Barvais L, Engelman E, Eba JM, Coussaert E, Cantraine F, Kenny GN: Effect site concentrations of remifentanil and pupil response to noxious stimulation. Br.J.Anaesth. 2003; 91: 347–52.

29. Constant I, Nghe MC, Boudet L, Berniere J, Schrayer S, Seeman R, Murat I: Reflex pupillary dilatation in response to skin incision and alfentanil in children anaesthetized with sevoflurane: a more sensitive measure of noxious stimulation than the commonly used variables. Br.J.Anaesth. 2006; 96: 614–19.

30. Guglielminotti J, Grillot N, Paule M, Mentre F, Servin F, Montravers P, Longrois D: Prediction of movement to surgical stimulation by the pupillary dilatation reflex amplitude evoked by a standardized noxious test. Anesthesiology. 2015; 122: 985–93.

31. Isnardon S, Vinclair M, Genty C, Hebrard A, Albaladejo P, Payen JF: Pupillometry to detect pain response during general anaesthesia following unilateral popliteal sciatic nerve block: a prospective, observational study. Eur.J.Anaesthesiol. 2013; 30: 429–34.

32. Storm H: Changes in skin conductance as a tool to monitor nociceptive stimulation and pain. Curr.Opin. Anaesthesiol. 2008; 21: 796–804.

33. Ledowski T, Pascoe E, Ang B, Schmarbeck T, Clarke MW, Fuller C, Kapoor V: Monitoring of intra-operative nociception: skin conductance and surgical stress index versus stress hormone plasma levels. Anaesthesia. 2010; 65: 1001–6.

34. Ledowski T, Bromilow J, Paech MJ, Storm H, Hacking R, Schug SA: Monitoring of skin conductance to assess postoperative pain intensity. Br.J.Anaesth. 2006; 97: 862–5.

35. Ledowski T, Bromilow J, Wu J, Paech MJ, Storm H, Schug SA: The assessment of postoperative pain by monitoring skin conductance: results of a prospective study. Anaesthesia. 2007; 62: 989–93.

36. Hullett B, Chambers N, Preuss J, Zamudio I, Lange J, Pascoe E, Ledowski T. Monitoring electrical skin conductance: a tool for the assessment of postoperative pain in children? Anesthesiology. 2009; 111: 513–17.

37. Ledowski T, Bromilow J, Paech MJ, Storm H, Hacking R, Schug SA. Skin conductance monitoring compared with Bispectral Index to assess emergence from total i.v. anaesthesia using propofol and remifentanil. Br.J.Anaesth. 2006; 97: 817–21.

38. Ledowski T, Preuss J, Ford A, Paech MJ, McTernan C, Kapila R, Schug SA: New parameters of skin conductance compared with Bispectral Index monitoring to assess emergence from total intravenous anaesthesia. Br.J.Anaesth. 2007; 99: 547–51.

39. Ledowski T, Preuss J, Kapila R, Ford A: Skin conductance as a means to predict hypotension following spinal anaesthesia. Acta.Anaesthesiol.Scand. 2008; 52: 1342–7.

40. Ledowski T, Paech MJ, Browning R, Preuss J, Schug SA. An observational study of skin conductance monitoring as a means of predicting hypotension from spinal anaesthesia for caesarean delivery. Int.J.Obstet. Anesth.2010; 19: 282–6.

41. Huiku M, Uutela K, van Gils M, Korhonen I, Kymalainen M, Merilainen P, Paloheimo M, Rantanen M, Takala P, Viertio-Oja H, Yli-Hankala A: Assessment of surgical stress during general anaesthesia. Br.J.Anaesth. 2007; 98: 447–55.

42. Struys MM, Vanpeteghem C, Huiku M, Uutela K, Blyaert NB, Mortier EP: Changes in a surgical stress index in response to standardized pain stimuli during propofol-remifentanil infusion. Br.J.Anaesth. 2007; 99: 359–67.

43. Bonhomme V, Uutela K, Hans G, Maquoi I, Born JD, Brichant JF, Lamy M, Hans P: Comparison of the surgical Pleth Index with haemodynamic variables to assess nociception-anti-nociception balance during general anaesthesia. Br.J.Anaesth. 2011; 106: 101–11.

44. Chen X, Thee C, Gruenewald M, Wnent J, Illies C, Hoecker J, Hanss R, Steinfath M, Bein B: Comparison of surgical stress index-guided analgesia with standard clinical practice during routine general anesthesia: a pilot study. Anesthesiology. 2010; 112: 1175–83.

45. Bergmann I, Gohner A, Crozier TA, Hesjedal B, Wiese CH, Popov AF, Bauer M, Hinz JM: Surgical pleth index-guided remifentanil administration reduces remifentanil and propofol consumption and shortens recovery times in outpatient anaesthesia. Br.J.Anaesth 2013; 110: 622–8.

46. Ben-Israel N, Kliger M, Zuckerman G, Katz Y, Edry R: Monitoring the nociception level: a multi-parameter approach. J.Clin.Monit.Comput. 2013;

47. Martini CH, Boon M, Broens SJ, Hekkelman EF, Oudhoff LA, Buddeke AW, Dahan A: Ability of the nociception level, a multiparameter composite of autonomic signals, to detect noxious stimuli during propofol-remifentanil anesthesia. Anesthesiology. 2015; 123: 524–34.

48. Edry R, Recea V, Dikust Y, Sessler DI: Preliminary intraoperative validation of the Nociception Level Index: A noninvasive nociception monitor. Anesthesiology. 2016; 125: 193–203.

49. Luginbuhl M, Schumacher PM, Vuilleumier P, Vereecke H, Heyse B, Bouillon TW, Struys MM: Noxious stimulation response index: a novel anesthetic state index based on hypnotic-opioid interaction. Anesthesiology. 2010; 112: 872–80.

50. De Jonckheere J, Delecroix M, Jeanne M, Keribedj A, Couturier N, Logier R: Automated analgesic drugs delivery guided by vagal tone evaluation: interest of the Analgesia Nociception Index (ANI). Conf.Proc.IEEE. Eng.Med.Biol.Soc. 2013; 2013: 1952–5.

Personalized Sedation and Analgesia

Michael M. Beck, Jeffrey B. Horn and Ken B. Johnson

Introduction

The practice of medicine often requires procedures that cause pain and anxiety. With the advent of modern anaesthesia these procedures have become commonplace and tolerable. Procedures with the greatest degree of pain are frequently accomplished during a state of general anaesthesia. Many procedures, however, are performed under sedation and analgesia. In contrast to general anaesthesia, sedation and analgesia use short acting medications to alleviate pain and anxiety while leaving patients capable of maintaining their airway and basic physiological functions.

This chapter discusses goals, terminology, key elements and challenges of procedural sedation and analgesia (PSA). It also reviews application of existing drug delivery technology to enhance sedation practice and selected innovations that have the potential to better personalize sedation and analgesia. Existing drug delivery technologies in sedation practice include manually controlled and target-controlled infusions (TCI) and patient controlled sedation and analgesia. Selected innovations include the introduction of drug display technologies that provide real-time visualization of sedative–analgesic interactions and the development of a computer assisted personalized sedation (CAPS) device for moderate sedation.

Goals of Sedation and Analgesia

There are several objectives when providing sedation and analgesia, some of which may be in opposition to one another. The primary objective, keeping a patient safe (e.g. oxygenated and ventilated), can conflict with the goals of providing amnesia, relaxation (immobility) and analgesia to optimize surgical conditions for a successful procedure. Thus, providing sedation and analgesia is a delicate and occasionally dangerous endeavour that mandates the need for practitioners with specialized training in the realm of anaesthesiology.

Patient Safety

As healthcare costs continue to rise, proceduralists seek opportunities to perform increasingly complex surgical procedures out-of-the-operating-room (OOR) with the use of PSA. With an ageing population and the potential serious concomitant comorbidities, sedation practitioners must be adept at patient selection, drug choice and recognizing the dangers associated with deeper than intended sedation.

Patient safety can be defined as the avoidance of adverse events during PSA. Adverse events that may occur during PSA include apnoea, airway obstruction, haemodynamic instability, cardiac arrhythmia or arrest, permanent neurological deficits and death. OOR procedures continue to be performed with minimal uniformity in guidelines by healthcare providers often with no accredited training in anaesthesiology and a wide range of sedation training and experience. Because of this, it is difficult to collect data on the frequency of adverse events during PSA. Although recommended by many authors, no standard in reporting adverse events during PSA exists.

Patient Comfort

While secondary to patient safety, patient comfort is an important goal of PSA. Patient comfort begins with communication prior to beginning sedation or the procedure. The sedation practitioner and proceduralist should explain to the patient what to expect and the sedation practitioner should elicit the patient's expectations as well. The goal is to provide an agreed upon level of anxiolysis, amnesia and analgesia while maintaining patient safety.

Generally, these goals are largely achieved through medications; however, it is important to consider non-pharmacological adjuncts as well. Ensuring that the patient is in a comfortable position that is also acceptable to the proceduralist before initiating sedation can avoid difficulties later during the procedure. With paediatric patients, it can be beneficial to consider the benefit of the presence or absence of a parent or caregiver.

Procedure Optimization

A final goal of PSA is to optimize conditions for safe completion of the procedure. Key elements include (1) minimizing patient movement and providing patient relaxation and (2) communication between the proceduralist and sedation practitioner and between the sedation practitioner and the patient to adjust dosing of sedatives and analgesics as needed.

Terminology

The Sedation Continuum

Although the accepted definition of sedation is easily interpreted as a decreased level of consciousness or awareness, a clinically relevant definition has yet to be elucidated or accepted. The historically popular term 'Conscious Sedation' has fallen out of favour while many other terms continue to be used interchangeably in the literature, including: monitored anaesthesia care (MAC), monitored sedation, procedural sedation, deep sedation, moderate sedation, light sedation, sedation and analgesia, and anxiolysis.

Standardized terminology provides a basis for improving sedation quality and patient safety, and reporting adverse outcomes. Due to incongruent regulations and guidelines, patients, proceduralists and sedation practitioners adhere to a wide range of sedation expectations. Patients may expect no pain or awareness during a procedure. Proceduralists may expect patients to lie still during critical segments of a procedure. Sedation practitioners may expect their patient to respond to verbal prompts and breathe spontaneously. A succinct description of sedation levels in characterizing the goals of these competing expectations is therefore needed.

In 1999, the American Society of Anesthesiologists (ASA) published a sedation continuum as part of their practice guidelines for sedation and analgesia by non-anaesthesiologists [1] (Table 9.1). The continuum separates sedation and analgesia into four distinct yet subtle phases: (1) minimal sedation, (2) moderate sedation and analgesia, (3) deep sedation and analgesia and (4) general anaesthesia. Each phase is characterized by the impact on patient responsiveness, airway patency, ventilatory drive and cardiovascular function, which is followed by a brief summary of the rescue skills a non-anaesthesiologist should have when targeting a desired phase of PSA.

A couple of important points of this sedation continuum merit additional explanation. First, labels of moderate and deep sedation include both 'sedation and analgesia'. This is a more accurate representation that reflects the common practice of combining sedatives and analgesics for procedures associated with brief intermittent painful stimuli. Second, while under moderate sedation and analgesia, patients should maintain capability of responding to verbal and tactile stimuli, breathe spontaneously and maintain cardiovascular function. This feature makes moderate sedation attractive to sedation practitioners with limited airway skills and experience in managing cardiac or ventilatory depression. Given that patients remain responsive to verbal and tactile stimuli, one disadvantage of moderate sedation is the possibility of experiencing awareness and/or pain during portions of a procedure.

Deep sedation and analgesia is defined as a patient responsive to verbal and painful stimuli. It may be associated with impaired ventilatory function that may require airway manipulation and manual ventilatory support. Patients are less likely to be aware and/or perceive portions during their procedure. This is an

Table 9.1. The sedation continuum.

	Minimal Sedation (Anxiolysis)	Moderate Sedation/Analgesia (Conscious Sedation)	Deep Sedation/Analgesia	General Anaesthesia
Responsiveness	Normal response to verbal stimulation	Purposeful* response to verbal or tactile stimulation	Purposeful* response after repeated or painful stimulation	Unarousable, even with painful stimulus
Airway	Unaffected	No intervention required	Intervention may be required	Intervention often required
Spontaneous ventilation	Unaffected	Adequate	May be inadequate	Frequently inadequate
Cardiovascular function	Unaffected	Usually maintained	Usually maintained	May be impaired

* Reflex withdrawal from a painful stimulus is not considered a purposeful response.

Developed by the American Society of Anesthesiologists; approved by the ASA House of Delegates 13 October, 1999.

attractive feature to patients that wish to be unaware of the procedure; however, deep sedation necessitates practitioners to possess advanced airway management skills, provide life-saving temporary ventilatory support, and have the capability of recognizing and treating subtle changes in cardiovascular function (e.g. high or low blood pressure, fast or slow heart rate).

Sedation practitioners with limited experience in airway management and cardiopulmonary support may intend to deliver moderate sedation, but for various reasons, administer a deeper plane of sedation that may require rescue manoeuvres beyond their skill or experience level. Reasons for unintended deeper plane of sedation may include excessive drug administration, perceived patient awareness or pain, or requests from proceduralists to provide additional sedation and analgesia. A crucial element of sedation practice is the ability to recognize deeper than intended sedation while undertaking life-saving measures to lighten the depth of sedation.

Finally, the transition from one phase of sedation to another can be subtle. Detection of a transition to deeper than intended level of sedation requires heightened vigilance with repeated assessments of responsiveness, airway patency and ventilatory function in order to provide timely rescue manoeuvres.

Self-Rescue and Loss of Responsiveness

Loss of responsiveness to verbal and tactile stimulation marks an important transition from moderate to deep sedation. This crucial transition is associated with an increased likelihood of adverse cardiopulmonary events. Responsive patients can 'self-rescue' from a partial or complete airway obstruction as well as hypoventilation when prompted to breathe. Once a patient is rendered unresponsive, the burden of rescue has transitioned to the sedation practitioner. Rescue manoeuvres may require advanced airway skills and prompt pharmacological intervention. Provider rescue may involve calling for help, stopping delivery of sedatives and analgesics, administration of reversal agents if appropriate, positioning the patient to optimize airway management, returning the patient to the intended sedation state and communication with the proceduralist regarding the most prudent course of action (e.g. cancelling the procedure if unsafe or difficult to complete at the intended sedation state, or proceeding to a general anaesthetic).

Sedation practitioners may tolerate brief periods of loss of responsiveness as long as pulmonary function is not compromised. A major concern with sedatives, especially propofol, is the relaxation of oropharyngeal

structures that increases the likelihood of partial or complete airway obstruction. Dosing to achieve moderate but not deep sedation is advised when non-anaesthesia trained practitioners administer PSA. If patients cannot tolerate a procedure with moderate sedation, then a physician anaesthesiologist may be required to provide deep sedation and/or general anaesthesia. As always, sedation practitioners should practise within their scope of credentialing, experience and clinical skills.

Key Elements of Sedation

Key elements of a safe sedation practice include a dedicated sedation practitioner who is a distinctive person from the proceduralist, appropriate sedation practitioner training and qualifications, careful patient selection, use of appropriate patient monitors, and a working knowledge of the clinical pharmacology of sedatives and analgesics. Additional detail regarding patient monitoring and the clinical pharmacology of sedatives and analgesics is presented below.

Patient Monitoring

Patient monitoring during sedation and analgesia is primarily directed at detecting adverse cardiopulmonary events [2, 3]. Monitoring standards [1] for sedation recommend frequent assessment of responsiveness, blood pressure, respiratory rate, temperature and oxygen-haemoglobin saturation. In addition, continuous monitoring of the electrocardiogram is recommended along with the ability to detect common arrhythmias. Emergency airway equipment, supplemental oxygen and reversal agents should be immediately available in the procedural suite and post-procedural care area [1]. This section will briefly review monitoring of oxygenation, ventilation, capnography and circulation.

Oxygenation

Assessments of oxygenation include skin colour and pulse oximetry. Pulse oximetry is a standard of care throughout the world and mandated by numerous agencies [4]. Randomized controlled trials [5, 6], however, have reported earlier identification and response to hypoxia, but have failed to demonstrate a reduction in adverse events or an improvement in patient outcomes. Although there are conflicting findings in the literature, pulse oximetry is an innocuous monitor that allows earlier detection of hypoxia compared to no pulse oximetry monitoring.

One limitation of pulse oximetry is the delay between the onset of apnoea, hypopnoea or airway obstruction and a decrease in oxygen-haemoglobin saturation. While breathing room air, healthy individuals can take several minutes before their oxygen saturation drops. Supplemental oxygen only prolongs that delay. For this reason, some sedation practitioners elect not to provide supplemental oxygen. Capnography, by contrast, can detect a decrease or absence of exhaled carbon dioxide much sooner than a decrease in oxygen saturation.

Ventilation

Assessments of ventilatory function include visual observation of chest rise, facemask fogging, impedance measurements of respiratory rate via the electrocardiogram leads, and presence of exhaled carbon dioxide. Detection of inadequate ventilation can be difficult in a sedation setting. Patients may exhibit chest wall movement yet have inadequate ventilation due to partial or complete airway obstruction.

Capnography

In 2011, the ASA added capnography to the recommended list of required monitors for moderate and deep sedation. The aim was to improve monitoring of ventilatory function through continuous detection of exhaled carbon dioxide. Capnography can be more effective at detecting apnoea and/or hypopnoea than pulse oximetry or even direct patient observation.

Capnography may also help sedation practitioners detect partial obstruction even in the presence of chest wall movement. Sedatives can produce airway obstruction before they substantially impair ventilatory drive. In this condition, patients exhibit chest wall movement, but do not ventilate the lungs. This can lead to a paradoxical chest wall movement (a dyssynchronous movement of the chest and abdomen) that, with the abdominal wall and chest covered by the procedure drapes, may appear as normal ventilatory effort.

Proper interpretation of the capnogram may warrant some additional considerations. First, some upper endoscopy procedures may use carbon dioxide to distend the gastrointestinal tract to better visualize tissues. Capnography signals in this case do not represent lung exhalation and do not confirm adequate ventilation. Second, if using high oxygen flows near the carbon dioxide sampling line, exhaled carbon dioxide may be washed away and go undetected or be detected intermittently. Third, most capnography monitors are designed to report a value for the end-tidal carbon dioxide level. The monitor assumes that the signal source is an endotracheal tube or supraglottic airway. When used in sedation practice, there is no endotracheal tube or supraglottic airway present, and the capnography sensor is placed within a face mask or nasal cannula. The gas analyser thus will not be exclusively sampling end-expired gas, but a mixture of end-expired gas and gas from the immediate environment. Consequently, when used in this configuration, the sampled gas does not represent end-tidal gas, and may provide spurious respiratory rates because sampling of these mixed gases may cause CO_2 oscillations that are interpreted as consecutive respiratory efforts. To sedation practitioners unfamiliar with this nuance, the capnograph can be difficult to interpret. Capnography monitors should be configured to present the presence or absence of carbon dioxide, not quantify it, and may not accurately present the respiratory rate.

Selected professional societies (The American Society for Gastrointestinal Endoscopy, ASGE, the American Gastroenterological Association, AGA, and the American College of Gastroenterology, ACG) and various studies [7, 8] have pointed out insufficient or conflicting data demonstrating improved clinical outcomes with the use of capnography. The ASGE, AGA and ACG suggest that the use of capnography will lead to excess cost without a proven benefit. Additionally, without standardized definitions and appropriate clinical responses to capnography findings, the use of this technology for PSA is claimed to be questionable. These professional groups do, however, endorse further collaboration with the ASA to develop and validate definitions and appropriate interventions based on capnography. Although the literature presents conflicting outcomes, the authors recommend the use of capnography in all patients undergoing PSA and affirm that it will provide indispensable and timely information to avert preventable sources of morbidity and mortality including hypoxic neurological damage and death. Clinical assessments [2, 9] or a single monitor of ventilation may be misleading and unreliable [10, 11]. To fully monitor ventilatory function (O_2 delivery and CO_2 removal), complementary measures (pulse oximetry and capnography) should be used.

Chapter 10 discusses the pathophysiology of respiratory depression in anaesthesia and a full discussion of monitoring systems to quantify it.

Circulation

Haemodynamic monitoring during sedation and analgesia includes continuous electrocardiography, non-invasive blood pressure and heart rate. Monitoring standards recommend that the blood pressure be measured at 5-minute intervals while the heart rate and electrocardiogram be continuously monitored [1]. It is important to keep in mind that these parameters are a surrogate of end-organ perfusion and should be used with procedures that require sedation.

Clinical Pharmacology of Sedatives and Analgesics

The pharmacological profiles of selected common sedative and analgesic drugs are presented in Table 9.2 [12, 13]. Approaches to drug delivery for sedation and analgesia include intermittent boluses and continuous infusions. Infusions can be manually controlled, target controlled or patient controlled. Several core principles of clinical pharmacology are important to

Table 9.2. Pharmacological profile of selected sedatives and analgesics [12, 13].

Drug Name	Mechanism of Action	Onset of Action (min)	Time to Peak Effect (min)	Duration of Action (min)	Sedative/ Analgesic Dosing Titrate to Effect	Antagonist/ Reversal Agent	Side Effect Profile
Benzodiazepines							
Midazolam	GABA agonist	1–2	3–4	30–80	0.02–0.03 mg/kg	Flumazenil	Dose-dependent respiratory depression
Diazepam		2–3	3–5	360	5–15 mg		Hypotension
Opiods							
Remifentanil	μ-receptor agonist	1–3	3–5	3–10	0.5–3 μg/kg	Naloxone	Dose-dependent respirator depression Nausea/Vomiting
Fentanyl		1–2	3–5	30–60	0.5–2 μg/kg		Dose-dependent respiratory depression Nausea/Vomiting Bradycardia Muscle rigidity
Meperidine		3–6	5–7	60–180	5–10 mg		Dose-dependent respiratory depression Nausea/Vomiting Active metabolite [Twitching] Interaction with MAOI
Other							
Dexmeditomidine	α_2-Agonist	3–5	15	Unknown	0.5–1 μg/kg over 10 minutes	None	Hypotension Bradycardia
Ketamine	NMDA antagonist	<1	1	10–15	1–2 mg/kg		Hallucination Laryngospasm
Propofol	GABA agonist	<1	1–2	4–8	0.25–1 mg/kg		Dose-dependent respiratory depression Cardiovascular instability Pain on injection
Antagonists/Reversal Agents							
Naloxone	μ-receptor antagonist	1–2	5	30–45	Overdose: 0.4–2 mg Respiratory depression: 0.04–0.4 mg	None	Hypertension Tachycardia
Flumazenil	GABA antagonist	1–2	3	60	0.2 mg every 1 minute Not to exceed 1 mg		Agitation Flushing Headache Muscle tension

consider when formulating a safe and effective dosing regimen. These include time to peak effect, titration and opioid–sedative interactions. The reader is also referred to Chapters 1 and 3 for further discussion of pharmacological concepts.

Time to Peak Effect

Perhaps the safest approach to sedation is the titration of small boluses over time to achieve a desired effect using the least amount of drug possible. This approach requires an understanding of the time to peak effect, which can be longer than expected for selected drugs used in sedation practice. Initial bolus doses are based on observations in patient populations. Subsequent bolus doses are titrated based on individual patient responses. Large bolus doses used to achieve a desired effect quickly have the disadvantage of excessive effect leading to deeper than intended sedation. The times to peak effect for selected sedatives and analgesics are presented in Table 9.3. A few clinical nuances of these times to peak effect include the following:

- Remifentanil has a substantially faster time to peak effect than fentanyl or morphine. Central ventilatory depression can be more pronounced with remifentanil. Its rapid onset limits the amount of time for blood carbon dioxide levels to rise and offset opioid ventilatory depression.
- The long time to peak effect for morphine is important to consider for procedures of brief duration and a planned same day discharge. It will reach peak effect long after the procedure has been completed and will likely still have an effect even after discharge to home.
- The time to onset of anxiolysis for midazolam is rapid (seconds) and may be misconstrued as

the peak effect. Sedation practitioners should keep in mind the time to peak effect may be up to 5 minutes after the first manifestation of anxiolysis.

- When titrating midazolam and propofol, patients may exhibit a biphasic response. This manifests as an excitatory disinhibition at lower effect-site concentrations followed by decreased responsiveness or unresponsiveness at higher effect-site concentrations. The time to peak effect is important to consider when administering additional bolus doses to achieve the desired level of sedation. This can be challenging when providing sedation for brief but stimulating procedures.
- Patients that chronically consume opioids and/ or benzodiazepines may require larger doses to achieve desired effects. The concentration–effect relationship in this patient group is difficult to ascertain. Suggested initial bolus doses based on prior observations in otherwise healthy patient populations can be ineffective. Accounting for the time to peak effect can be useful when carefully titrating to effect in this patient group.

Titration

Careful titration is used to achieve desired effects (sedation and analgesia) while minimizing adverse effects (unresponsiveness, ventilatory depression). Titration consists of many small doses rather than one large one. As an example, consider Fig. 9.1. It presents two dosing schemes for the same amount of propofol, 75 mg, based on published propofol dosing regimens for endoscopy procedures [12]. Administering the 75 mg in four divided doses separated by three minutes produces a much different profile in the probability of unresponsiveness than administering all 75 mg at once.

This simulation illustrates that larger propofol boluses can lead to a high probability of unresponsiveness for several minutes. When unresponsive, the ability of a patient to self-rescue with prompting is lost. As mentioned above, this represents an important transition from moderate to deep sedation or general anaesthesia where patient rescue is entirely up to the sedation practitioner.

Opioid–Sedative Interactions

Opioid–sedative interactions for several drug effects (e.g. sedation, ventilatory depression, loss of responsiveness, etc.) are synergistic, meaning that when an opioid is combined with a sedative, they accentuate the effects of one another. Opioids act primarily

Table 9.3. Simulations of time to peak effect for bolus doses of select sedatives and analgesics.

Drug	Time to Peak Effect (minutes)
Sedatives	
Propofol	1–1.5
Midazolam	6–9
Ketamine	2–10
Opioids	
Remifentanil	1–1.5
Sufentanil	1–3
Fentanyl	3–5
Morphine	75–90

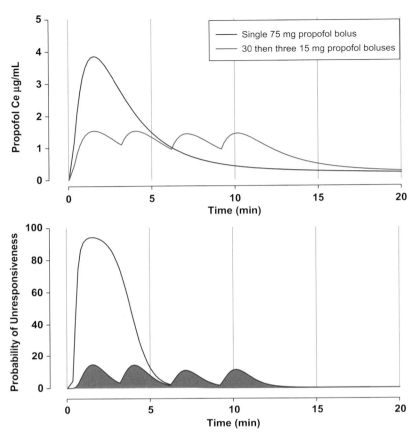

Fig. 9.1 Simulations of predicted propofol effect site concentrations (C_e) and the probability of unresponsiveness over time using two dosing schemes using suggested propofol bolus dosing to achieve sedation during endoscopy procedures [12]. The first regimen is a single 75 mg bolus. The second regimen is a series of four intermittent boluses of 30, 15, 15 and 15 mg separated by three minutes. Both deliver the same amount of drug (75 mg). The single bolus dose yields a high probability of unresponsiveness (greater than 50%) for up to four minutes whereas the intermittent small boluses yield a low probability of unresponsiveness (less than 20%) for over ten minutes.

at opioid receptors to produce analgesia. High doses are required to render a patient unresponsive. By contrast, common sedatives act via gamma-aminobutyric acid receptors and have little analgesic effect. When administering either a sedative or an opioid without the other, large doses are required to achieve desired therapeutic effects for both analgesia and sedation. For example, if using a sedative, in order to tolerate painful procedures, large doses are required to the point where patients may become unresponsive. If using an opioid, patients may better tolerate painful stimuli, but are likely to experience ventilatory depression. When combined, sedatives and analgesics achieve therapeutic goals yet minimize many of the adverse effects from dosing them as a single agent.

Figure 9.2 presents a simulation of fentanyl co-administered with propofol adapted from suggested doses of each for sedation during brief endoscopy procedures [14]. The dosing regimen consists of a simultaneous bolus of propofol 0.3 mg/kg and fentanyl 1 μg/kg. The simulation predicts both the drug effect-site

concentrations and selected drug effects to include predictions of unresponsiveness, sedation, analgesia, and ventilatory depression. It also presents the predicted effects from each drug individually.

Important points from this simulation include:

- When co-administered at the same time, propofol reaches peak effect faster than fentanyl by up to two minutes.

- The probability of unresponsiveness (defined as no response to verbal and painful tactile stimuli) is low, but not inconsequential. For two minutes, there is up to a 20% probability that a patient will not respond. This may be of concern with patients that require prompting to breathe to maintain their oxygenation.

- As dosed, the probability of sedation reaches up to 60% for several minutes (in other words, up to six out of ten people will be sedated for this period of time). Sedation was defined as loss of verbal response to name combined with a non-painful tactile stimulus.

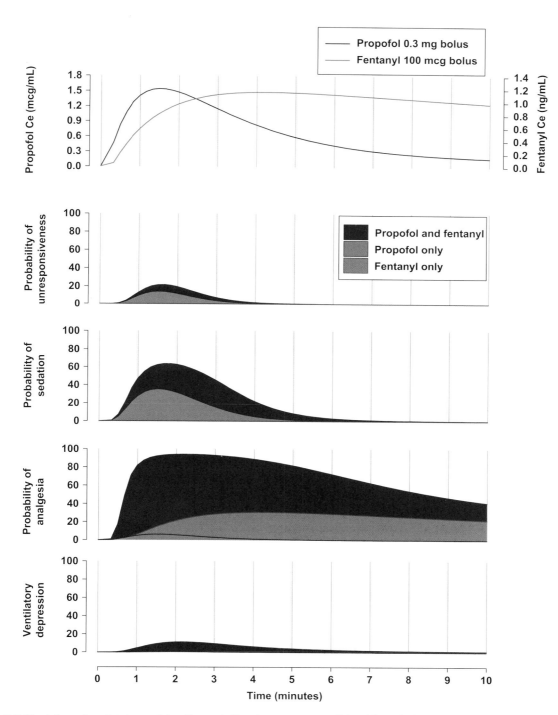

Fig. 9.2 Simulations of predicted propofol and fentanyl effect-site concentrations (C_e) and the probabilities of unresponsiveness, sedation, analgesia and ventilatory depression over time using a suggested dosing scheme for sedation during endoscopy procedures [14]. The regimen consists of a 0.3 mg/kg propofol bolus and a 1 μg/kg fentanyl bolus administered simultaneously. The single bolus dose yields a high probability of ventilatory depression in an un-stimulated state. Each simulation of drug effects plots the individual effect from propofol alone (light blue), fentanyl alone (red) and fentanyl combined with propofol (dark blue). Patient demographics and definitions of each predicted effect are presented in Table 9.4.

- With only propofol, the probability of sedation reaches up to 40% for a few minutes with no significant analgesic effect.
- With only fentanyl, the probability of analgesia reaches up to 30% for several minutes with no significant sedative effect.
- As dosed, the probability of analgesia is up to 95% and can last for over ten minutes (in other words, up to 19 out of 20 people will be sedated for this period). Analgesia was defined as no response to a moderately painful stimulus.
- Thus, with this dosing regimen, although patients may experience less sedation, when combining opioids and hypnotics, the likelihood a patient will tolerate a moderately painful stimulus is high.
- This dosing regimen is likely to be inadequate for long moderately painful procedures.

- Predictions of ventilatory depression from both drugs were low (less than 12%) for approximately three minutes, but not inconsequential.

Drug Delivery Technology in Sedation Practice

Perhaps the technology that has contributed most to drug delivery in sedation practice is the continuous infusion pump. Popular uses include manually controlled, target controlled and patient controlled infusions. By way of comparison to intermittent bolus dosing, continuous infusions offer several advantages. They provide more consistent effect-site concentrations offering more predictable drug effects over time. They are better suited for delivery of drugs that have a rapid PK profile. To illustrate this point, consider

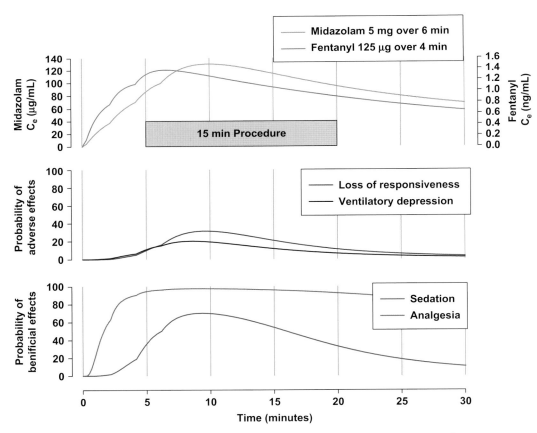

Fig. 9.3 Simulations of predicted midazolam and fentanyl effect-site concentrations (C_e) and the probabilities of unresponsiveness, sedation, analgesia and ventilatory depression over time using suggested intermittent bolus doses for sedation during endoscopy procedures [12, 14]. The regimen consists of 2 mg of midazolam and 75 μg of fentanyl followed by 1 mg of midazolam and 25 mcg of fentanyl two and four minutes later and 1 mg of midazolam six minutes later. Total midazolam was 5 mg over six minutes. Total fentanyl was 125 mcg over four minutes. This simulation assumes a 15-minute procedure associated with intermittent moderately painful stimuli. Table 9.4 presents definitions of 'adequate sedation and analgesia', patient demographics and definitions of predicted effects.

simulations of intermittent bolus dosing and continuous infusion dosing to provide sedation and analgesia for a 15-minute procedure associated with a moderately painful stimulus (Figs. 9.3–9.5).

Figure 9.3 presents intermittent bolus dosing with midazolam and fentanyl using suggested doses for endoscopy procedures [12, 14]. Doses were administered every two minutes for six minutes for a total of 5 mg of midazolam and 125 mcg of fentanyl. This simulation presents estimates of drug effect-site concentrations, the duration of loss of responsiveness, ventilatory depression, sedation, and analgesia. As dosed, fentanyl and midazolam effect-site concentrations reach their respective peaks in eight to ten minutes.

It is useful to critique this and other techniques with several questions: (1) How much time was required to achieve conditions suitable to conduct a procedure? (2) Were conditions adequate throughout the duration of the procedure? (3) Once the procedure was completed, what time was required before the risk of adverse effects (ventilatory depression and loss of responsiveness) dissipated? (4) Once the procedure was completed, what was the time required before the sedation and analgesia dissipated?

With this technique, midazolam and fentanyl were administered five minutes prior to the procedure, yet, as dosed, did not reach peak effect until nearly three minutes after the procedure started. In this condition, a sedation practitioner may be tempted to administer more drug if the patient or proceduralist complained. Without waiting until reaching the peak effect, additional doses may lead to deeper than intended sedation. Once achieved, the concentrations begin to decline yet the beneficial effects persisted throughout the remainder of the procedure. Once the procedure was completed, there was a small risk of both ventilatory depression and loss of

Table 9.4. Patient demographics, models, definitions, assumptions and limitations of pharmacology simulations.

Patient Demographics	
Age: 50	
Gender: Male	
Height: 173 cm	
Weight: 80 kg	
BMI = 26 kg/m²	
PK Models	Predicted Effect
Fentanyl	C_e [20]
Midazolam	C_e [21]
Propofol	C_e [22, 23]
Remifentanil	C_e [24, 25]
PD Interaction Models	Predicted Effect
Loss of Responsiveness*	OAA/S < 2 [26]
Ventilatory Depression	Respiratory rate < four breaths per minute [27]
Analgesia	No response to a moderately painful stimulus [28]
Sedation	OAA/S < 4 [26]
Definitions	
Analgesia to moderately painful stimulus	Loss of response to 30 pounds of focused pressure on the tibia, a moderately painful stimulus
OAA/S < 2	No response to a verbal and painful stimulus
OAA/S < 4	Responds to verbal and tactile stimuli

Table 9.4. (cont.)

Loss of 'Self Rescue'	Probabilities of loss of responsiveness and ventilatory depression both > 10%
Ventilatory Depression	Respiratory rate less than four breaths per minute in an otherwise healthy individual in the absence of any painful stimuli
Adequate Sedation and Analgesia	Probabilities of sedation and analgesia both > 50%
Assumptions	
Normal cardiac output and intravascular volume	
No chronic consumption of opioids and benzodiazepines	
Limitations	
Predictions of ventilatory depression assume absence of painful stimuli	
Not all models properly account for height, weight, gender and age	

BMI = Body Mass Index. C_e = Effect site concentration. OAA/S indicates Observer's Assessment of Alertness/Sedation. *No model of consciousness or awareness exists; only models of responsiveness. Previously published PD models used to illustrate the profiles of anaesthetic drugs in sedation practice are inherently wrong and are unlikely to consistently predict an individual patient's response. However, they are useful to visualize anaesthetic behaviour as it pertains to sedation. Model assumptions and limitations, presented above, should be considered when interpreting model predictions.

responsiveness (< 5%), but the sedation and analgesic effects persisted long after the procedure had ended. As described above, the loss of responsiveness combined with ventilatory depression is an important transition from moderate to deep sedation or even general anaesthesia. In this condition, patients are likely to require provider-rescue, as they are unable to self-rescue with prompts to breathe. Given the relatively slow kinetic profile of midazolam, when administered in combination with fentanyl, the synergistic interaction can lead to prolonged profound ventilatory depression and hypoxia if not recognized. Without proper rescue, this can lead to hypoxic brain injury or death, as was experienced when midazolam was initially introduced.

Manually Controlled Infusions

Manual infusions are often used to provide sedation. By comparison to a bolus technique using fentanyl and midazolam, Figure. 9.4 presents a simulation of manual controlled infusions of remifentanil and propofol for sedation and analgesia. To quickly achieve therapeutic concentrations, before starting the infusions, a small bolus is administered of each drug (0.25 mg/kg of propofol and 0.25 µg/kg remifentanil). This is followed by continuous infusions of 40 and 0.04 µg/kg/min for propofol and remifentanil, respectively. For comparison purposes, the simulations were repeated without the bolus to visualize the impact the boluses had on achieving conditions suitable for a moderately painful procedure.

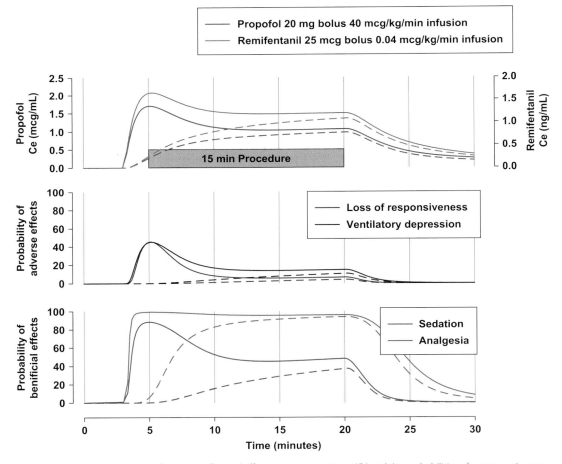

Fig. 9.4 Simulations of predicted propofol and remifentanil effect-site concentrations (C_e) and the probabilities of unresponsiveness, sedation, analgesia and ventilatory depression over time using bolus doses followed by manually controlled continuous infusions. The regimen consists of propofol 0.25 mg/kg and remifentanil 0.25 µg/kg boluses followed by continuous infusions of 40 and 0.04 µg/kg/min respectively. The dotted lines represent the predicted concentrations and effects with no bolus dose of either propofol or remifentanil. This simulation assumes a 15-minute procedure associated with intermittent moderately painful stimuli. Table 9.4 presents definitions of 'adequate sedation and analgesia', patient demographics and definitions of predicted effects.

With this technique, propofol and remifentanil were administered two minutes prior to the procedure. As dosed, they reached near peak effect in less than two minutes. Once maximal effect was achieved, the concentrations declined over the next few minutes and then stabilized throughout the remainder of the procedure. The associated beneficial effects were adequate with a high probability of sedation and analgesia throughout the duration of the procedure. Of note, the probability of analgesia was higher than the probability of sedation. Although there is some concern that there may be inadequate sedation (probability ranged between 50% and 80% throughout the procedure), there was a consistent high probability of analgesia (above 95% throughout). If analgesic, the sedation requirements may be less. This is one of the major advantages of combining an opioid with a sedative.

Once the procedure was completed, there was a risk of both ventilatory depression and loss of responsiveness (15–20%), but it quickly dissipated within two to three minutes of turning off the infusions at the end of the procedure. With the infusions turned off, the sedation and analgesic effects also quickly dissipated and were nearly fully dissipated within ten minutes. This illustrates a key advantage to using propofol and remifentanil for moderately painful procedures that are associated with little to no postoperative pain.

In addition, without the boluses, the infusions require up to ten minutes after the procedure started to achieve therapeutic effects (see dotted lines). Thus, without the dotted lines, infusions alone may not be useful for procedures of this nature and duration. Although both propofol and remifentanil have rapid PK, when administered as continuous infusions, they

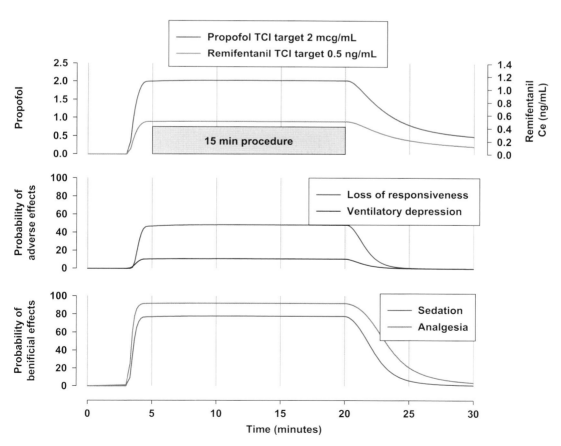

Fig. 9.5 Simulations of predicted propofol and remifentanil effect-site concentrations (C_e) and the probabilities of unresponsiveness sedation, analgesia and ventilatory depression over time using target controlled infusions. The regimen consists of propofol and remifentanil target controlled infusions set to maintain targets of 2 µg/mL and 0.5 ng/mL respectively based on published target concentrations for sedation–analgesia during endoscopic procedures [15]. This simulation assumes a 15-minute procedure associated with intermittent moderately painful stimuli. Table 9.4 presents definitions of 'adequate sedation and analgesia', patient demographics and definitions of predicted effects.

require 10–15 minutes to reach a near steady state. That also holds true when adjusting to a new infusion rate.

Although in some ways easier to use, infusion pumps do carry some inherent risk to patients, and safe use of these devices requires understanding of important principles of intravenous drug behaviour. Sedation practitioners who consider using infusions should have the appropriate training to properly address these concerns.

Target Controlled Infusions

An even more sophisticated approach to infusion delivery of sedation and analgesia is TCI. TCI targets and maintains drug concentrations at a desired level. Figure 9.5 presents a simulation of TCI used for a 15-minute intermittently painful procedure. The dosing regimen consists of two target controlled infusions, for propofol and remifentanil. Target effect-site, concentrations were set at 2 µg/mL and 0.5 ng/mL for propofol and remifentanil respectively. Target effect-site concentrations were selected from published target concentrations for sedation–analgesia during endoscopic procedures [15].

With TCI, propofol and remifentanil were started two minutes prior to the procedure. They reached their target effects in less than two minutes. By comparison to the bolus followed by infusion technique, there was very little change in the resultant effect-site concentrations throughout the procedure. The associated beneficial effects were adequate with a high probability of sedation and analgesia throughout the duration of the procedure. Again, as with the other simulations of propofol and remifentanil, and midazolam and fentanyl, the probability of analgesia was higher than the probability of sedation.

Once the procedure was completed, there was a risk of both ventilatory depression and loss of responsiveness (up to 50%), but it quickly dissipated within three to four minutes of turning off the infusions at the end of the procedure. With the infusions turned off, the sedation and analgesic effects also quickly dissipated and were nearly fully dissipated within ten minutes.

An important advantage of TCI over the manual infusion technique is that there is no need to administer a bolus prior to starting the infusion. Also, should a sedation practitioner desire a higher target concentration, a TCI pump will quickly achieve the new target in a time frame similar to what was observed with the original target (~90 sec). This feature, however, does not hold when decreasing the target concentration.

With decreases or turning the TCI off, drug concentrations and effects will dissipate according to the PK properties of the drug.

One challenge with procedures associated with moderate to severe pain near the beginning of a procedure is to identify a dose that will blunt or even block the response to these painful stimuli while minimizing the risk of loss of responsiveness combined with ventilatory depression, an important transition point from 'self-rescue' to 'provider rescue'. One such procedure group are upper endoscopy and transesophageal echocardiography procedures. They are associated with a significant gag response when placing an endoscope over the posterior third of the tongue. Recent work by Borrat et al explored propofol and remifentanil TCI concentrations to achieve no gag response [16]. Using an up-down method, they found that a median propofol effect site concentration of 2.4 µg/mL in the presence of remifentanil set at 1 ng/mL was needed to block the gag response. Similarly, they found that a median remifentanil effect-site concentration of 0.7 ng/mL in the presence of propofol set to 3 µg/mL was needed to block the gag response. These concentration pairs are somewhat higher than those reported by others for lower and upper endoscopy procedures [12, 14]. To explain this discrepancy, it is likely that topicalization with local anaesthetic was used prior to endoscope insertion, or clinicians and patients tolerated some degree of gag response to endoscope insertion. In sum, it is difficult to achieve a complete block of the gag response without administering enough sedation and analgesia to achieve deep sedation.

Patient Controlled Sedation

Although not widely used, investigators have explored the use of patient controlled TCIs of propofol during upper endoscopy procedures. In a clinical trial comparing patient controlled propofol delivery (0.3 mg/kg bolus with a zero minute lockout) with intermittent midazolam dosing by an anaesthesiologist for colonoscopies in 88 patients, investigators found that the patient controlled propofol administration led to better patient and endoscopist satisfaction compared to anaesthesiologist-administered midazolam [17]. They reported that patients required a mean of 1.7 mg/kg for procedures that lasted a mean of nine minutes. Patients in the propofol group were more sedated during the procedure, but were more alert 30 minutes after the procedure was terminated.

In a preliminary study, 16 patients were allowed to alter the target propofol concentration by 0.2 μg/mL via a handset that they pushed over a 20 minute period prior to their upper endoscopy procedure [18]. Once pushed, there was a two-minute lockout to allow the TCI pump to achieve the new target concentration. The maximal target concentration was set at 3 μg/mL. If no button pushes were noted, the TCI concentration was decreased by 0.2 μg/mL. Of note, the oropharynx was topicalized with local anaesthetic prior to scope insertion. During the upper endoscopy, patients could continue to adjust their sedation. They observed that patients self-titrated to a range of propofol effect-site concentrations of 1.2 to 2.6 μg/mL. Three patients were inadequately sedated using this technique and required that the patient controlled TCI be abandoned.

These studies suggest that patient controlled bolus or target controlled infusions are feasible for endoscopy procedures. This approach, however, has not achieved widespread use. Based on the simulations presented above, it is likely these techniques might have been more successful if an opioid was added either as a fentanyl bolus or as a remifentanil infusion.

Concerns of Continuous Infusions Administered by Non-anaesthesiologist Sedation Practitioners

Continuous infusions of sedatives alone or in combination with analgesics require expertise that many non-anaesthesiologist sedation practitioners may not possess. The infusion techniques described above increase the risk of unrecognized entry into deeper-than-intended sedation states. There are a number of concerns: (1) With infusions, the level of vigilance in assessing a patient's responsiveness and ventilatory function may be diminished. (2) If using infusions only, patients and proceduralists may become impatient and request additional drugs before the existing dosing regimen reaches peak effect. (3) During an adverse event, sedation practitioners may be distracted to the point where they inadvertently do not turn off the infusion.

Innovations that May Improve Sedation Practice

Drug Displays of Sedative–Analgesic Interactions

Through recent advances in characterizing sedative–analgesic interactions, medical device engineers have developed drug displays for use at the point of care. Available drug displays estimate several effects of common sedatives and analgesics (e.g. propofol, midazolam, fentanyl, remifentanil) in terms of sedation, loss of responsiveness, analgesia and ventilatory depression. They use complex models to provide clinicians with estimates of drug concentrations and their effects. Clinicians can use a real-time drug display alongside a physiological monitor. The display is based on what researchers have observed from dosing anaesthetic medications, measuring resultant drug concentrations and effects, and using the data to build mathematical models of drug behaviour [19]. There is a high potential for application of drug display systems in sedation. Chapter 6 thoroughly reviews the topic.

Computer Assisted Personalized Sedation

Computer assisted personalized sedation (CAPS) technology has been recently developed for the administration of propofol by a slow loading dose followed by an infusion to achieve and maintain moderate sedation for brief endoscopy procedures. The target user group is endoscopists and their sedation teams. It was not designed to be used by anaesthesia care providers with advanced airway skills and intimate familiarity with propofol. CAPS uses capnography, pulse oximetry and cardiovascular monitors to frequently assess cardiopulmonary status and patient responsiveness.

A novel sensor added to a CAPS system called SEDASYS® uses a patient response assessment technology. The patient response system intermittently assesses patient responsiveness with a prompt to squeeze a hand-held button. When decreased responsiveness or decreased respiratory function is detected, SEDASYS® turns down or turns off propofol delivery. It is intended as a tool to avoid deeper than intended sedation.

A pivotal trial evaluated this technology in 496 patients undergoing colonoscopy and upper endoscopy procedures [14]. Endoscopist–sedation nurse teams successfully provided minimal to moderate sedation for these procedures using SEDASYS®. SEDASYS® was recently approved for clinical use by the USA Food and Drug Administration and is labelled only for use in American Society of Anesthesiologist PS I–II patients undergoing routine upper endoscopy and colonoscopy procedures. Unfortunately, after only a few years on the market, the manufacture of SEDASYS® removed the system from the market after successful use in thousands of patients.

This system takes advantage of the synergistic relationship between fentanyl and propofol, minimizing the amount of propofol required to achieve sedation during brief noxious stimuli. Figure. 9.6 presents a simulation of a fentanyl–propofol dosing scheme used in a CAPS system. Propofol is administered as a slow loading dose over three minutes followed by an infusion for the remainder of a brief procedure (less than

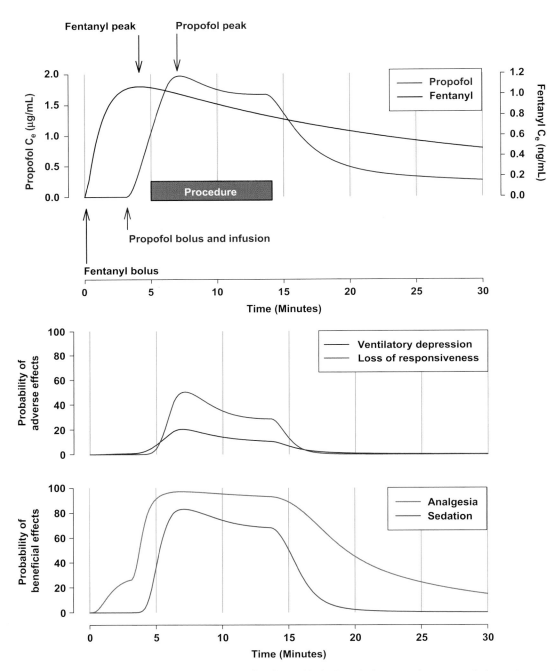

Fig. 9.6 Simulations of effect-site concentrations (C_e, top plot) for a fentanyl bolus (75 µg) administered intravenously three minutes prior to the start of a slow propofol loading dose (0.5 mg/kg) over three minutes followed by a propofol infusion (75 µg/kg/min) for seven minutes. In the middle and bottom plots, the predictions of adverse and beneficial drug effects on a probability range of 1% to 100%. In the presence of a noxious stimulus (e.g. colonoscopy), these simulations likely overestimate the probability of effect. Simulations assume a patient undergoing a colonoscopy where the propofol was turned off after reaching the caecum, the most uncomfortable part of the procedure.

ten minutes). Fentanyl is administered three minutes before propofol.

This simulation illustrates the following points: (1) fentanyl somewhat enhances the sedative effects of propofol and propofol markedly enhances the analgesic effects of propofol. This allows sedation practitioners to administer less of each drug, minimizing oversedation with propofol and respiratory depression with fentanyl. (2) Because fentanyl takes longer to reach peak effect, it is prudent to administer fentanyl early so that fentanyl and the propofol loading dose reach their peak effects at different times, minimizing the risk of respiratory depression. The slow propofol loading dose is administered over three minutes. (3) If an adverse effect (i.e. ventilatory depression) is detected, propofol administration is automatically decreased or terminated. (4) Once the propofol infusion is turned off, the rate of decline in concentration is rapid, offering an advantage over midazolam.

By way of comparison to Figs. 9.4 and 9.5, the time to onset of effect is slower because propofol is administered as a loading dose instead of a bolus. This is done by design to avoid the potentially unwanted loss of responsiveness and partial and complete airway obstruction commonly observed with propofol. This dosing approach required approximately six minutes to achieve maximal effect. During the induction period, to account for patient variability, sedation practitioners were allowed to provide 0.25 mg/kg propofol boluses as needed.

With this dosing regimen, the associated beneficial effects were adequate with a high probability of sedation and analgesia throughout the procedure. Once the procedure was completed, there was a risk of both ventilatory depression and loss of responsiveness (up to 35%), but it quickly dissipated within two to three minutes of turning off the infusions at the end of the procedure. With the infusions turned off, the sedation and analgesic effects also quickly dissipated and had nearly fully dissipated within ten minutes.

Summary

In summary, important guiding principles in personalizing PSA include: (1) With a spontaneously breathing patient, weight normalized slow loading doses and continuous infusions are less likely than rapid large boluses to produce conditions that lead to unresponsiveness in combination with significant ventilatory depression even if the overall doses are the same. (2) Accounting for the synergistic interaction between

sedatives and opioids for desired (e.g. analgesia and sedation) and adverse (e.g. ventilatory depression and unresponsiveness) effects, opioids can be combined with sedatives to administer less of each drug and provide adequate sedation with rapid return to a non-sedated state. (3) Drugs that have a more rapid kinetic profile (e.g. propofol, remifentanil, fentanyl) may be better suited to weight normalized infusions than drugs with slower kinetic profiles (midazolam, morphine, diazepam, etc.).

Advances in drug display technology and infusion pumps may provide sedation practitioners with more sophisticated approaches to delivery of sedatives and analgesics (e.g. TCI, PCAs) as well as a means to visualize predicted drug concentrations and effects (e.g. Smart Pilot and Navigator). Additional advances in automated assessment of patient responsiveness, as has been developed in computer-assisted personalized sedation, may in the future provide an additional layer of personalized safety in guiding the administration of sedatives and analgesics.

Finally, sedation and analgesia is a complex discipline spanning a wide range of healthcare providers with an ever-growing number of procedures being performed OOR. As this practice continues to emerge, it is important to consider key principles of safe sedation practice. These include: (1) Sedation practitioners should target a sedation state that is commensurate with their rescue skill set and credentialing. If trained and credentialed to provide minimal and moderate sedation, targeting one of those sedation states should always be the goal. (2) If the goal is to tolerate the procedure regardless of the sedation state, then a provider with advanced airway skills and the proper training to administer general anaesthesia should provide the sedation. (3) If the patient is unable to tolerate a procedure with moderate sedation and the sedation practitioner is not trained or credentialed to provide deep sedation or general anaesthesia, then the procedure should be postponed until an anaesthesia provider is available. (4) Anaesthesiologists should take the lead in the development of practice guidelines and credentialing requirements at their institutions to ensure safe and effective sedation practices.

References

1. American Society of Anesthesiologists Task Force on S, Analgesia by N-A. Practice guidelines for sedation and analgesia by non-anesthesiologists. Anesthesiology. 2002; 96 (4): 1004–17. PubMed PMID: 11964611.

2. Cohen LB, Wecsler JS, Gaetano JN, Benson AA, Miller KM, Durkalski V, Aisenberg J: Endoscopic sedation in the United States: results from a nationwide survey. Am.J.Gastroenterol. 2006; 101 (5): 967–74. doi:10.1111/j.1572-0241.2006.00500.x. PubMed PMID: 16573781.

3. Krauss B, Green SM: Sedation and analgesia for procedures in children. N.Engl.J.Med. 2000; 342 (13): 938–45. doi:10.1056/NEJM200003303421306. PubMed PMID: 10738053.

4. Shah A, Shelley KH: Is pulse oximetry an essential tool or just another distraction? The role of the pulse oximeter in modern anesthesia care. J.Clin.Monit. Comput. 2013; 27 (3): 235–42. doi:10.1007/s10877-013-9428-7. PubMed PMID: 23314807.

5. Moller JT, Johannessen NW, Espersen K, Ravlo O, Pedersen BD, Jensen PF, Rasmussen NH, Rasmussen LS, Pedersen T, Cooper JB, et al: Randomized evaluation of pulse oximetry in 20,802 patients: II. Perioperative events and postoperative complications. Anesthesiology. 1993; 78 (3): 445–53. PubMed PMID: 8457045.

6. Moller JT, Pedersen T, Rasmussen LS, Jensen PF, Pedersen BD, Ravlo O, Rasmussen NH, Espersen K, Johannessen NW, Cooper JB, et al: Randomized evaluation of pulse oximetry in 20,802 patients: I. Design, demography, pulse oximetry failure rate, and overall complication rate. Anesthesiology. 1993; 78 (3): 436–44. PubMed PMID: 8457044.

7. Mehta P, Kochhar G, Albeldawi M, Kirsh B, Rizk M, Putka B, John B, Wang Y, Breslaw N, Vargo JJ: Capnographic monitoring does not improve detection of hypoxemia in colonoscopy with moderate sedation. A randomized, controlled trial. American College of Gastroenterology; Philadelphia, 2014.

8. Waugh JB, Epps CA, Khodneva YA: Capnography enhances surveillance of respiratory events during procedural sedation: a meta-analysis. J. Clin.Anesth. 2011; 23 (3): 189–96. doi:10.1016/j. jclinane.2010.08.012. PubMed PMID: 21497076.

9. Van de Velde M, Roofthooft E, Kuypers M: Risk and safety of anaesthesia outside the operating room. Curr. Opin.Anaesthesiol. 2008; 21 (4): 486–7. doi:10.1097/ ACO.0b013e328304d95e. PubMed PMID: 18660658.

10. Tanaka PP, Tanaka M, Drover DR: Detection of respiratory compromise by acoustic monitoring, capnography, and brain function monitoring during monitored anesthesia care. J.Clin.Monit.Comput. 2014; 28 (6): 561–6. doi:10.1007/s10877-014-9556-8. PubMed PMID: 24420342.

11. Vargo JJ, Zuccaro G, Jr., Dumot JA, Conwell DL, Morrow JB, Shay SS: Automated graphic assessment of respiratory activity is superior to pulse oximetry and visual assessment for the detection of early respiratory depression during therapeutic upper endoscopy. Gastrointest.Endosc. 2002; 55 (7): 826–31. PubMed PMID: 12024135.

12. Cohen S, Lhuillier F, Mouloua Y, Vignal B, Favetta P, Guitton J: Quantitative measurement of propofol and main glucuroconjugate metabolites in human plasma using solid phase extraction-liquid chromatography-tandem mass spectrometry. J.Chromatogr.B.Analyt. Technol.Biomed.Life.Sci. 2007; 854 (1–2): 165–72. doi:10.1016/j.jchromb.2007.04.021. PubMed PMID: 17485254.

13. Gahart BL, Nazzareno AR, Qrtega MQ: *Intravenous Medications: A Handbook for Nurses and Health Professionals.* Amsterdam: Elsevier, 2019.

14. Pambianco DJ, Whitten CJ, Moerman A, Struys MM, Martin JF: An assessment of computer-assisted personalized sedation: a sedation delivery system to administer propofol for gastrointestinal endoscopy. Gastrointest.Endosc. 2008; 68 (3): 542–7. doi:10.1016/j. gie.2008.02.011. PubMed PMID: 18511048.

15. Gambus PL, Jensen EW, Jospin M, Borrat X, Martinez Palli G, Fernandez-Candil J, Valencia JF, Barba X, Caminal P, Troconiz IF: Modeling the effect of propofol and remifentanil combinations for sedation-analgesia in endoscopic procedures using an Adaptive Neuro Fuzzy Inference System (ANFIS). Anaesth.Analg. 2011; 112 (2): 331–9. doi:10.1213/ANE.0b013e3182025a70. PubMed PMID: 21131550.

16. Borrat X, Valencia JF, Magrans R, Gimenez-Mila M, Mellado R, Sendino O, Perez M, Nunez M, Jospin M, Jensen EW, Troconiz I, Gambus PL: Sedation-analgesia with propofol and remifentanil: concentrations required to avoid gag reflex in upper gastrointestinal endoscopy. Anaesth.Analg. 2015; 121 (1): 90–6. doi:10.1213/ANE.0000000000000756. PubMed PMID: 25902320.

17. Ng JM, Kong CF, Nyam D: Patient-controlled sedation with propofol for colonoscopy. Gastrointest.Endosc. 2001; 54 (1): 8–13. doi:10.1067/mge.2001.116110. PubMed PMID: 11427834.

18. Gillham MJ, Hutchinson RC, Carter R, Kenny GN: Patient-maintained sedation for ERCP with a target-controlled infusion of propofol: a pilot study. Gastrointest.Endosc. 2001; 54 (1): 14–17. doi:10.1067/ mge.2001.116358. PubMed PMID: 11427835.

19. Syroid ND, Agutter J, Drews FA, Westenskow DR, Albert RW, Bermudez JC, Strayer DL, Prenzel H, Loeb RG, Weinger MB: Development and evaluation of a graphical anesthesia drug display. Anesthesiology. 2002; 96 (3): 565–75. PubMed PMID: 11873029.

20. Shafer SL, Varvel JR, Aziz N, Scott JC: Pharmacokinetics of fentanyl administered by computer-controlled infusion pump. Anesthesiology. 1990; 73 (6): 1091–102. PubMed PMID: 2248388.

21. Albrecht S, Ihmsen H, Hering W, Geisslinger G, Dingemanse J, Schwilden H, Schuttler J: The effect of age on the pharmacokinetics and pharmacodynamics of midazolam. Clin.Pharmacol.Ther. 1999; 65 (6): 630–9. Epub 1999/ 07/03. doi:S0009923699000727 [pii] 10.1016/S0009-9236(99)90084-X. PubMed PMID: 10391668.

22. Schnider TW, Minto CF, Gambus PL, Andresen C, Goodale DB, Shafer SL, Youngs EJ: The influence of method of administration and covariates on the pharmacokinetics of propofol in adult volunteers. Anesthesiology. 1998; 88 (5): 1170–82. PubMed PMID: 9605675.

23. Schnider TW, Minto CF, Shafer SL, Gambus PL, Andresen C, Goodale DB, Youngs EJ: The influence of age on propofol pharmacodynamics. Anesthesiology. 1999; 90 (6): 1502–16. PubMed PMID: 10360845.

24. Minto CF, Schnider TW, Egan TD, Youngs E, Lemmens HJ, Gambus PL, Billard V, Hoke JF, Moore KH, Hermann DJ, Muir KT, Mandema JW, Shafer SL: Influence of age and gender on the pharmacokinetics and pharmacodynamics of remifentanil. I. Model development. Anesthesiology. 1997; 86 (1): 10–23. PubMed PMID: 9009935.

25. Minto CF, Schnider TW, Shafer SL: Pharmacokinetics and pharmacodynamics of remifentanil. II. Model application. Anesthesiology. 1997; 86 (1): 24–33. PubMed PMID: 9009936.

26. Kern SE, Xie G, White JL, Egan TD: A response surface analysis of propofol-remifentanil pharmacodynamic interaction in volunteers. Anesthesiology. 2004; 100 (6): 1373–81. PubMed PMID: 15166554.

27. LaPierre CD, Johnson KB, Randall BR, White JL, Egan TD: An exploration of remifentanil-propofol combinations that lead to a loss of response to esophageal instrumentation, a loss of responsiveness, and/or onset of intolerable ventilatory depression. Anesth.Analg. 2011; 113 (3): 490–9. doi:10.1213/ ANE.0b013e318210fc45. PubMed PMID: 21415430.

28. Johnson KB, Syroid ND, Gupta DK, Manyam SC, Egan TD, Huntington J, White JL, Tyler D, Westenskow DR: An evaluation of remifentanil propofol response surfaces for loss of responsiveness, loss of response to surrogates of painful stimuli and laryngoscopy in patients undergoing elective surgery. Anesth.Analg. 2008; 106 (2): 471–9. doi:10.1213/ ane.0b013e3181606c62. PubMed PMID: 18227302; PMCID: 3050649.

Chapter 10

Respiratory Depression

Malin Jonsson Fagerlund

Introduction

Respiratory depression is a common and unwanted side-effect of anaesthetics, sedatives and analgesics. It has been known since the end of the 18th century that anaesthesia has pronounced effects on control of respiration, however the effects are highly specific depending on the drug and drug concentration.

Respiratory depression in the perioperative context is a drug-induced depression of breathing, resulting in a reduction in minute ventilation and a subsequent rise in P_aCO_2 (arterial CO_2 partial pressure). Often, this is detected as a low respiratory rate or as a desaturation. Notably, desaturation is a late sign of respiratory depression, especially if the patients are on supplemental oxygen (e.g. nasal cannula) so pulse oximetry, although extensively used, is not an optimal way of monitoring respiratory depression. Monitoring of respiratory frequency or carbon dioxide gives more precise measurements of respiratory depression.

A small percentage of patients undergoing surgery will need an intervention at the postoperative ward for treatment of respiratory depression [e.g. arousal, verbal or mechanical stimulation, continuous positive airway pressure (CPAP)]. It can be notoriously difficult to predict and identify which patients will be at risk for postoperative respiratory depression. Therefore, knowledge about the physiological mechanisms behind respiratory depression and the pharmacological effects of the drugs used in anaesthesia is crucial to understand the complexity of respiratory depression in the perioperative period. For each individual patient, the physiology, pharmacology but also comorbidities, effects of acute illness etc. have to be taken into account. There are groups of patients that are extra vulnerable to respiratory depression, such as patients with obstructive sleep apnoea, morbidly obese patients, patients with neuromuscular disorders, very young (neonates) and very old patients as well as very sick patients (ASA IV–V).

During anaesthesia the patient is closely monitored in the operating room by an anaesthesiologist or anaesthesia nurse in the room. Because respiratory depression and apnoea are to be expected, everyone is well prepared to manage this departure from normal physiology. The real challenge of respiratory depression starts during emergence from anaesthesia and in the early and late postoperative period, especially at the surgical ward, where the frequency and quality of monitoring for respiratory depression vary.

Overview of Control of Respiration

Control of breathing is of crucial importance for adequate oxygenation and removal of CO_2. It is based on chemical and behavioural control. Regulation of breathing is tightly controlled by autonomic mechanisms. In addition, during wakefulness, we can use our neocortex to voluntarily adjust ventilation to override the autonomic drive if it would be insufficient or to enable speech, diving, singing and the response to pain. Deviation from chemical equilibrium at the cellular level will elicit a compensatory response (e.g. changes in respiratory rate and tidal volume) to restore homeostasis. Anaesthesia and sedation interact with key components of regulation of breathing, ultimately causing various degrees of respiratory depression. In order to understand this, basic knowledge about regulation of breathing is needed.

Regulation of breathing is coordinated in the brainstem. After afferent input from various sensors, the central breathing pattern may be adjusted, causing efferent signals to be transmitted to effectors such as the respiratory muscles (Fig. 10.1).

Respiration is generated and controlled by the respiratory neurons of the medulla that receive afferent input from central chemoreceptors located in the central nervous system (CNS) and from peripheral chemoreceptors in the carotid bodies. There are also peripheral chemoreceptors in the aortic bodies, but these seem to be of less importance in humans. Afferent input also comes from peripheral stretch receptors in

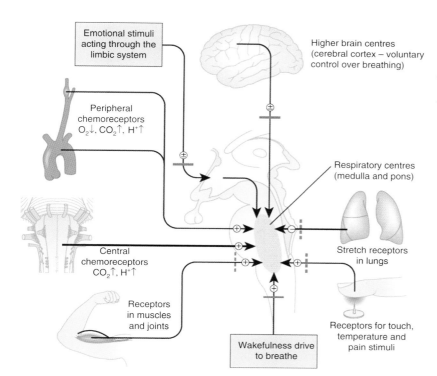

Fig. 10.1 Afferent input that interacts with control of breathing. (From Eckert DJ and Butler JE (2017) Respiratory Physiology: Understanding the Control of Ventilation. In M Kryger, T Roth and WC Dement, eds., *Principles and Practice of Sleep Medicine* (Sixth Edition), Elsevier, pp. 167–173.e4.)

the lung, from receptors in muscles and tendons, and from afferent signals from pain, touch and temperature receptors.

The respiratory neurons in the medulla can be divided into the ventral and dorsal respiratory group, based on their anatomical localization. The dorsal respiratory group contains the nucleus tractus solitarius (nTS), the key cardiorespiratory integrator. The ventral respiratory group consists of four nuclei and includes the pre-Bötzinger complex that is the major respiratory pacemaker. Close to the ventral respiratory group lies the retrotrapezoid nucleus that has important connections to the dorsal respiratory group and the key respiratory control centre, the nTS. The retrotrapezoid nucleus is an important area for central chemoreception. Thus, the respiratory neurons of the respiratory centre and the central chemoreceptors are both located in the medulla, but are clearly separated entities.

Central chemoreceptors tightly control the arterial CO_2 partial pressure by sensing the pH-changes in cerebrospinal fluid. Because the blood–brain barrier is impermeable to polar molecules such as hydrogen ions and bicarbonate, a decrease in blood pH cannot affect the central chemoreceptors. In contrast, CO_2 readily passes the blood–brain barrier, and a rise in arterial pCO_2 therefore causes a similar rise in the pCO_2 of the

cerebrospinal fluid (CSF) (however the pCO_2 in CSF is approximately 1.3 kPa higher than the arterial). An elevation of pCO_2 (CSF) increases the concentration of hydrogen ions in CSF and subsequently reduces the pH in the CSF:

$$CO_2 + H_2O <-> H_2CO_3 <-> HCO_{3^-} + H^+$$
(increased H^+ -> decrease in pH)   (1)

The resulting decrease in pH stimulates the central chemoreceptor neurons by a mechanism that is still not fully understood. Approximately 70% of the ventilatory response to CO_2 arises from the central chemoreceptors, and 30% from the peripheral chemoreceptors. Notably, the central chemoreceptors do not respond to hypoxia.

The response of the central chemoreceptors to changes in CSF PCO_2/H^+ can take up to one minute, in contrast to the rapidly responding peripheral chemoreceptors in the carotid bodies that responds to hypoxia but also to a lesser degree to, for example, hypercarbia and low pH.

During resting ventilation, the central chemoreceptors modulate breathing, and the peripheral chemoreceptors remain mostly silent (unless exposed to hypoxia). An increased activity in the peripheral chemoreceptors in the carotid bodies is transferred via the glossopharyngeal nerve to the nTS, where it modulates respiration. The efferent arc of breathing control is mediated via the phrenic nerve and respiratory muscles, and results in an increased work of breathing.

Ventilatory Responses to Hypercapnia

During normal circumstances, arterial P_aCO_2 controls ventilation. Therefore, the ventilatory response to hypercapnia has often been used as a measure to investigate the effect of drugs on respiration. An increase in inhaled CO_2 causes a linear increase in ventilation which can be described in terms of a slope (S, l/min) and the X-axis intercept B at zero ventilation (kPa):

$$Ventilation = S(P_aCO_2 - B) \qquad (2)$$

B is the apnoeic threshold, the P_aCO_2 value below which ventilation ceases. The bold line in Fig. 10.2 displays a normal ventilation curve with a slope of 15 L/min and an intercept (apnoeic threshold) at 4.8 kPa.

There is wide inter-individual variation in the P_aCO_2/ventilatory response. The response is linear up to approximately 10 kPa, but at higher CO_2 partial pressures central respiratory neurons become depressed and the ventilation decreases. The linear P_aCO_2/ventilation slope is steeper during hypoxia and less steep during hyperoxia (Fig. 10.2). As shown in Fig. 10.2, respiratory depression may be caused by a shift of the P_aCO_2/ventilatory response curve to the right, or a decrease in slope, or both.

Hypercapnia arouses and stimulates the respiratory centre. When patients are waking up from anaesthesia, we use this physiological process: we allow the end-tidal CO_2 and thus P_aCO_2 to rise to stimulate the respiratory centre, thereby increasing the likelihood that the patient will start breathing spontaneously. Vice versa, hyperventilation may lower P_aCO_2 below the apnoeic threshold, causing the patient to cease any spontaneous breathing efforts.

Ventilatory Responses to Hypoxia

The ventilatory response to hypoxia is an immediate reaction to hypoxaemia in arterial blood that aims to restore normoxia. In a healthy adult breathing room air, desaturation and subsequent hypoxaemia occur within a few minutes if apnoea occurs and even faster in patients with comorbidities. The hypoxic ventilatory response is illustrated below (Fig. 10.3).

Minute ventilation increases within seconds after hypoxia (the hypoxic ventilatory response). The degree of the response is dependent on whether there are isocapnic or poikilocapnic conditions. But after two to five minutes, the hypoxic ventilatory decline (HVD) sets in, caused by hypoxia-induced depression of the respiratory neurons in the brainstem. If hypoxia persists, a new balance will occur and (during isocapnia) ventilation will gradually increase again. Under normal conditions, the ventilatory response to hypoxia only contributes a small part to resting ventilation, but its contribution may become crucial in situations where the central chemoreceptors are affected, i.e.

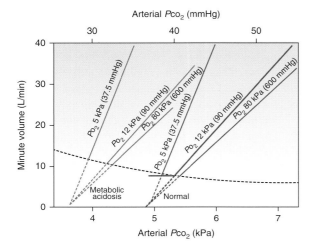

Fig. 10.2 The ventilatory response to hypercapnia during various physiological conditions. (From A. B. Lumb, *Nunn's Applied Respiratory Physiology* 8th Edition, 2017.)

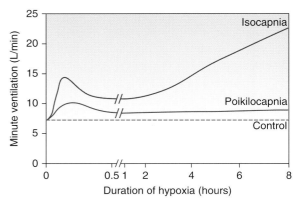

Fig. 10.3 The hypoxic ventilatory response. Hypoxia initially causes an acute increase in minute ventilation (the acute hypoxic ventilatory response or HVR), but this is followed after two to five minutes by a decline in ventilation (the hypoxic ventilatory decline or HVD). (From A. B. Lumb, *Nunn's Applied Respiratory Physiology* 8th Edition, 2017.)

after opioid administration, in patients with chronically high pCO_2 etc. – in fact, approximately 10% of the population lacks the ventilatory response to hypoxia. Patients that have undergone bilateral neck dissection and to some extent also those that underwent bilateral carotid surgery and thus had their carotid bodies removed, totally lack the ventilatory response to hypoxia. In animals this response restores with time, probably due to compensatory mechanisms in the *aortic* bodies, but in humans this is irreversible due to the lack of clinical effect by the aortic bodies [1].

If progressive hypoxia is applied during 15 minutes, ventilation progressively increases. This pO_2/ventilation curve has the shape of a rectangular hyperbola (Fig. 10.4).

Hypoxic ventilation can also be tested with the Dejour's test: in a healthy adult, administration of 100% oxygen for a short period will silence the chemoreceptive cells in the carotid body and transiently reduce basal ventilation. Patients that are exposed to chronic or intermittent hypoxia such as COPD or obstructive sleep apnoea (OSA) will have a disturbed response to hypoxia.

Effects of Anaesthetics, Sedatives and Analgesics on Control of Breathing

General anaesthesia impairs control of breathing. Different drug classes differently affect the various parts of control of breathing, i.e. resting ventilation and the hypercapnic and hypoxic ventilatory response.

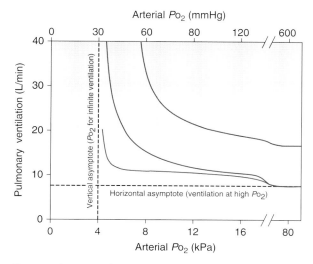

Fig. 10.4 Progressive hypoxia, the pO_2/ventilation curve. (From A. B. Lumb, *Nunn's Applied Respiratory Physiology* 8th Edition, 2017.)

Inhaled anaesthetics: Resting ventilation is affected by inhaled anaesthetics in a partial pressure dependent manner. At low partial pressures, there are only minimal effects on the minute volume: tidal volume will gradually decrease, but this is compensated by an increase in respiratory frequency. Importantly, anaesthesia per se can reduce metabolic demand and thereby cause a decrease in CO_2 production. At higher partial pressures of the inhaled anaesthetic, the respiratory frequency slows down and the spontaneous minute ventilation can become very low. The subsequent rise in P_aCO_2 may partly counteract the reduction in ventilation. Since monotherapy with inhaled anaesthetics rarely causes apnoea during spontaneous ventilation up to 2MAC but does depress airway reflexes around 1.5MAC, inhaled anaesthetics have been used for 'awake' fibreoptic intubation in patients with compromised airways.

Inhaled anaesthetics dose-dependently attenuate the response to hypoxia; at subanaesthetic concentrations, such as those that can be seen in the postoperative period or in an awake sedated patient, the ventilatory response to hypoxia is reduced by approximately 30–50% and at anaesthetic concentrations the response is virtually *abolished* [2, 3, 4]. The ventilatory response to increased CO_2 during subanaesthetic concentrations of inhaled anaesthetics is reduced, but to a lesser extent than the hypoxic response [3].

Propofol: Propofol is a well recognized respiratory depressant. Resting ventilation is reduced in a dose-dependent manner: with increasing concentrations, minute ventilation is reduced, mainly due to a reduced tidal volume, and a subsequent rise in P_aCO_2 occurs. Apnoea after induction with propofol is common. The ventilatory response to hypoxia is reduced by 50% during moderate sedation. There is a similar 50% reduction in hypercapnic ventilatory response with increased doses of propofol [5, 6, 7].

α2-agonists such as clonidine and dexmedetomidine have minimal effects on resting ventilation in both sedative and anaesthetic doses and have therefore been put forward as a sedative/anaesthetics with minimal effect on ventilation. However, when dexmedetomidine is given as a bolus dose of 1–2 µg/kg over ten minutes, a short apnoea might occur, and minute ventilation can be slightly decreased [8]. Oral clonidine causes a reduction in the ventilatory response [9] and, recently, it was demonstrated that dexmedetomidine in sedative doses reduces both hypoxic and hypercapnic ventilatory response in healthy volunteers [7].

Ketamine is an intravenous anaesthetic that causes dissociative anaesthesia, and in contrast to other intravenous anaesthetics is characterized by maintaining more stable respiration. Low doses of ketamine (< 0.5 mg/kg) *stimulate* the respiratory centre, causing an increase in frequency and tidal volume that results in an increase in minute ventilation [3]. Anaesthetic doses of ketamine (1–2 mg/kg) depress ventilation. The ventilatory response to increased CO_2 is also reduced, with a right-shift in the CO_2 response curve (i.e. a parallel shift and no change in slope). Ketamine inhibits NMDA-receptors but in addition works as a μ-opioid receptor agonist, and studies involving μ-opioid receptor knock-out mice indicate that the respiratory depressant effect of ketamine most likely is related to its effect on the μ-opioid receptor [3]. There have not been any human studies on the effect of ketamine on hypoxic ventilatory response.

Benzodiazepines and more specifically **midazolam** dose-dependently depress ventilation. Resting ventilation is reduced by a reduction in tidal volume. Induction of anaesthesia with midazolam can cause apnoea. Furthermore, midazolam attenuates the ventilatory response to both hypoxia and hypercarbia [3].

While non-opioid analgesics such as non-steroidal anti-inflammatory drugs (e.g. paracetamol) have minimal effect on control of breathing, **opioids** are the classical example of a respiratory depressant drug. The most commonly used opioids during anaesthesia are morphine, fentanyl, alfentanil, sufentanil and remifentanil. Opioids target μ-, κ- and δ-opioid receptors, but it is now clear that it is the interaction with the μ-opioid receptors at respiratory neurons in the respiratory centre of the brainstem that is responsible for opioid-induced respiratory depression. Importantly, the μ-opioid receptor antagonist naloxone can reverse opioid-induced ventilatory depression. It is however critical to consider the duration of action of the administered opioid in relation to the duration of action of naloxone. Currently, alternative approaches to avoid opioid-induced respiratory depression are being investigated, e.g. biased μ-opioid receptor ligands that selectively target a non-β-Arrestin signalling pathway associated with the G-protein of the μ-opioid receptor [10].

Synergy for Opioids, Hypnotics and Benzodiazepines

Modern anaesthesia and sedation strategies are based on so-called balanced anaesthesia, i.e. a combination of a hypnotic/sedative with an opioid and a muscle relaxant, in order to achieve desirable levels of hypnosis/sedation, analgesia and immobility without cardiovascular compromise. Importantly, drug synergy may cause profound respiratory depression. With all anaesthetics, the respiratory depressant effect is augmented (or synergistic) if an opioid is added.

If a *low* dose of ketamine is combined with a low dose of propofol, midazolam or opioid, the respiratory stimulant effect of ketamine will prevent the respiratory depressant action of these drugs; with *higher* doses of ketamine though, respiratory depression is augmented. Sedative doses of propofol in combination with low doses of opioids (e.g. remifentanil) cause synergistic depression of resting ventilation, increase resting P_aCO_2 and decrease the ventilatory response to CO_2 [11]. It is speculated that this is due to an interaction with chemoreceptors (by propofol) and a simultaneous inhibition of behavioural control of breathing (by remifentanil) [11].

Patient Breathing Spontaneously: Sedation for Procedure

Procedural sedation is a challenge that differs from general anaesthesia in many aspects. First, it is often done outside the operating room in an environment that differs from what we are used to; (2) it may be hard to achieve a stable depth of sedation; (3) there is a lack of validated monitoring tools for sedation; and (4) it is easy to underestimate the risk associated with sedation – there is actually a much higher risk for an anaesthesia-related complication during sedation than during general anaesthesia. A common indirect way of measuring depth of sedation related to control of breathing is to monitor SpO_2 and respiratory rate. If the SpO_2 is decreasing or the respiratory rate is going down, the sedation is too deep, and vice versa (with the prerequisite of healthy lungs so that a decrease in SpO_2 reflects a lower minute ventilation). In order to monitor the effect of 'true' respiration, i.e. minute ventilation, it is recommended to use an indirect CO_2 monitor such as a nasal cannula that monitors CO_2, a transcutaneous CO_2 monitor, etc. The combination of sedative/anaesthetic and opioid needs to be carefully considered since some of the drugs display a clear and occasionally very pronounced synergy for respiratory depression. It is also important to avoid rapid peaks in plasma concentrations from boluses because these have a higher risk of causing apnoea as the CO_2 has not yet accumulated in that situation. Moreover, during sedation it is critical to avoid a rapid loss of wakefulness because that affects behavioural control of breathing which can lead to respiratory depression and apnoea [3]. Based on the above considerations, and in order to achieve a stable sedation without a roller-coaster pattern for sedation and subsequently control of respiration, it is recommended to avoid boluses and rather use a continuous infusion of sedatives and/or analgesics. More details are provided in Chapter 9.

Respiratory Depression during Postoperative Analgesia

Postoperative analgesia can be accomplished with various drugs, but a multimodal approach is often recommended in the hope that targeting various components of the pain signalling pathway minimizes side effects. Typical postoperative analgesics other than opioids include paracetamol, non-steroidal anti-inflammatory drugs (NSAIDs), selective cyclooxygenase inhibitors (COX2 inhibitors), α_2-agonists and low dose ketamine. Of these, opioids (morphine, oxycodone, fentanyl, etc. administered via various routes) are the drugs causing respiratory depression. The respiratory depressant effect of opioids depends on the type of drug, the administration route, the frequency of administration and also on whether or not they are combined with other medications such as sedatives or other analgetics (NSAIDs, acetaminophen, α_2-agonists etc.).

Monitoring of Respiratory Depression

The gold standard to monitor respiration is minute ventilation, because it defines how much the patient breathes. However, it is also important to consider metabolic rate (anaesthesia, for example, may lower it), because the alveolar partial pressure $F_ACO_2 = VCO_2/V_A$ ($VCO_2 = CO_2$ production; V_A = alveolar ventilation). In those circumstances where VCO_2 may change, measurement of CO_2 partial pressure is important. Below is an overview of different techniques that can be used to measure ventilation.

Minute Ventilation, Respiratory Rate, Tidal Volume

If the patient is connected to a ventilator/anaesthesia machine or non-invasive ventilation tool, the tidal volume, respiratory rate and minute ventilation will be measured or calculated based on other parameters. In the spontaneously breathing patient not connected to such machines, respiratory rate can be used as a surrogate for minute ventilation and the depth and quality of

breathing can be assessed. In that case, respiratory rate is often derived from transthoracic impedance measurements (e.g. from ECG electrodes) or from the capnograph. Electric impedance tomography will provide both tidal volume and respiratory rate.

Measurement of Oxygen Saturation

Adequate oxygenation is essential for aerobic life, and therefore the body tightly controls these processes. The adequacy of oxygenation can be non-invasively measured by the oxygen saturation (SaO_2), the percentage of haemoglobin molecules that are saturated with oxygen. Blood oxygen saturation (SaO_2) is measured photometrically with four wavelengths, allowing oxygenated, deoxygenated, carboxy-, and methaemoglobin to be measured. Conventional pulse oximetry (SpO_2) only uses two wavelengths, only allowing an approximation of the SaO_2 measured by blood oximetry; in the presence of carbon monoxide or methaemoglobin, the displayed SpO_2 will not match SaO_2.

It is well known that intermittent SpO_2 measurements at the ward underestimate and miss many episodes of desaturation [12]. Moreover, in patients with obstructive sleep apnoea who can have 20–60 desaturations per hour of sleep, traditional monitoring of SpO_2 will miss the rapid and intermittent episodes of desaturation. In order to detect those desaturations, special pulse oximeters have been developed that can calculate the O_2 desaturation index (ODI), the number of desaturation episodes below 3% of baseline SpO_2 per hour. Finally, it is important to remind the reader that, when a high F_IO_2 is administered, PaO_2 can decrease significantly before SaO_2 starts to decrease.

Measurement of CO_2

The CO_2 partial pressure can be measured at various locations in the body. To be able to correctly interpret the absolute value, it is of crucial importance to keep in mind where the CO_2 has been measured. Arterial PCO_2 is the place of measurement that most often is referred to, but CO_2 partial pressure is also commonly measured as end-tidal CO_2, venous CO_2 or transcutanous CO_2.

The arterial CO_2 partial pressure (P_aCO_2) is measured by intermittent sampling of arterial blood gases that are analysed in a blood gas machine, sometimes by a Severinghaus electrode. The reference range for arterial PCO_2 is 5.1 ± 1.0 kPa, but 5% of the population will be outside of this range.

Transcutaneous CO_2. When heat is applied locally to the skin, the capillary beds become arterialized, and arterial CO_2 can be measured transcutaneously by Stow–Severinghaus electrodes. The partial pressures measured with non-invasive plastic electrodes correlate well with P_aCO_2 in normally perfused patients. Interpretation should be done cautiously if perfusion is abnormal (sepsis, shock, etc).

Venous CO_2. The PCO_2 in a sample from a peripheral vein will be higher than in the arterial blood because it will also contain the amount of CO_2 produced in the tissues that the blood drains. The venous PCO_2 is therefore generally approximately 1.3 kPa higher than in the arterial blood. The absolute values can be difficult to interpret since they are dependent on those factors that influence CO_2 production and elimination. Still, in a specific situation, venous PCO_2 can be used for trending of CO_2. The measurement technique is the same as for arterial CO_2.

End-tidal CO_2 and capnography. End-tidal or end-expiratory CO_2 corresponds to alveolar CO_2 in normal, healthy individuals under the prerequisite that all parts of the alveoli are ventilated and perfused (i.e. if no dead-space is present). The normal arterial/end-tidal CO_2 gradient is between 0.7 and 1.3 kPa. End-tidal CO_2 is most commonly measured by infra-red gas analysis.

Portable CO_2 monitors (used in the prehospital setting or during unplanned intubations at the ward) are based on chemical or spectrophotometric methods.

A capnogram displays the partial pressure of end-tidal CO_2 against time. Capnography is the gold standard to confirm that the endotracheal tube is placed correctly in the trachea and not in the oesophagus. Patients that are intubated or have a subglottic device or laryngeal mask in place should be monitored by capnography. The capnogram monitors both the patient and anaesthesia machine and provides important information about airway patency, ventilation, cardiac output and inhaled CO_2 (which may, for example, indicate CO_2 absorber exhaustion), etc.

Quantitative and Modelling Information

During the last 20 years, there have been some attempts to quantify the degree and speed of respiratory depression by propofol and/or the opioids alfentanil or remifentanil. It would indeed be desirable to be able to predict the effect of different concentrations and combinations of sedatives/anaesthetics and opioids on respiration. It is now acknowledged that in order to predict the effects of sedatives/anaesthetics and/or analgesics, the P_aCO_2 is a crucial player. Different

pharmacokinetic/pharmacodynamic (PKPD) models have been proposed involving the drug effect-site concentration and P_aCO_2. Bouillon and co-workers have created a PKPD indirect response model. The model predicts the ventilatory response time to rapidly acting agents such as propofol and remifentanil [13, 14]. The Bouillon model explains why the speed of injection of a potent respiratory depressant drug is of importance: the compensatory increase in P_aCO_2 is not fast enough to ensure it remains above the apnoeic threshold, thus apnoea can ensue. This explains why a rapid bolus of propofol causes apnoea, while spontaneous breathing can be maintained during a long term infusion. This is illustrated in Fig. 10.5.

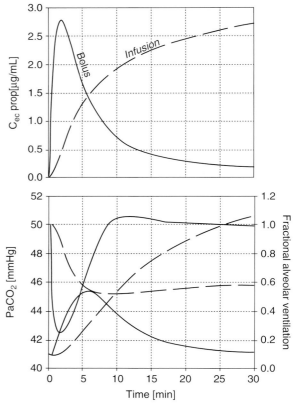

Fig. 10.5 The concentration–effect relation of propofol for respiratory depression depends on the administration rate. The top panel displays the propofol effect-site concentration (C_e) after a 100 mg bolus and during an infusion, the lower panel the corresponding changes in P_aCO_2 and fractional alveolar ventilation (i.e. change relative to baseline). A bolus causes a transient peak in C_e that is followed by a short period of profound hypoventilation resulting in a transient increase in P_aCO_2. An infusion causes C_e to rise gradually, resulting in a more gradual onset of respiratory depression and hypoventilation, which will cause (and allow) P_aCO_2 to rise more gradually, thus partially offsetting the more profound hypoventilation seen after bolus administration (from [14]).

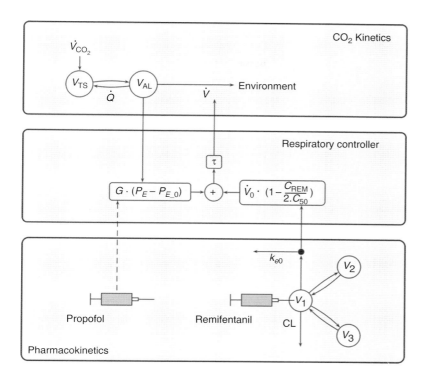

Fig. 10.6 Overview of the indirect response model for remifentanil in the awake state or during propofol sedation. For details, see [18].

Dahan and co-workers have been using steady-state response surface modelling on various combinations of drugs (sevoflurane and alfentanil, propofol and remifentanil). With this approach, a three dimensional graph displays the effect of the different drugs and their combinations on various ventilatory parameters such as resting end-tidal CO_2, resting minute ventilation and the response to CO_2 [15, 16].

More recently, Olofsen and co-workers extended their previous work [17] with steady-state models to a non-steady-state model describing the effects of remifentanil in the awake state and during propofol sedation [18]. The model assumes a linear relationship between ventilation and P_aCO_2 and is being described as an indirect response model [18]. Shown is a schematic overview of the model (Fig. 10.6) and an illustration of the linear relationship between remifentanil concentration and ventilation (Fig. 10.7).

The disadvantage of the previously described models is that they have been evaluated in healthy volunteers and/or during limited conditions. Recently, Hannam and co-workers developed an indirect-effect model with system feedback in patients undergoing sedation with propofol and remifentanil for gastroscopy (see Fig. 10.8) [19]. Transcutaneous PCO_2 was used as an objective biomarker of respiratory depression. It was clear that age was an important covariate in

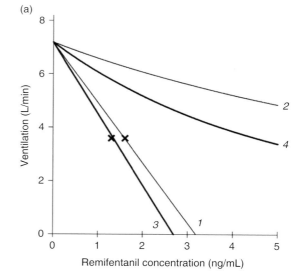

(b)

$$\dot{V}(C_{REM}) = \dot{V}_0 \cdot \left(1 - \frac{C_{REM}}{2 \cdot C_{50}} \right) + G \cdot (P_E - P_{E\_0}).$$

Fig. 10.7 Relationship between remifentanil concentration and ventilation using the equation above. When there has been no accumulation in P_aCO_2 (as during boluses), response 1 is seen for the awake state and line 3 for the propofol sedated state. When CO_2 accumulates, a steady state occurs, which is represented by line 2 for the awake state and line 4 during propofol sedation. The crosses represent C_{50} values (i.e. the steady-state concentration of remifentanil causing 50% respiratory depression) (from [18]).

this model whereas noxious stimuli or genotype for a μ-opioid receptor were not.

Define the Optimal Physiological Ranges

Optimal Ranges for Respiratory Rate, Tidal Volume

A respiratory rate lower than 12 breaths/minute (bradypnoea) is considered as respiratory depression, whereas a respiratory rate above 20 breaths/minute is considered as tachypnoea. It should be noted that not only the respiratory rate is of importance, but also the breathing pattern. Patients with sleep apnoea for example can have a normal respiratory rate but an abnormal breathing pattern. A normal tidal volume is approximately 8 mL/kg (ideal body weight) but this is definitively influenced by weight, height, body position, etc. The intraoperative use of protective lung ventilation is an active research field.

Optimal Ranges for SpO$_2$, Its Meaning, and Its Dynamic Range or Fast Response

The normal range for S$_p$O$_2$ in adult healthy patients is 94–100%, but it can be significantly lower in very young and very old patients as well as in sick patients. It is important to acknowledge that when the oxygen stores in the lungs (i.e. reduced functional residual capacity) are depleted, the drop in saturation is very rapid. The time it takes for desaturation to occur depends on several factors such as ongoing oxygen administration, obesity, metabolic demand and whether the patient breathes or is apnoeic. The optimal range for SpO$_2$ in perioperative patients can vary, depending on comorbidities such as COPD but also on the factors referred to above, and it is therefore difficult to define an optimal range – that will be a clinical decision based upon assessment of the individual patient. It is important to consider the properties of the oxyhaemoglobin dissociation curve – it is sigmoid in shape (with S$_a$O$_2$ varying linearly with P$_a$O$_2$ over the 40–60 mmHg range) and how it is affected by changes in for example pH, P$_a$CO$_2$, temperature, etc. The accuracy of pulse oximetry (SpO$_2$) as an indicator of SaO$_2$ drops below 70–80%.

Optimal Ranges of PCO$_2$: Clinical Narcosis

As described above, the CO$_2$ partial pressure is tightly regulated in order to guarantee stable breathing and to avoid hypo- and hypercapnia. Hypocapnia results from excessive alveolar ventilation. The most common causes of acute hypocapnia in this context are artificial ventilation by an anaesthesia machine or ICU-ventilator, or psychological factors during spontaneous breathing, such as procedure anxiety or pain. Metabolic acidosis can cause chronic hypocapnia due to an increased respiratory drive and compensatory

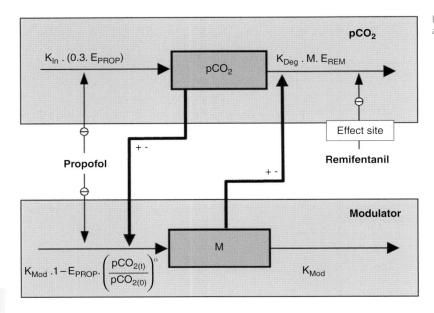

Fig. 10.8 Model of the effects of propofol and remifentanil on pCO$_2$ (see [19]).

hyperventilation (e.g. in diabetic ketoacidosis) in order to keep the arterial pH within the physiological range. If the patient is unable to compensate (i.e. hyperventilate) a deleterious rapid fall in pH occurs, ultimately resulting in circulatory collapse. Hypoxia is also a common cause of hyperventilation. Neurological conditions such as subarachnoidal or intracranial haemorrhage with subsequent blood in the CSF can also cause hyperventilation.

Hypercapnia is *un*common in a healthy individual. A P_aCO_2 above 6.1 kPa should be considered abnormal except during breath holding when it can even be slightly higher. There are four major causes of hypercapnia: hypoventilation, increased production of CO_2, increased deadspace, or an increased inhaled CO_2 partial pressure. In clinical anaesthesia/ICU, the clinician may decide to tolerate a higher than normal P_aCO_2 (permissive hypercapnia), e.g. in patients with acute respiratory distress syndrome (ARDS) where the use of lower tidal volumes has been shown to increase survival and reduce morbidity. The use of lower tidal volumes (6–8 mL/min) as part of a protective lung ventilation mode during anaesthesia is currently being widely explored.

A slightly elevated P_aCO_2 during anaesthesia can be accepted as long as it remains controlled within reasonable limits. During laparoscopic surgery, CO_2 is used to inflate the peritoneal space, and while this may mandate an increase in ventilation, it can also be combined with moderate degrees of permissive hypercapnia.

Recently, a new method to provide apnoeic oxygenation during anaesthesia for ENT surgery was introduced. It uses high flow transnasal oxygen with flows up to 70 L/min, a technique entitled trans-nasal humidified rapid insufflation ventilatory exchange (THRIVE). While securing a difficult airway or during short laryngeal procedures [20, 21], oxygenation can be well maintained with degrees of hypercapnia that are lower with THRIVE than with traditional apnoeic oxygenation and with a slower rate of rise of the P_aCO_2 (0.25 kPa/min instead of 0.4–0.5 kPa/min with the conventional approach). This makes it possible to extend the duration of apnoea while still ensuring acceptable P_aCO_2 levels. The CO_2 partial pressure has to be measured via an arterial line or transcutaneously because the end-tidal CO_2 obviously is unavailable. The normal rate of rise of the P_aCO_2 during apnoea with normal metabolism is approximately 0.4–0.8 kPa, with a slightly faster rise in the first minutes. An increase in P_aCO_2 stimulates ventilation up to a certain maximum; with a higher P_aCO_2 still, respiratory fatigue and ultimately CO_2 narcosis will ensue.

Summary

In summary, sedation and anaesthesia cause respiratory depression to a degree that depends on the drug, speed of administration and combinations of drugs. Respiratory depression is best monitored by minute volume or arterial CO_2. In the future, we hope for even shorter acting drugs that are target specific, such as the biased μ-opioid receptor ligands.

References

1. Teppema LJ, Dahan A: The ventilatory response to hypoxia in mammals: mechanisms, measurement, and analysis. Physiol.Rev. 2010; 90 (2): 675–754.

2. Eriksson LI: The effects of residual neuromuscular blockade and volatile anesthetics on the control of ventilation. Anesth.Analg. 1999; 89 (1): 243–51.

3. Stuth EA, Stucke AG, Zuperku EJ: Effects of anesthetics, sedatives, and opioids on ventilatory control. Compr. Physiol. 2012; 2 (4): 2281–367.

4. Pandit JJ: Volatile anaesthetic depression of the carotid body chemoreflex-mediated ventilatory response to hypoxia: directions for future research. Scientifica. (Cairo). 2014; X: 394270.

5. Blouin RT, Seifert HA, Babenco HD, Conard PF, Gross JB: Propofol depresses the hypoxic ventilatory response during conscious sedation and isohypercapnia. Anesthesiology. 1993; 79 (6): 1177–82.

6. Nieuwenhuijs D, Sarton E, Teppema L, Dahan A: Propofol for monitored anesthesia care: implications on hypoxic control of cardiorespiratory responses. Anesthesiology. 2000; 92 (1): 46–54.

7. Lodenius A, Ebberyd A, Hardemark Cedborg A, Hagel E, Mkrtchian S, Christensson E, Ullman J, Scheinin M, Eriksson LI, Jonsson Fagerlund M: Sedation with dexmedetomidine or propofol impairs hypoxic control of breathing in healthy male volunteers: a nonblinded, randomized crossover study. Anesthesiology. 2016; 125 (4): 700–15.

8. Belleville JP, Ward DS, Bloor BC, Maze M: Effects of intravenous dexmedetomidine in humans. I. Sedation, ventilation, and metabolic rate. Anesthesiology. 1992; 77 (6): 1125–33.

9. Foo IT, Warren PM, Drummond GB: Influence of oral clonidine on the ventilatory response to acute and sustained isocapnic hypoxia in human males. Br.J.Anaesth. 1996; 76 (2): 214–20.

10. Siuda ER, Carr R, 3rd, Rominger DH, Violin JD: Biased mu-opioid receptor ligands: a promising new

generation of pain therapeutics. Curr.Opin.Pharmacol. 2017; 32: 77–84.

11. Dahan A, Teppema LJ: Influence of anaesthesia and analgesia on the control of breathing. Br.J.Anaesth. 2003; 91 (1): 40–9.

12. Taenzer AH, Pyke J, Herrick MD, Dodds TM, McGrath SP: A comparison of oxygen saturation data in inpatients with low oxygen saturation using automated continuous monitoring and intermittent manual data charting. Anesth.Analg. 2014; 118 (2): 326–31.

13. Bouillon T, Schmidt C, Garstka G, Heimbach D, Stafforst D, Schwilden H, Hoeft A: Pharmacokinetic-pharmacodynamic modeling of the respiratory depressant effect of alfentanil. Anesthesiology. 1999; 91 (1): 144–55.

14. Bouillon TW, Bruhn J, Radulescu L, Andresen C, Shafer TJ, Cohane C, Shafer SL: Pharmacodynamic interaction between propofol and remifentanil regarding hypnosis, tolerance of laryngoscopy, bispectral index, and electroencephalographic approximate entropy. Anesthesiology. 2004; 100 (6): 1353–72.

15. Dahan A, Nieuwenhuijs D, Olofsen E, Sarton E, Romberg R, Teppema L: Response surface modeling of alfentanil-sevoflurane interaction on cardiorespiratory control and bispectral index. Anesthesiology. 2001; 94 (6): 982–91.

16. Nieuwenhuijs DJ, Olofsen E, Romberg RR, Sarton E, Ward D, Engbers F, Vuyk J, Mooren R, Teppema LJ, Dahan A: Response surface modeling of remifentanil-propofol interaction on cardiorespiratory control and bispectral index. Anesthesiology. 2003; 98 (2): 312–22.

17. Romberg R, Olofsen E, Sarton E, den Hartigh J, Taschner PE, Dahan A: Pharmacokinetic-pharmacodynamic modeling of morphine-6-glucuronide-induced analgesia in healthy volunteers: absence of sex differences. Anesthesiology. 2004; 100 (1): 120–33.

18. Olofsen E, Boom M, Nieuwenhuijs D, Sarton E, Teppema L, Aarts L, Dahan A: Modeling the non-steady state respiratory effects of remifentanil in awake and propofol-sedated healthy volunteers. Anesthesiology. 2010; 112 (6): 1382–95.

19. Hannam JA, Borrat X, Troconiz IF, Valencia JF, Jensen EW, Pedroso A, Munoz J, Castellvi-Bel S, Castells A, Gambus PL: Modeling respiratory depression induced by remifentanil and propofol during sedation and analgesia using a continuous noninvasive measurement of pCO_2. J.Pharmacol.Exp.Ther. 2016; 356 (3): 563–73.

20. Patel A, Nouraei SA: Transnasal Humidified Rapid-Insufflation Ventilatory Exchange (THRIVE): a physiological method of increasing apnoea time in patients with difficult airways. Anaesthesia. 2015; 70 (3): 323–9.

21. Gustafsson IM, Lodenius A, Tunelli J, Ullman J, Jonsson Fagerlund M: Apnoeic oxygenation in adults under general anaesthesia using Transnasal Humidified Rapid-Insufflation Ventilatory Exchange (THRIVE) – a physiological study. Br.J.Anaesth. 2017; 118 (4): 610–17.

Immobility

Klaus T. Olkkola and Douglas J. Eleveld

Muscle Relaxation and Neuromuscular Block

Surgical anaesthesia usually requires hypnosis, antinociception (ensuring blood pressure and heart rate control) and immobility with varying degrees of muscle relaxation. However, the relative contribution of these three components to the state of anaesthesia may vary between different anaesthesias and surgical procedures. While volatile anaesthetics may be used to produce anaesthesia in and by themselves, most often anaesthesia is produced by a combination of drugs. Anaesthesia produced by the concomitant use of hypnotics, analgesics and neuromuscular blocking drugs is called 'balanced anaesthesia'.

The degree of neuromuscular block induced by neuromuscular blocking drugs and the depth of anaesthesia (induced by other drugs) both affect muscle relaxation [1]. While in the early days of our profession deep ether anaesthesia alone provided sufficient muscle relaxation for many procedures, the introduction of neuromuscular blocking drugs nowadays allows us to target specific degrees of muscle relaxation in an easy and safe manner. Provided the airway is secured and adequate ventilation and hypnosis are ensured, adverse effects of neuromuscular blocking drugs are few.

After briefly reviewing pertinent physiology, the different degrees of neuromuscular block depth are defined and the tools to measure them are described. The chapter then focuses on the properties of modern neuromuscular blocking drugs (only cisatracurium, mivacurium and rocuronium will be discussed) and suxamethonium. Finally, the clinically optimal neuromuscular block is defined, and the different routes to achieve this goal are explored.

Neuromuscular Junction

An action potential causes synaptic vesicles of the motor nerve endings containing the neurotransmitter acetylcholine to fuse with the plasma membrane and release their content into the neuromuscular junction.

Acetylcholine then binds to postjunctional nicotinic acetylcholine receptors on the motor endplate. These receptors consist of two alpha and one beta, delta and epsilon subunits. They are directly linked to ion channels. If acetylcholine is bound to both alpha subunits, the permeability of the ion channel for Na^+ and K^+ ions increases, depolarizing the muscle cell [2]. Subsequent calcium release causes contraction of the cell, and if a sufficient number of muscle cells are depolarized simultaneously, muscle contraction ensues.

In addition to the postjunctional receptors, there are also prejunctional acetylcholine receptors that are involved in the modulation of acetylcholine release in the neuromuscular junction. They consist of three alpha and two beta subunits. While clinically used non-depolarizing neuromuscular blocking drugs have affinity for these presynaptic receptors, the only available depolarizing neuromuscular blocking drug, suxamethonium, does not [3]. Because a non-depolarizing neuromuscular block displays fade after train-of-four stimulation (see further) while a suxamethonium induced neuromuscular block does not, it is plausible to explain this by the aforementioned different effects on presynaptic nicotinic acetylcholine receptors. Fade is used to quantify the degree of neuromuscular block elicited by the non-depolarizing neuromuscular blocking drugs.

Quantification of Neuromuscular Block

Because the individual response to neuromuscular blocking drugs varies to such an extent that it becomes unpredictable in the individual patient, neuromuscular function has to be measured continually during anaesthesia. Fortunately, of all components making up anaesthesia, the degree of the neuromuscular block is the one that can be measured most easily by applying a supramaximal electrical stimulus to a peripheral motor nerve and quantifying the subsequent muscle contraction (or other muscle response). A complete or partial neuromuscular block is said to exist if no or some (but not a full) response is present, respectively.

After administration of a neuromuscular blocking drug, the degree of neuromuscular block is not uniform in all muscles throughout the body. For example, laryngeal muscles achieve peak effect faster than peripheral muscles but the effect there also dissipates faster. Both pharmacokinetic (PK) (e.g. blood flow) and pharmacodynamic (PD) (sensitivity) factors account for these differences. These differences have to be taken into account when monitoring neuromuscular block in one muscle (e.g. because of ease of access) to get an idea of the neuromuscular block in another muscle that may be the more relevant one to ensure optimal surgical conditions – it explains why the quantification of neuromuscular block at the hand is not perfectly informative for neuromuscular block at diaphragm or abdominal wall [4].

Stimulation Patterns

While quantifying the muscle response following electrical stimulation of a motor nerve seems straightforward, in reality it is a rather complex subject.

While a number of stimulation patterns are in widespread use, the type of electrical stimulation is often quite similar. Typically, a unipolar constant-current pulse is used, and this current has to be strong enough to evoke a supramaximal response from the muscle. The reason for the need of supramaximal stimulation is to ensure that the magnitude of muscle contraction is independent of the intensity of the electrical stimulation. If all of the motor units innervated by the stimulated nerve are recruited, then we have supramaximal stimulation. The magnitude of the contraction then (ideally) becomes independent of the magnitude of the electrical stimulus. Under these conditions, the only limiting factor in muscle contraction is the neuromuscular transmission, which is the characteristic of interest. This method also reduces the dependence of muscle contraction on stimulating electrode conditions which can vary during the surgical procedure. Moisture or gel under the electrodes changes the electrical properties of the skin under the electrodes. Typically, constant-current pulses of up to 50–60 milliamperes are used with duration of 200–300 microseconds.

Ideally, both the stimulation site, i.e. the site where electrodes are placed, and the monitoring site, i.e. the site where muscle response is registered, have to remain easily accessible throughout the surgical procedure. Because during most surgical procedures at least one hand is accessible, the ulnar nerve at the wrist and the adductor pollicis it innervates are the most commonly used monitoring sites. When this site is not accessible, the orbicularis oculi or corrugator supercilii at the eye, and the flexor hallucis brevis at the foot can be used. Accessibility of the area of the motor nerve is important for the initial electrode placement, but once the electrodes are placed, often the site does not need repeated access.

Single-twitch Stimulation

Single-twitch stimulation refers to the application of a single electrical pulse to a motor nerve, with quantification of the resulting muscle contraction called 'single-twitch response'. Before the administration of neuromuscular blocking drugs, a 'control twitch' is determined that serves as the baseline muscle contraction to which subsequent twitches are referenced. A value of 0% indicates complete neuromuscular block, and 100% indicates no neuromuscular block. While single-twitch stimulation has been used extensively in older research, it has only been rarely applied in routine clinical practice. A proper understanding of this method helps the clinician to gain insight into much of the research on neuromuscular blocking drugs.

The interpretation of the single-twitch stimulation response is confounded by 'twitch potentiation', a physiological phenomenon whereby repetitive stimulation can cause a gradual increase in twitch response that ultimately plateaus. To make matters even more complex, the magnitude of the control twitch response may also depend on the stimulation pattern. Because intraoperative neuromuscular transmission monitoring requires repetitive stimulation of the nerve, post-relaxation twitch responses, defined as the responses during and after the recovery of neuromuscular block, will be potentiated and plateau at some higher value. If insufficient time is taken for twitch response stabilization prior to the administration of neuromuscular blocking drugs, twitch potentiation during and after recovery of a drug-induced neuromuscular block can result in a twitch response that exceeds the control twitch, obtained prior to the administration of neuromuscular blocking drugs, by 150–180%. In these conditions, a twitch response of 100% of the control twitch will falsely indicate full recovery and underestimate a residual block that may still cause the patient to experience clinical signs of residual neuromuscular block.

'Pre-relaxation twitch stabilization' will eliminate 'twitch potentiation' as a confounding factor when interpreting twitch responses after the administration of neuromuscular blocking drugs, but reaching a plateau can require up to 30 min of 0.1-Hz single-twitch simulation. Increasing the stimulation frequency can speed up the rate at which a plateau is reached but may also affect the ultimate plateau height as well. Careful balancing of these effects can be helpful in achieving a stable 'control' twitch response before the administration of neuromuscular blocking drugs. A two-second 50-Hz tetanic stimulus followed by two minutes of 0.1-Hz stimulus has been suggested for reasonably rapid twitch stabilization [5, 6]. Some researchers create a mathematical model of the postsynaptic process that causes a rise towards a plateau and incorporate it in their models of muscle relaxation [7].

Train-of-four Stimulation Pattern

The difficulties of obtaining and interpreting the 'control-twitch' for single-twitch stimulation have led to the development of the train-of-four (TOF) stimulation pattern. This stimulation pattern consists of four electrical pulses separated by 0.5 seconds, with each train usually separated by 12–20 seconds. As the depth of a non-depolarizing neuromuscular block increases, the fourth twitch will diminish first because the previous three stimuli have depleted the acetylcholine content of the presynaptic vesicles, causing a preponderance of the competitive inhibitor at the neuromuscular junction. As the concentration of the competitive inhibitor (the non-depolarizing neuromuscular blocking drug) further increases and the block deepens, the third, second and first twitch responses also decrease (in that sequence, because less and less acetylcholine is available during each subsequent pulse in the TOF sequence). The origin of the TOF 'fade' is thought to be a prejunctional effect of non-depolarizing neuromuscular blocking drugs.

The TOF stimulation pattern eliminates the need for a pre-relaxation control twitch because it references the magnitude of the fourth to the first twitch and uses this ratio to quantify the depth of a neuromuscular block. This ratio is known as the TOF ratio. A TOF ratio of 100% indicates the absence of neuromuscular block and 0% indicates that the fourth twitch has disappeared, suggesting a moderately deep level of neuromuscular block. At deeper levels, the third, second and first twitches become progressively smaller and ultimately disappear. As recovery from neuromuscular block occurs, the twitches reappear in order and when the fourth twitch reappears the TOF ratio can be again calculated. Even with a TOF ratio of one, a significant number of acetylcholine receptors may be blocked. It reflects the considerable margin of safety of neuromuscular transmission: up to 80% of receptors may be blocked without a noticeable effect on muscle strength. It also explains why the top-up dose of a neuromuscular

blocking drug to maintain a certain block is only a fraction of the initial dose (see further).

When the fourth twitch disappears and the so-called TOF count becomes three (out of four) and the TOF ratio becomes 0%, a 'moderately deep' block is said to exist. Once the TOF ratio becomes zero, the ratio itself cannot be used to quantify deeper blocks, and the clinician reverts to counting the number of detectable twitch responses after TOF stimulation, with a TOF count of three, two, one and zero indicating a progressively deeper block. A TOF count of zero or one corresponds to moderately deep neuromuscular block and indicates that considerable time must elapse before the fourth twitch will reappear and a TOF ratio can be calculated.

Tetanic Stimulation Pattern

Even when the TOF count is zero, deeper levels of neuromuscular block can be monitored still with a post-tetanic count (PTC) stimulation pattern. To obtain a PTC, a supra-maximal tetanic stimulation pattern of 50 Hz for five seconds is followed by a three-second pause, after which a single-twitch 1 Hz stimulus is applied for 15 seconds. The number of muscle responses to the 1 Hz stimuli is related to the time of reappearance of the first twitch of a TOF stimulus [8].

Tetanic stimulation overcomes a deep non-depolarizing block by inducing by a process called 'post-tetanic facilitation': tetanic stimulus induced exhaustion of presynaptic vesicles accelerates recycling and synthesis of acetylcholine in the prejunctional synapse, a process that actually overshoots in the sense that a larger than normal amount of acetylcholine is released after a subsequent single twitch. This excessive amount of acetylcholine succeeds in overcoming a deep (competitive, non-depolarizing) neuromuscular block. Very deep levels of neuromuscular block can be quantified in this manner. A PTC of one to two suggests that considerable time is still needed before reappearance of the first twitch response to a TOF stimulus. The PTC pattern is typically preceded by a number of TOF stimulations and the tetanic stimulation of the PTC is only applied if no detectable responses are observed.

Quantification of the Response to Stimulation: The Muscle Response

Following stimulation of a motor nerve, muscle response can be detected and quantified in a number of ways. Each method has various advantages and disadvantages.

Manual or Visual Estimation

The clinician can simply feel or observe the muscle contraction. However, manual estimation is not particularly accurate – even experienced researchers cannot observe fade at TOF ratios higher than about 40% [9]. Because current standards mandate that TOF ratios exceed 90% [10, 11] at the end of a procedure, manual or visual estimation is insufficient to judge whether recovery is adequate. Manual estimation is acceptable to monitor deep levels of neuromuscular block with the PTC stimulation pattern. It is generally accepted though that state-of-the-art neuromuscular monitoring requires objective quantification of muscle contraction.

Mechanomyography

Mechanomyography (MMG) measures the peak isometric muscle force after supramaximal neuromuscular stimulation. MMG is considered the 'gold standard' of neuromuscular monitoring because it is the generation of muscle force that maintains the airway and effective contraction of the diaphragm [12]. However, despite its importance, there are no commercially available devices that use isometric MMG neuromuscular monitoring. MMG has been used for research purposes though.

Typically, the peak isometric muscle force of the thumb's adductor pollicis is measured after stimulating the ulnar nerve at the elbow or at the wrist. MMG requires the associated limb to remain immobile. The thumb is held immobile by fixing the forearm to an armboard, and force is measured using a strain gauge at the thumb [13]. The resting tension of the muscle or 'preload' influences the muscle force that is generated – it is generally accepted that a preload associated muscle length of 100–125% of resting length generates maximum muscle force. At the adductor pollicis, this corresponds to a preload of approximately 200 grams, and ideally this should vary less than 25% throughout the period of neuromuscular monitoring. Obviously, the force of the preload is not exclusively conveyed to the muscle – some force is transferred to connective tissues as well. The geometry of any joints of the system also plays a role in the force produced. A drawback of the arm-board system is that subtle changes in patient positioning can change the placement of the forearm within the armboard, which changes the resting tension, which in turn affects interpretation of the observed muscle force.

Non-isometric Mechanomyography

Related to MMG monitoring is mechanical sensing of the muscle response. In this approach muscle contraction causes bending or compression of a piezoelectric sensor. It is used in the clinically widely applied NMT MechanoSensor® (GE Healthcare, Finland) (Fig. 11.1). The transducer is available in adult and paediatric sizes. Muscle preload cannot be evaluated because this depends on the mechanical properties of the transducer and how it matches with the individual anatomy. However, this approach does make attaching the device to the patient considerably simpler than for isometric systems, is much less sensitive to variation in patient positioning, and – even though it does not measure isometric muscle force – is sufficiently accurate for clinical applications.

Acceleromyographic Measures

If the limb associated with a muscle is free to move when the motor nerve is stimulated, then the movement of the limb can be also used to quantify muscle response. Acceleration is related to muscle force through Newton's second law, force = mass × acceleration. Because mass remains constant, the peak acceleration must be proportional to the peak muscle force resulting from the activation of the motor nerve. Accelerometers are robust, wear and tear free, and inexpensive to manufacture, making them well suited for the harsh clinical environment. They are also small, allowing considerable flexibility in how they can be placed: even though most are commonly used to measure thumb adduction, they can also be applied to the obicularis occuli, corrugator supercilii and the flexor hallucis brevis muscles. Many patient monitors have integrated modules which quantify the degree of neuromuscular block with accelerometry.

Electromyographic Measures

Prior to generating force, action potentials propagate throughout the muscle, initiating calcium release from the sarcoplasmic reticulum. These action potentials

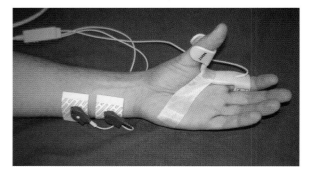

Fig. 11.1 Monitoring of neuromuscuslar block with the Mechanosensor® is based on bending of a piezoelectric sensor.

can also be detected and used to quantify the muscle's response to neuromuscular stimulation. The summation of the action potentials can be recorded using electrodes placed over the belly of the activated muscle. The peak-to-peak amplitude or the integration of the surface underneath the electromyographic (EMG) signal can be used to quantify muscle response. The ulnar nerve is stimulated at the elbow or wrist and the EMG response captured with electrodes placed over the adductor pollicis (at the thenar eminence), the abductor digiti minimi (at the hypothenar eminence), or at the first dorsal interosseus muscle. An active recording electrode should be placed over the muscle and a ground electrode between the stimulation and the recording electrodes. Sources of artefacts are multiple. External pressure on or moving of the electrodes and the arm can make the EMG quantification unreliable, but can be avoided by properly shielding and immobilizing the arm and electrodes. Changes in temperature, electrode conditions (due to, for example, absorption of electrode gel and sweating) and monopolar diathermy can all interfere with EMG monitoring.

Neuromuscular diseases can make EMG neuromuscular monitoring problematic. Volatile anaesthetics can impair muscle function and force generation without having an effect on the EMG signal [14, 15]. In general, MMG and AMG rather than EMG are often preferred as techniques to monitor the degree of a neuromuscular block because they measure the actual movement in muscles.

Pharmacology of Neuromuscular Blocking Drugs

Several drugs can prevent the contraction of skeletal muscles at the neuromuscular junction by inhibiting the synthesis or release of acetylcholine or by blocking its actions at the postjunctional membrane. Clinically used neuromuscular blocking drugs mainly act by the latter mechanism, inhibition of the postjunctional actions of acetylcholine at the nicotinic acetylcholine receptor. Two classes of neuromuscular blocking drugs exist, non-depolarizing and depolarizing. Only one depolarizing drug is clinically used, suxamethonium (also called succinylcholine). These two drug classes have different properties.

All neuromuscular blocking drugs are quaternary ammonium compounds that hold acetylcholine somewhere in their chemical structure. The quaternary ammonium (NH_{4+}) prevents their absorption from the gastrointestinal tract, placenta and into the cerebrospinal fluid (CSF). Because of these chemical properties, neuromuscular blocking drugs are not widely distributed in the body and their volume of distribution (0.1–0.5 L/kg) is rather close to the volume of extracellular fluid [17].

Non-depolarizing Neuromuscular Blocking Drugs

Mechanism of Action

Chemically, non-depolarizing neuromuscular blocking drugs are either benzylisoquinolones (cisatracurium, mivacurium) or aminosteroid derivatives (rocuronium). They are competitive inhibitors of acetylcholine at the postjunctional nicotinic receptor. If they occupy one or both alpha subunits, ion channel opening is prevented and neuromuscular transmission becomes impaired. At higher concentrations they can also block the channel directly, in a non-competitive action. However, this so-called 'channel block' is of minor clinical significance [16].

Adverse Effects

The action of non-depolarizing neuromuscular blocking drugs on nicotinic receptors outside the neuromuscular endplate or on muscarinic receptors explains many of their adverse effects. Cisatracurium, mivacurium and rocuronium have essentially no effects on nicotinic receptors in the autonomic ganglia (Table 11.1). Via an effect on the vagal nerve, rocuronium can activate cardiac muscarinic receptors, but tachycardia will only ensue at a dose which is three- to five-fold higher than a usual dose for endotracheal intubation. Benzylisoquinolones can cause serosal mast cells to release histamine, but this effect is mild with mivacurium and absent with cisatracurium. Overall, the incidence of serious adverse effects is low. However, of all intraoperative life-threatening anaphylactic or anaphylactoid reactions (1 in 10,000 to 20,000 anaesthetics in a French study), 60% are caused by neuromuscular blocking drugs [17].

ED_{95} is the dose which is required to induce a 95% neuromuscular block (the height of the first twitch in the TOF sequence reaches 5% of the height of the control twitch obtained before the administration of neuromuscular blocking drugs).

Pharmacokinetics and Pharmacodynamics of Non-depolarizing Neuromuscular Blocking Drugs

Essential basic PK/PD characteristics are summarized in Table 11.1. Renal clearance accounts for 10–25% of the elimination of rocuronium [18], with the remainder

Table 11.1. Effect of commonly used neuromuscular blocking drugs on the autonomic nervous system and histamine release and their basic PK and PD properties.

| Drug | Chemical structure | Autonomic Nervous System and Histamine Release | | | | Basic PK and PD Properties | | |
		Autonomic ganglia	Cardiac muscarinic receptor	Histamine release	ED$_{95}$ (mg/kg)	Rate of infusion required to maintain neuromuscular block at 95% (µg/kg/min)	Time to peak effect following 2 × ED$_{95}$ (min)	Time to T1 = 25% of control following 2 × ED$_{95}$ (min)	Renal clearance (% total clearance)
Cisatracurium	Benzylisoquinoline	None	None	None	0.05	1–2	5.2	20–50	16
Mivacurium	Benzylisoquinoline	None	None	Slight	0.08	3–15	3	10–20	<5
Rocuronium	Aminosteroid	None	Blocks weakly	None	0.3	9–12	1.5	20–50	10–25
Suxamethonium	Diacetylcholine	Stimulates	Stimulates	Slight	0.3	–	1.4	<10	<2

being excreted into bile unchanged or after metabolism by the liver. While its metabolism remains poorly understood, increased rocuronium requirements in patients ingesting enzyme inducing drugs indicate that rocuronium is at least partly metabolized by the inducible microsomal enzymes in the liver. Cisatracurium is degraded by Hoffman elimination, a chemical process independent of renal or hepatic function. Mivacurium is metabolized by plasma pseudocholinesterase, which explains why its plasma clearance (5 L/min in healthy adults) exceeds liver blood flow.

Simultaneous PK/PD modelling has been used to give a full description of the pharmacological properties of neuromuscular blocking drugs. Population modelling is a powerful tool to identify quantitatively which factors affect the PK/PD of various drugs. The major strength of the population approach is that

useful information can be extracted even from sparse data using blood samples and pharmacological monitoring during routine efficacy studies conducted during the development of a drug. Table 11.2 shows the population PK/PD variables for non-depolarizing neuromuscular blocking drugs.

The model parameters shown in Table 11.2 allow computer simulations to be performed of the behaviour of neuromuscular blocking drugs following any proposed administration regime. Compartmental volumes V1 (central), V2 and V3 (peripheral) represent drug distribution volumes, where the drug is administered (central) and where it can diffuse or be transported while in the body. These may have vague associations with different tissues in the body due to various factors such as differing solubilites and other drug–tissue interactions. In any case they represent a

Table 11.2. Population pharmacokinetic and pharmacodynamic variables for non-depolarizing neuromuscular blocking drugs.

	Author	Subgroup	Pharmacokinetics		Pharmacodynamics
Cisatracurium	Schmith [54]		V1=0.0457·WGT l V2=0.0988·WGT l	CL=0.00457·WGT L/min Q2=0.00569·WGT L/min	keo=0.0575 L/min C_e50=141 ng/mL λ=4.01
	Lui [55]	Control group	V1=0.0583·WGT l V2=0.0428·WGT l	CL=0.00642·WGT L/min Q2=0.0180·WGT	keo=0.14 L/min C_e50=198.8 ng/mL λ=6.96
	Tran [56]		V1=0.035·WGT l V2=0.0511·WGT l	CL=0.0037·WGT L/min Q2=0.00367·WGT L/min	keo=0.054 L/min C_e50=153 ng/mL λ=6.9
Mivacurium	Schiere et al [19]		V1=0.0397·WGT l V2=0.0194·WGT l	CL=0.031·WGT L/min Q2=0.00464·WGT L/min	kip=0.374 L/min (plasma-interstitial) kei=0.151 L/min (interstitial-effect) C_e50=98 mg/mL λ=3.7
Rocuronium	Ploeger [51]	Caucasians	V1=3.58 l V2=3.26 l V3=7.64 l	CL=0.353 L/min Q2=0.565 L/min Q3=0.134 L/min	keo=0.655 L/min C_e50=720 ng/mL λ=6.57
		Japanese	V1=2.56 l V2=3.26 l V3=4.42 l	CL=0.252 L/min Q2=0.354 L/min Q3=0.0584 L/min	
	Kleijn [52]		$V1_{ct}$·4.74·WGT/70 V_{ct}=exp (-0.00143·(CR-119)) $V2_{age}$·6.76·WGT/70 $V2_{age}$=exp(0.00613·(AGE-43))	Cl_{age}·0.269·(WGT/70)$^{.75}$ Cl_{age}=1– 0.00678·(AGE-43) Q2rac·0.279· (WGT/70)$^{.75}$ Q2rac=1-(Asian)0.212	keo=Ksev·0.134· (WGT/70)$^{-0.25}$ L/min Ksev=1-(Sev)0.567 C_e50=Esev·1.62 μM Esev=1-(Sev)0.395 λ=7.52
	Proost [53]		V1=0.0372·WGT V2=0.0370·WGT V3=0.114*WGT	CL=0.00422*WGT Q2=0.00617·WGT Q3=0.00185·WGT	keo=0.137 L/min C_e50=1257 mg/mL λ=3.68

WGT=bodyweight in kg; AGE=age is years; CR=creatinine clearance in mL/min; Asian=1 for asian, 0 otherwise; Sev=1 for Sevoflurane anaesthesia, 0 otherwise.
For explanation of the PK and PD variables, see the body of the text.

rather extreme simplification of the complex biological processes underlying drug distribution.

Model clearance parameters such as CL (elimination), Q2 and Q3 (inter-compartmental) represent drug transport between the various compartments, with CL being a special case of drug transport from the central compartment out of the body or otherwise made inactive. Drugs with a higher CL tend to have shorter duration of action in a straightforward manner. Interestingly, they also tend to provide a more rapid onset of paralysis because these drugs allow greater initial doses, creating a stronger driving force for drug distribution to the effect compartment. The rate of drug distribution to the effect site, described as k_{eo}, also plays an essential role in determining a drug's potential for rapid onset of effect. A slow k_{eo} limits the rate of onset of action. While a simple first-order rate constant is often sufficient to describe drug transport to the effect site, mivacurium is an exception to this, requiring modelling of an interstitial compartment for

accurate prediction of PD [19]. Other PD parameters describe various characteristics of drug effect. *Ce50* describes the effect-site concentration at which 50% of drug effect is achieved. Lower values for *Ce50* indicate higher drug potency. Parameter λ describes the slope of the sigmoidal E_{max} PD model. High values of λ indicate that drug effect changes rapidly over a low range of drug concentrations, creating an 'on–off switch' like drug effect. Lower values of λ describe a more gradual relationship between effect-site concentration and drug effect.

To highlight the PK/PD differences between two neuromuscular blocking drugs with an intermediate duration of action, we have simulated the course of effect-site concentrations after the administration of one ED_{95} dose of either rocuronium or cisatracurium. We also simulated context-sensitive 50% effect decrement times as a function of the duration of infusion which maintained neuromuscular block (and effect-site concentration) constant (Fig. 11.2).

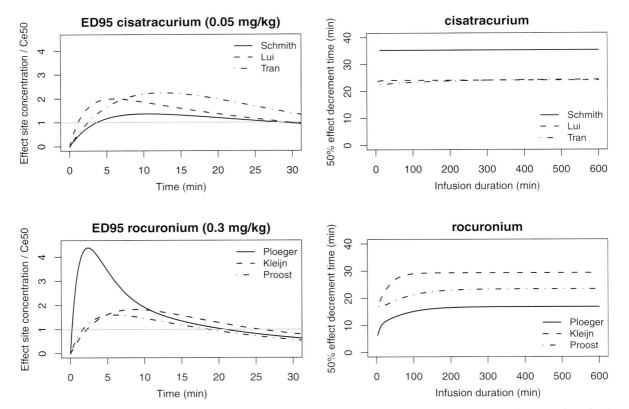

Fig. 11.2 Left panel: Simulated effect-site concentrations of rocuronium and cisatracurium after the administration of one ED_{95} dose of each drug. Right panel: Context-sensitive 50% effect decrement times as a function of the duration of rocuronium and cisatracurium infusions which maintained neuromuscular block (and effect-site concentration) constant. Simulations were based on the parameters obtained from Ploeger [51], Kleijn [52], Proost [53], Schmith [54], Liu [55], and Tran [56].

Clinical Pharmacology of Non-depolarizing Neuromuscular Blocking Drugs

Mivacurium has a shorter duration of action than rocuronium and cisatracurium, whose durations of action are considered 'intermediate' (Table 11.1). However, because rocuronium has the shortest onset of action of all three drugs, it is the more frequently used drug, especially if rapid endotracheal intubation is required.

While cisatracurium has often been considered the drug of choice in patients having severe renal and/or hepatic dysfunction because of its organ-independent elimination, rocuronium can be used as well if the degree of neuromuscular block is monitored properly.

Non-depolarizing neuromuscular blocking drugs are most often used to achieve neuromuscular block during balanced anaesthesia. Provided hypnosis is induced by other means, they may also be used to provide immobility during diagnostic procedures or during transportation of critically ill patients, and occasionally to facilitate ventilation during intensive care.

Depolarizing Neuromuscular Blocking Drugs
Mechanism of Action

The onset of action of suxamethonium is fast. Stimulation of the acetylcholine receptors usually results in visible fasciculations before the onset of muscle relaxation. Suxamethonium causes a long-lasting depolarization which prevents the muscular contraction. Experimentally, a similar effect can be produced by the administration of acetylcholine and anticholinesterases. Anticholinesterases augment the action of suxamethonium [2].

Adverse Effects

Because suxamethonium consists of two acetylcholine molecules (diacetylcholine), it is understandable that its adverse effects mimic those of acetylcholine. Suxamethonium has effects on cholinergic receptors all over the body, including striated muscle and the autonomic nervous system (Table 11.1). Suxamethonium has effects on both autonomic ganglia and cardiac muscarinic receptors. Depending on the actual status of the patient's autonomic nervous system, it may cause bradycardia, tachycardia or other arrhythmias, and hypo- or hypertension. These effects can be prevented by administration of anticholinergic drugs such as atropine or glycopyrrolate.

Suxamethonium typically causes fasciculations before the onset of neuromuscular block. Many

patients also have muscle pains, which are more common in young muscular adults. They can be rather effectively prevented with a small dose of non-depolarizing neuromuscular drug.

Hyperkalaemia and malignant hyperthermia are two life-threatening adverse effects. Plasma potassium concentrations often rise, but without clinical consequences in otherwise healthy patients. However, in patients with upper or lower motoneuron lesions, trauma, burns or immobilization, the number of extrajunctional acetylcholine receptors may be increased so much that their activation causes life-threatening hyperkalaemia. Suxamethonium can trigger malignant hyperthermia, a rare autosomal dominant condition that may be fatal without prompt administration of dantrolene and effective symptomatic treatment.

Large doses or prolonged administration of suxamethonium may cause a transition of typical depolarizing block to phase II block which resembles the block produced by non-depolarizing neuromuscular drugs. Phase II block is not observed following an intubation dose of suxamethonium.

Pharmacokinetics/Pharmacodynamics of Suxamethonium

The duration of action of suxamethonium is four to 12 minutes following an intubation dose because it is rapidly metabolized by plasma pseudocholinesterase. Actually, only a small fraction of the administered dose reaches the neuromuscular endplate. The drug is thus not metabolized at the neuromuscular junction itself: in order to terminate its effect, it must diffuse back out of the neuromuscular junction into systemic circulation, where plasma pseudocholinesterase degrades it into choline and succinylmonocholine (with the latter being further metabolized to choline and succinic acid) [2]. Several genetically determined forms of plasma pseudocholinesterase exist, and this may affect the duration of action of suxamethonium. Approximately 2.5–4% of the population is carrying one abnormal gene allele, which prolongs the action of suxamethonium by 50% to 100%. Another 0.04% of the population is carrying two abnormal gene alleles, and this prolongs the duration of neuromuscular block to two to six hours [20].

Clinical Pharmacology of Suxamethonium

Because of its numerous adverse effects, the clinical use of suxamethonium has been declining. It is mainly used to facilitate endotracheal intubation, and for rapid sequence inductions in particular because it has the fastest, most reliable onset (with a consistent deep block). However, many authorities nowadays consider rocuronium [21] a suitable alternative even for rapid sequence induction because it can easily and rapidly be reversed with sugammadex if necessary (see below). Suxamethonium also continues to be used for short-lasting muscle relaxation needed during electroconvulsive therapy or for the reposition of dislocated joints, and to treat laryngospams.

Optimal Level of Neuromuscular Block

Immobility is an essential part of balanced anaesthesia. Regardless of the surgical procedure, the patient should not move after a noxious stimulus. It is impossible to perform surgery if the patient is wiggling around and trying to escape the operating table. For some types of surgery, it is imperative the patient does not move because it would cause irreparable harm, e.g. during intra-ocular or intra-cranial surgery.

Muscle relaxation is needed when the force or pressure generated by that force makes it impossible to complete the surgical procedure, the typical example being intra-abdominal surgery. The high intra-abdominal pressures resulting from the force generated by the diaphragm and abdominal wall muscles make it impossible to perform open abdominal surgery and (somewhat more controversial, see further) laparoscopic intra-abdominal surgery. Similarly, relocation of a hip prosthesis may need relaxation.

Although immobility can be produced very selectively with neuromuscular blocking drugs, the question remains of how much neuromuscular block is enough to provide immobility and surgical relaxation. What is regarded as adequate surgical relaxation is dependent on a multitude of factors. It is not only the degree of neuromuscular block that determines the adequacy of muscle relaxation – depth of anaesthesia, type of surgery and surgical skill all have an influence. For superficial surgery, immobility is obviously required but the surgery itself does not require any significant muscle relaxation. For intra-abdominal surgery, deeper muscle relaxation may be required. What degree of neuromuscular block is needed to provide adequate surgical relaxation for what procedure has been poorly explored and is only beginning to be studied in randomized controlled trials.

For many surgical procedures, balanced anaesthesia does not need to entail the use of neuromuscular blocking drugs. Fast track cardiac surgery has been performed without muscle relaxants once the airway has been secured [22]. Surgeons rated operating conditions in the 87 patients as satisfactory, and no reversing agents were needed because the TOF ratio had recovered spontaneously to 0.90 by the end of the operation.

In accordance with the previous study, suxamethonium for facilitating endotracheal intubation was the only neuromuscular blocking drug which was needed in 86 patients undergoing spinal surgery with total intravenous anaesthesia [23]: muscle relaxation was deemed sufficient and the surgery was successful, regardless of whether atracurium was used later during surgery or not. An isoflurane–fentanyl anaesthetic alone produced also good to excellent surgical field conditions in approximately two-thirds of patients undergoing radical retropubic prostatectomy without the use of neuromuscular blocking drug. Thus, the authors concluded that the routine use of muscle relaxants in adequately anaesthetized patients undergoing this procedure may not be indicated [24].

During laparoscopic abdominal surgery, a CO_2 pneumoperitoneum is usually needed to allow the surgeon to visualize the abdominal contents and to provide sufficient working space. Because the pressure generated by the abdominal wall muscles and diaphragm is believed to reduce the space provided by the pressurized CO_2, neuromuscular blocking drugs are administered in the belief that it increases abdominal wall compliance. However, there are few studies that convincingly prove that.

One study that did find a difference (i.e. better surgical conditions with a deep [25] versus shallow block) was criticized because depth in the control group was not tightly controlled and because the average quality of the visual field did not differ [26]. Another study claiming 'marginally better' surgical space conditions with deep rather than moderate muscle relaxation during laparoscopic cholecystectomy [27] suffered from similar flaws, with the authors basically comparing deep versus very shallow or minimal block for a considerable portion of the surgical procedure. When patients were randomized to a deep (PTC 2–3) or a moderate neuromuscular block (TOF count 1–2) during laparoscopic bariatric surgery [28], a deep neuromuscular block was associated with better surgical visualization and lower pain scores in the immediate postoperative period (p = 0.03) (see Fig. 11.3).

Two recent systematic reviews tried to clarify whether surgical conditions and patient outcome are related to the degree of neuromuscular block during surgery. Interestingly, the two reviews arrived at

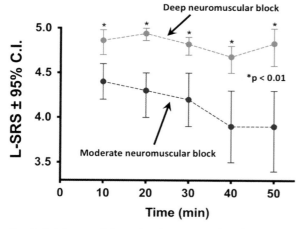

Fig. 11.3 Influence of deep relaxation on surgical conditions scored with Leiden-surgical rating scale (L-SRS, mean with 95% CI) from 1 (extremely poor) to 5 (optimal conditions) in laparoscopic bariatric surgery. *Mann–Whitney U test p < 0.01 versus moderate block.

different conclusions. While Madsen et al concluded that deep neuromuscular block may improve surgical conditions in laparoscopic and open abdominal surgery [29], Kopman and Naguib [30] stated that there are few objective data to demonstrate that a deep neuromuscular block (PTC ≥ 1 with TOF twitch count = 0) improves surgical conditions or patient outcome compared to a moderate block (TOF twitch count = 1–3). Kopman and Naquib were also concerned about the economic consequences of the increasing use of sugammadex which cannot be avoided if a deep neuromuscular block is deemed necessary until the very end of surgery. More information can be found in two editorials that discuss the relationship between surgical muscle relaxation and degree of neuromuscular block and that try to define 'adequacy of muscle relaxation' [31, 32].

To summarize, for many surgical procedures no consensus has been reached regarding the optimal level of neuromuscular drug-induced block. While different types of operations need different levels of muscle relaxation, it is important to realize this depends on both the depth of anaesthesia and the degree of neuromuscular block: deeper levels of anaesthesia may allow shallower neuromuscular block to obtain the same degree of relaxation. The price to pay for using a deep level of anaesthesia as an essential component of muscle relaxation is prolonged emergence. If surgery requires deep muscle relaxation until the very end of surgery and if this is accomplished by a deep level of drug-induced neuromuscular block (e.g. a PTC of 1–3), sugammadex can be used to antagonize the

block, but this comes with a price tag; the only alternative under these conditions is to wait for the spontaneous recovery.

Factors Affecting the Requirements of Neuromuscular Blocking Drugs

The dose of neuromuscular blocking drugs obviously depends on the desired degree of neuromuscular block. However, there are other factors that affect the requirements of neuromuscular blocking drugs.

Drug–Drug Interactions

Drugs that inhibit plasma cholinesterase may delay neuromuscular recovery after suxamethonium administration. These drugs include anticholinesterase inhibitors (donepezil, ecothiopate, neostigmine, pyridostigmine, rivastigmine, etc.), the antineoplastic drug cyclophosphamide, bambuterol and the monoamine oxidase inhibitor phenelzine [33].

Enzyme inducing drugs like rifampicin and older antiepileptic drugs antagonize the neuromuscular blocking effects of rocuronium, probably by enhancing their hepatic elimination (although other mechanisms may also contribute) [34]. The mechanism by which phenytoin and carbamazepine antagonize cisatracurium is not known [35, 36]. Enzyme induction or inhibition does not affect mivacurium [37].

Volatile anaesthetics potentiate the effects of nondepolarizing muscle relaxants in a dose-dependent manner, an effect most pronounced with desflurane (Fig. 11.4) [38]. The underlying mechanism remains controversial, and several factors have been invoked: increased muscle blood flow, increased sensitivity of

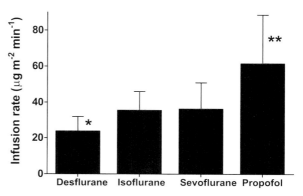

Fig. 11.4 The rate of infusion of cisatracurium maintaining neuromuscular block constant at 90% in patients anaesthetized with desflurane, isoflurane, sevoflurane or propofol. *P < 0.02 as compared to the other groups, **P < 0.002 as compared to patients with volatile anaesthetics.

the motor endplate, decreased release of acetylcholine, change of ion-channel conductance, or other effects at the central nervous system.

Aminoglycosides, polymyxins, lincomycin and clindamycin all can potentiate a neuromuscular block [33] by inhibiting the prejunctional release of acetylcholine and by depressing postjunctional acetylcholine receptor sensitivity to acetylcholine.

Hypothermia

Hypothermia affects the PK and/or PD of nondepolarizing neuromuscular blocking drugs [39]. Hypothermia at 30.4 °C causes a 50% reduction in rocuronium plasma clearance, reducing rocuronium requirements in a hypothermic patient [40]. Hypothermia also reduces the Hoffman elimination process, which prolongs the action of cisatracurium [41, 42]. Hypothermia also affects the neuromuscular monitoring process itself: if the monitored arm becomes hypothermic, the onset and duration of action of the drugs will become slower and longer, respectively, than in the more centrally located muscles (e.g. abdominal wall and diaphragm) at normal core temperature [43].

Dosing of Neuromuscular Blocking Drugs

Initial Administration

A relative overdose administered as an intravenous bolus achieves the most rapid onset of neuromuscular block during induction of anaesthesia. The blood rapidly transports the drug to the neuromuscular junctions of the body where its pharmacological effects take place. The initial dose is higher than that required to attain those peak concentration levels needed at the

neuromuscular junction to facilitate endotracheal intubation. Typically, the initial dose is two to four times the ED_{95}. ED_{95} is the dose which is required to induce a 95% neuromuscular block (the height of the first twitch in the TOF sequence reaches 5% of the height of the control twitch obtained before the administration of neuromuscular blocking drugs). In general, the accompanying overshoot is not deleterious because a moderate overdose of modern competitive neuromuscular blocking drugs has little or no adverse effects. However, the prolonged duration of drug effect can be problematic for short procedures.

Intermittent Bolus Dosing

Most often, a neuromuscular block is maintained by repeated bolus doses. Because of the large margin of safety (or neuromuscular reserve) of the neuromuscular junction, the maintenance dose is considerably smaller than the induction dose: even though monitoring shows the block induced by the loading dose is recovering, up to 70% of the postjunctional nicotinic receptors may still be blocked, a condition under which even a small top-up dose can have a profound effect on the twitch response. Fig. 11.5 shows the time course of neuromuscular block following intermittent bolus doses. The degree of neuromuscular block varies throughout the procedure, reaching barely adequate levels just before administration of the maintenance dose and usually achieving complete block for a period thereafter.

Continuous Infusion

One way to improve stability of the neuromuscular block over time is to start an infusion once the muscle starts to recover from the induction dose (Fig. 11.6). The infusion rates of most neuromuscular blocking drugs to accomplish this have been published. Typical

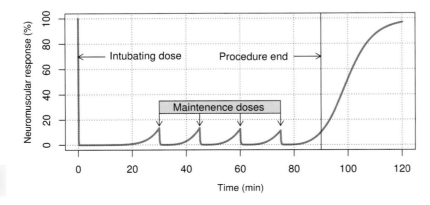

Fig. 11.5 Maintenance of neuromuscular block using intermittent bolus dosing. The degree of neuromuscular block varies throughout the procedure between barely adequate and complete neuromuscular block.

values for rates of infusion required to maintain neuromuscular block constant at 95% are given in Table 11.1. However, because of major inter-individual differences, it is important to quantify the degree of neuromuscular block repetitively and adjust the rate of infusion accordingly.

Computer-controlled Infusion

Short-acting neuromuscular blocking drugs can also be administered via a computer-controlled infusion. Both target-controlled and closed-loop controlled systems have been described. At least theoretically, target-controlled infusion (TCI) systems are able to attain and maintain the desired concentration of the neuromuscular blocking drug. Vermeyen et al and Motamed et al have described a target-controlled infusion system for the continuous administration of rocuronium [44, 45] and Ma et al [46] for cisatracurium.

Although the TCI of neuromuscular blocking drugs can obviously maintain the concentrations at a reasonably constant level, they cannot be used without the monitoring of neuromuscular block. Without adaptation of the model parameters during drug administration, the control of neuromuscular block is far from optimal as compared to closed-loop control of neuromuscular block. The values for median performance error and median absolute performance error (expressed as median with range) during TCI of rocuronium were 9.7 (−35, 40) and 23.6 (5, 40)% without adaptation of the model parameters and 14.8 (11, 44) and 16 (13, 44)% with Bayesian forecasting of parameters [45]. These figures are far from the values of median performance error and median absolute performance error obtained for closed-loop control of rocuronium infusion. For instance, Kansanaho and Olkkola [47] observed that the values of median performance error and median absolute performance error (expressed as median with 25th and 75th percentile) were 0.5 (0.0, 0.9) and 1.3 (1.1, 1.7)%, respectively.

Figure 11.7 depicts the typical course of neuromuscular block during closed-loop control. The closed-loop system can be started any time after the initial bolus, and will deliver only that amount of drug needed to achieve the target neuromuscular block level. Theoretically, it should be able to render a neuromuscular block even more stable than with continuous

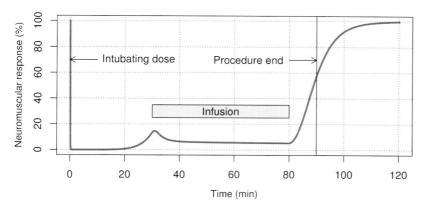

Fig. 11.6 Maintenance of neuromuscular block using a continuous infusion. Compared to the intermittent bolus dosing, the degree of neuromuscular block varies considerably less throughout the procedure.

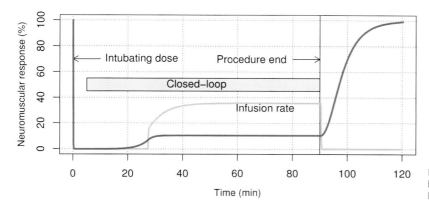

Fig. 11.7 Maintenance of neuromuscular block using a computer-controlled, 'closed-loop' system.

infusions. Long-acting drugs are less suitable for use with closed-computer-controlled infusion because fewer dose adjustments will be needed – and it is precisely that which a computer-controlled infusion is well suited for. While it could be applied during long-term sedation in the intensive care unit, any benefit should be weighed against that of using short-acting drugs in this context, a benefit not likely to be clinically relevant.

A closed-loop system is used to steer drug delivery by the computer-controlled pump. Actually, neuromuscular blocking drugs were amongst the first anaesthetic drugs to be administered with this technology (see below). The first component is a signal quantifying a patient's neuromuscular block. The signal obtained automatically and repeatedly is fed back to a controller where it is compared to a desired 'target'. The computer then applies algorithms on the various inputs it receives from the actual and desired states of neuromuscular block. Time and time-differences can also be used as inputs for the algorithm. Next, the computer adjusts the injection rate of syringe pump loaded with neuromuscular blocking drugs to achieve the desired block.

The advantages of closed-loop infusions of neuromuscular blocking drugs are several-fold. First, it allows anaesthesiologists to focus on other aspects of care by freeing up time that may otherwise be needed for tedious repetitive dose calculations. It may also avoid 'cognitive-overload' in particularly complex cases. Second, complex control algorithms can be implemented, allowing one to achieve a more stable neuromuscular block more rapidly than is possible with direct human control. Finally, control algorithms can more accurately monitor dosing histories, provide feedback, or trigger alarms to warn the anaesthesiologist about potential over- or underdosing.

Of course, these systems have disadvantages as well. First, some systems require time and attention to be set up. This includes entering patient covariates (weight, age, etc.) and neuromuscular block targets, and filling and placement of syringes. For some systems, these tasks have to be completed before anaesthesia can be started. This increases clinical workload during the busy induction period, precisely when clinicians need to focus on a host of other factors. Second, increased technical complexity may introduce new sources of error and failure. Patient information can be entered incorrectly, syringes can be empty and/or

need replacement, syringes can be incorrectly filled, etc. Understanding potential workflow errors and their consequences for patient care (as well as preventing them) is a complex undertaking.

Despite the fact that closed-loop control of neuromuscular blocking drugs has a surprisingly long history, and despite a plethora of closed-loop systems described in anaesthesia research, no such systems have found broad commercial application. One reason for this is the limitations inherent in many of the control algorithms. For example, adaptive and model-based systems 'learn' individual characteristics based on the history of applied doses and recorded responses, which means the computer needs to have all dosing information. This precludes clinicians from dosing 'alongside' a control system because doses given by the clinician outside of the control algorithm may be interpreted by the algorithm as increased sensitivity of the patient to neuromuscular blocking drugs. The algorithm may consequently administer lower drug doses than needed to maintain the desired effect, because it will rely on this (incorrect) high sensitivity and decrease the injection rate. Complex stability issues can occur, causing poor performance resulting in a clinically insufficient neuromuscular block.

Avoiding the potential issues with complex control algorithms requires abandoning some degrees of 'adaptation' in the control algorithm. This has been successful in some ways: a simple non-adaptive proportional-integrative-derivative controller combined with a lookup-table for TOF counts has been shown to achieve good stability in muscle relaxation, while maintaining adequate performance despite relaxant dosing 'alongside' the control algorithm [48]. The system even performed adequately during power-cycling (switching it off and then on again) during the surgical procedure. Despite some initial system development, the proposed system was never offered commercially.

Reversal of Neuromuscular Block

If the effect of neuromuscular blocking drugs is not monitored with objective methods, the patient is at risk for residual neuromuscular block at the end of the procedure. If the patient is extubated before the TOF ratio has reached at least 0.9, there is an increased risk for reduced acute hypoxic ventilatory response and aspiration (the laryngeal muscles that prevent this from happening are very sensitive to neuromuscular blocking drugs). Because the risk of postoperative complications is markedly increased in patients with a postoperative residual neuromuscular block [49], a residual neuromuscular block has to be antagonized. The action of suxamethonium cannot be reversed. If it would cause a prolonged block (e.g. in a patient with atypical pseudocholinesterases), the patient has to be ventilated until the block has worn off. Theoretically one could also administer fresh frozen plasma, but it is usually regarded safer to wait for the recovery of the neuromuscular block.

The action of non-depolarizing neuromuscular blocking drugs, however, can be pharmacologically reversed. The conventional way of antagonizing the neuromuscular block is the administration of anticholinesterases together with anticholinergic drugs. Because non-depolarizing neuromuscular drugs produce the block by competitive antagonism, the effect can be overcome and reversed by increasing the concentration of the agonist acetylcholine. The most commonly used anticholinesterases are neostigmine and edrophonium which are combined with glycopyrrolate or atropine to counteract the stimulation of muscarinic receptors. The onset time of neostigmine matches that of glycopyrrolate while the onset time of edrophonium matches that of atropine. When using anticholinesterases, reversal should not be attempted until the recovery of the neuromuscular junction can be observed. Deep neuromuscular block cannot be antagonized with anticholinesterases. At least two, but preferably three to four twitches should be observable in the TOF sequence. Anticholinesterases can be used to antagonize the block induced by any of the non-depolarizing neuromuscular drugs.

The action of the aminosteroid rocuronium can also be antagonized with the cyclodextrin derivative sugammadex. Sugammadex forms tight complexes with rocuronium. After administration of sugammadex the free concentration of rocuronium decreases rapidly. The resulting concentration gradient between plasma and neuromuscular junction rapidly decreases the concentration of rocuronium at the postjunctional nicotinic receptors, terminating rocuronium's neuromuscular blocking effect within minutes. The sugammadex–rocuronium complex is excreted unchanged into urine, and has an elimination half-life of approximately two hours. Sugammadex is effective at any depth of neuromuscular block; its efficacy is not affected by the type and depth of anaesthesia [50].

Prior administration of sugammadex affects subsequent rocuronium dosing requirements. According to the manufacturer's recommendation, after 4 mg/kg of sugammadex, rocuronium should not be given in the ensuing five minutes. If rocuronium were to be given within this five-minute period, the dose should be 1.2 mg/kg. Even then, the onset of neuromuscular block is delayed and the duration of action is likely to be markedly reduced. After 16 mg/kg of sugammadex, the manufacturer recommends not to use rocuronium for 24 hours. If a neuromuscular blocking drug is required soon after the administration of sugammadex, most anaesthesiologists would choose one of the benzylisoquinolone derivatives, because their action is not modified by sugammadex.

Conclusions and Recommendations

Immobility and sufficient surgical muscle relaxation are essential components of balanced anaesthesia. Although they can be accomplished selectively with neuromuscular blocking drugs, adequate muscle relaxation during anaesthesia also depends on the depth of anaesthesia.

Although neuromuscular blocking drugs have been administered by continuous infusion and with computer-controlled infusion, an intermittent bolus is the more frequently used administration method. The initial dose of non-depolarizing neuromuscular blocking drugs is normally two to four times the ED_{95} dose, followed by smaller doses to maintain the neuromuscular block.

The degree of neuromuscular block should always be measured with objective monitoring methods. Full neuromuscular recovery (TOF ratio > 0.90) must be ensured before the waking up of the patient at the end of the anaesthetic. Residual neuromuscular block considerably increases the risk for reduced acute hypoxic ventilatory response, aspiration and other serious postoperative complications.

References

1. Tammisto T, Olkkola KT: Dependence of the adequacy of muscle relaxation on the degree of neuromuscular block and depth of enflurane anesthesia during abdominal surgery. Anesth.Analg. 1995; 80: 543–7.

2. Hibbs RE, Zambon AC: Agents acting at the neuromuscular junction and autonomic ganglia. In: Brunton LL, Chabner BA, Knollmann BC. eds. *Goodman & Gilman's: The Pharmacological Basis of Therapeutics,*

12th Edition. New York, NY: McGraw-Hill. http://accessmedicine.mhmedical.com/content.aspx?bookid=1613&sectionid=102158134 [last accessed 15 June, 2019].

3. Bowman WC, Prior C, Marshall IG: Presynaptic receptors in the neuromuscular junction. Ann. NY.Acad.Sci. 1990; 604: 69–81.

4. Hemmerling TM, Donati F: Neuromuscular blockade at the larynx, the diaphragm and the corrugator supercilii muscle: a review. Can.J.Anesth. 2003; 50: 779–94.

5. Viby-Mogensen J, Engbaek J, Eriksson LI, Gramstad L, Jensen E, Jensen FS, Koscielniak-Nielsen Z, Skovgaard LT, Østergaard D: Good clinical research practice (GCRP) in pharmacodynamic studies of neuromuscular blocking agents. Acta.Anaesthesiol. Scand. 1996; 40: 59–74.

6. Fuchs-Buder T, Claudius C, Skovgaard LT, Eriksson LI, Mirakhur RK, Viby-Mogensen J: Good clinical research practice in pharmacodynamic studies of neuromuscular blocking agents II: the Stockholm revision. Acta.Anaesthesiol. Scand. 2007; 51: 789–808.

7. Eleveld DJ, Kopman AF, Proost JH, Wierda JM: Model to describe the degree of twitch potentiation during neuromuscular monitoring. Brit.J.Anaesth. 2004; 92: 373–80.

8. El-Orbany MI, Joseph NJ, Salem MR: The relationship of posttetanic count and train-of-four responses during recovery from intense cisatracurium-induced neuromuscular blockade. Anesth.Analg. 2003; 97: 80–4.

9. Viby-Mogensen J, Jensen NH, Engbaek J, Ording H, Skovgaard LT, Chraemmer-Jorgensen B: Tactile and visual evaluation of the response to train-of-four nerve stimulation. Anesthesiology. 1985; 63: 440–3.

10. Eikermann M, Groeben H, Husing J, Peters J. Predictive value of mechanomyography and accelerometry for pulmonary function in partially paralyzed volunteers. Acta.Anaesthesiol. Scand. 2004; 48: 365–70.

11. Capron F, Alla F, Hottier C, Meistelman C, Fuchs-Buder T: Can acceleromyography detect low levels of residual paralysis? A probability approach to detect a mechanomyographic train-of-four ratio of 0.9. Anesthesiology. 2004; 100: 1119–24.

12. Viby-Mogensen J, Engbaek J, Eriksson LI, Gramstad L, Jensen E, Jensen FS, Koscielniak-Nielsen Z, Skovgaard LT, Ostergaard D: Good clinical research practice (GCRP) in pharmacodynamic studies of neuromuscular blocking agents. Acta.Anaesthesiol. Scand. 1996; 40: 59–74.

13. Rowaan CJ, Vandenbrom RH, Wierda JM: The Relaxometer: a complete and comprehensive computer-controlled neuromuscular transmission measurement system developed for clinical research on muscle relaxants. J.Clin.Monit. 1993; 9: 38–44.

14. Weber S, Muravchick S: Monitoring technique affects measurement of recovery from succinylcholine. J.Clin. Monit. 1987; 3: 1–5.

15. Kopman AF: The relationship of evoked electromyographic and mechanical responses following atracurium in humans. Anesthesiology. 1985; 63: 208–11.

16. Colquhoun D, Dreyer F, Sheridan RE: The actions of tubocurarine at the frog neuromuscular junction. J. Physiol. 1979; 293: 247–84.

17. Mertes PM, Laxenaire PM, Alla F: Anaphylactic and anaphylactoid reactions occurring during anesthesia in France in 1999–2000. Anesthesiology. 2003; 99: 536–45.

18. Atherton DPL, Hunter JM: Clinical pharmacokinetics of the newer neuromuscular blocking drugs. Clin. Pharmacokinet. 1999; 36: 169–89.

19. Schiere S, Proost JH, Roggeveld J, Wierda M: An interstitial compartment is necessary to link the pharmacokinetics and pharmacodynamics of mivacurium. Eur.J.Anaesthesiol. 2004; 21 (11): 882–91.

20. Jensen FS, Viby-Mogensen J: Plasma cholinesterase and abnormal reaction to succinylcholine: twenty years' experience with the Danish Cholinesterase Research Unit. Acta.Anaesthesiol. Scand. 1995; 39: 150–6.

21. Andrews JI, Kumar N, van den Brom RHG, Olkkola KT, Roest GJ, Wright PMC: A large simple randomized trial of rocuronium versus succinylcholine in rapid sequence induction of anaesthesia along with propofol. Acta.Anaesthesiol. Scand. 1999; 43: 4–8.

22. Gueret G, Rossignol B, Kiss G, Wargnier JP, Miossec A, Spielman S, Arvieux CC: Is muscle relaxant necessary for cardiac surgery? Anesth.Analg. 2004; 99: 1330–3.

23. Li YL, Liu YL, Xu CM, Lv XH, Wan ZH: The effects of neuromuscular blockade on operating conditions during general anesthesia for spinal surgery. J. Neurosurg.Anesthesiol. 2014; 26: 45–9.

24. King M, Sujirattanawimol N, Danielson DR, Hall BA, Schroeder DR, Warner DO. Requirements for muscle relaxants during radical retropubic prostatectomy. Anesthesiology. 2000; 93: 1392–7.

25. Dubois PE, Putz L, Jamart J, Marotta ML, Gourdin M, Donnez O: Deep neuromuscular block improves surgical conditions during laparoscopic hysterectomy: a randomised controlled trial. Eur.J.Anaesthesiol. 2014; 31: 430–6.

26. Kopman AF, Naguib M: Laparoscopic surgery and muscle relaxants. Is deep block helpful? Anesth.Analg. 2015; 120: 51–8.

27. Staehr-Rye AK, Rasmussen LS, Rosenberg J, Juul P, Lindekaer AL, Riber C, Gätke MR: Surgical space conditions during low-pressure laparoscopic

cholecystectomy with deep versus moderate neuromuscular blockade: a randomized clinical study. Anesth.Analg. 2014; 119: 1084–92.

28. Torensma B, Martini CH, Boon M, Olofsen E, Veld B, Liem RS, Knook MT, Swank DJ, Dahan A: Deep neuromuscular block improves surgical conditions during bariatric surgery and reduces postoperative pain: a randomized double blind controlled trial. PLoS. One. 2016; 11: e0167907.

29. Madsen MV, Staehr-Rye AK, Gätke MR, Claudius C: Neuromuscular blockade for optimising surgical conditions during abdominal and gynaecological surgery: a systematic review. Acta.Anaesthesiol. Scand. 2015; 59: 1–16.

30. Kopman AF, Naguib M: Laparoscopic surgery and muscle relaxants. Is deep block helpful? Anesth.Analg. 2015; 120: 51–8.

31. Kopman AF, Naguib M: Is deep neuromuscular block beneficial in laparoscopic surgery? No, probably not. Acta.Anaesthesiol. Scand. 2016; 60: 717–22.

32. Madsen MV, Staehr-Rye AK, Claudius C, Gatke MR: Is deep neuromuscular blockade beneficial in laparoscopic surgery? Yes, probably. Acta.Anaesthesiol. Scand. 2016; 60: 710–16.

33. Aronson JK: *Meyler's Side Effects of Drugs*, 16th Edition. Amsterdam-Oxford: Elsevier, 2015.

34. Spacek A, Neiger FX, Krenn CG, Hoerauf K, Kress HG: Rocuronium-induced neuromuscular block is affected by chronic carbamazepine therapy. Anesthesiology. 1999; 90: 109–12.

35. Koenig MH, Edwards LT: Cisatracurium-induced neuromuscular blockade in anticonvulsant treated neurosurgical patients. J.Neurosurg.Anesthesiol. 2000; 12: 314–18.

36. Richard A, Girard F, Girard DC, Boudreault D, Chouinard P, Moumdjian R et al: Cisatracurium-induced neuromuscular blockade is affected by chronic phenytoin or carbamazepine treatment in neurosurgical patients. Anesth.Analg. 2005; 100: 538–44.

37. Spacek A, Neiger FX, Spiss CK, Kress HG: Chronic carbamazepine therapy does not influence mivacurium-induced neuromuscular block. Br.J.Anaesth. 1996; 77: 500–2.

38. Hemmerling TM, Schuettler J, Schwilden H: Desflurane reduces the effective therapeutic infusion rate (ETI) of cisatracurium more than isoflurane, sevoflurane, or propofol. Can.J.Anesth. 2001; 48: 532–7.

39. Caldwell JE, Heier T, Wright PM, Lin S, McCarthy G, Szenohradszky J, Sharma ML, Hing JP, Schroeder M, Sessler DI: Temperature-dependent pharmacokinetics and pharmacodynamics of vecuronium. Anesthesiology. 2000; 92: 84–93.

40. Beaufort AM, Wierda JM, Belopavlovic M, Nederveen PJ, Kleef UW, Agoston S: The influence of hypothermia (surface cooling) on the time-course of action and on the pharmacokinetics of rocuronium in humans. Eur.J.Anaesthesiol.Suppl. 1995; 11: 95–106.

41. Stenlake JB, Hughes R: In vitro degradation of atracurium in human plasma. Br.J.Anaesth. 1987; 59: 806–7.

42. Cammu G, Coddens J, Hendrickx J, Deloof T: Dose requirements of infusions of cisatracurium or rocuronium during hypothermic cardiopulmonary bypass. Br.J.Anaesth. 2000; 84: 587–90.

43. Eriksson LI, Viby-Mogensen J, Lennmarken C: The effect of peripheral hypothermia on vecuronium-induced neuromuscular block. Acta.Anaesthesiol. Scand. 1991; 35: 387–92.

44. Vermeyen KM, Hoffmann VL, Saldien V: Target controlled infusion of rocuronium: analysis of effect data to select a pharmacokinetic model. Br.J.Anaesth. 2003; 90: 183–8.

45. Motamed C, Devys J-M, Debaene B, Billard V: Influence of real-time Bayesian forecasting of pharmacokinetic parameters on the precision of a rocuronium target-controlled infusion. Eur.J.Clin. Pharmacol. 2012; 68: 1025–31.

46. Ma X-D, Yan J, Dai B-Z, Kong D-Q, Du S-Y, Li B-P: Comparative study: efficacy of closed-loop target controlled infusion of cisatracurium and other administration methods for spinal surgery of elderly patients. Eur.Rev.Med.Pharmacol.Sci. 2017; 21: 606–11.

47. Kansanaho M, Olkkola KT: Performance assessment of an adaptive model-based feedback controller: comparison between atracurium, mivacurium, rocuronium and vecuronium. Int.J.Clin.Monit. Comput. 1997; 13: 217–24.

48. Eleveld DJ, Proost JH, Wierda JM: Evaluation of a closed-loop muscle relaxation control system. Anesth. Analg. 2005; 101: 758–64.

49. Eriksson LI. Evidence-based practice and neuromuscular monitoring: it's time for routine quantitative assessment. Anesthesiology. 2003; 98: 1037–9.

50. Vanacker BF, Vermeyen KM, Struys MM, Rietbergen H, Vandermeersch E, Saldien V, Kalmar AF, Prins ME: Reversal of rocuronium-induced neuromuscular block with the novel drug sugammadex is equally effective under maintenance anesthesia with propofol or sevoflurane. Anesth.Analg. 2007; 104: 563–8.

51. Ploeger BA, Smeets J, Strougo A, Drenth HJ, Ruigt G, Houwing N, Danhof M. Pharmacokinetic-pharmacodynamic model for the reversal of neuromuscular blockade by sugammadex. Anesthesiology. 2009; 110 (1): 95–105

52. Kleijn HJ, Zollinger DP, van den Heuvel MW, Kerbusch T: Population pharmacokinetic–pharmacodynamic analysis for sugammadex-mediated reversal of rocuronium-induced neuromuscular blockade. Brit.J.Clin.Pharm. 2011; 72 (3): 415–33.

53. Proost JH, Schiere S, Eleveld DJ, Wierda JM: Simultaneous versus sequential pharmacokinetic-pharmacodynamic population analysis using an iterative two-stage Bayesian technique. Biopharm. Drug.Dispos. 2007; 28 (8): 455–73.

54. Schmith VD, Fiedler-Kelly J, Phillips L, Grasela TH: Prospective use of population pharmacokinetics/

pharmacodynamics in the development of cisatracurium. Pharm.Res. 1997; 14 (1): 91–7.

55. Liu J, Lu C, Zou Q, Wang S, Peng X: Altered pharmacodynamics and pharmacokinetics of cisatracurium in patients with severe mitral valve regurgitation during anaesthetic induction period. Brit.J.Clin.Pharm. 2017; 83 (2): 363–9.

56. Tran TV, Fiset P, Varin F: Pharmacokinetics and pharmacodynamics of cisatracurium after a short infusion in patients under propofol anesthesia. Anesth. Analg. 1998; 87 (5): 1158–63.

Chapter 12

Effects on Brain Function

Neus Fabregas and Adrian W. Gelb

Introduction

Surgery and anaesthesia alter the function of the brain and its control mechanisms. In the operating room, we daily observe the effects of anaesthetic agents during induction and recovery from anaesthesia: changes in the electroencephalogram, on consciousness, muscle tone as well as in the responses to different stimulations that immediately disappear after induction, and reappear gradually when anaesthetic effects wear off. To prevent short- or long-term functional changes of the brain, the parameters of its physiological defence mechanisms must be maintained within the patient's normal range. Failing to do so might lead to complications that can significantly alter patient outcome.

Every anaesthesiologist should be familiar with some basic concepts that may critically affect brain homeostasis, no matter what the surgical procedure is. The brain comprises only 2% of total body weight but receives approximately 12% of cardiac output. Cerebral blood flow (CBF) delivers oxygen and other substances like glucose which are essential to maintain normal brain function. CBF is determined by cerebral autoregulation, cardiac output, arterial CO_2 partial pressure ($PaCO_2$), arterial oxygen reactivity, body position and neurovascular coupling. Can we recommend a range of values for these physiological parameters that we should maintain perioperatively to prevent harm to the brain?

Anaesthesia itself can affect cerebral perfusion through three different mechanisms: (1) by suppressing cerebral metabolic activity; (2) by a direct effect of volatile anaesthetics on autoregulation (intrinsic cerebral vasodilation); and (3) by blunting the sympathetic nervous system activity which can alter systemic haemodynamics affecting CBF.

The interaction of CBF, arterial blood pressure (ABP), body position and anaesthesia in the perioperative setting has been well studied (Table 12.1 [1–20]).

This chapter will start by reviewing the physiology of cerebral haemodynamics and how to measure its defining parameters in the highly complex operating room environment. The next section will discuss normal, basal brain physiology and how it could be affected by anaesthetic drugs, surgical bleeding, hypothermia, and other events likely to occur in the perioperative phase. The last section of the chapter will discuss how the combined effects of surgery and anaesthesia might affect the basal conditions previously described.

Real-time Measuring of Cerebral Haemodynamics

Several methods have been described to measure blood inflow and outflow of the brain. We will consider cerebral oximetry and transcranial Doppler.

Cerebral Oximetry

Cerebral tissue oxygen saturation ($SctO_2$), also known as cerebral oximetry (rSO_2), estimates regional tissue oxygenation by transcutaneous illumination with 'near-infra-red' light in the area of the frontal cerebral cortex. Adhesive sensors applied to the forehead of the patient emit 'near-infra-red' light and detect the reflected waves via photodetectors, a process called 'near-infra-red' spectroscopy (NIRS). The waves are reflected from different tissue depths, including the cranial bone and any underlying cerebral tissue. The collected signal can be processed in different ways.

NIRS emits light of a certain frequency and amplitude, and the relative changes in light intensity of the reflected waves are related to changes in relative concentrations of haemoglobin through the modified Beer–Lambert equation. One of the factors needed to derive the absolute changes in haemoglobin concentration (THC = cerebral total haemoglobin concentration, the sum of oxy- and deoxy-haemoglobin, expressed in μmol) is the length of the path the reflected photon has travelled back. Continuous wave (CW) NIRS emits waves of constant frequency and amplitude. Because these do not allow the path length to be determined, CW NIRS can only be used as a trend monitor.

Table 12.1. Relevant clinical studies dealing with cerebral blood flow interactions with arterial pressure, body position and anaesthesia.

	Subject Numbers	Surgery	Body Position	Anaesthetic Agents	ETCO$_2$ Changes	Vasoactive Drugs Test	Haemodynamic Challenges	Bispectral Monitoring Target
Piechnik (1999)[1]	14 healthy volunteers	no	supine	no	hypercapnia vs hypocapnia (hyperventilation)	no	yes (Aaslid's cuffs tests)	no
McCulloch (2000)[2]	8	orthopaedic	supine	propofol vs sevoflurane	yes, ETCO$_2$ up to 40 mmHg and 50 mmHg and 5-mmHg increments until AR impairment	yes (phenylephrine)	no	no
Sharma (2010)[3]	35	craniotomy	supine	no, tests performed before an after surgery (awake tests)	yes (voluntary hyperventilation until ETCO$_2$ decrease 10 mmHg)	no	transient hyperaemic response test	no
Joshi (2010)[4]	127	cardiac during CBP rewarming	supine	isoflurane	no	no	no	no
Klein (2011) [5]	21 (CT)	craniotomy	supine	propofol + remifentanil	no	no	no	20 vs 40
Burkhart (2011) [6]	50 (18–40 yo vs > 65 yo)	major surgery	supine	sevoflurane	no	no	no	no
Joshi (2012) [7]	232	cardiac during CPB	supine	isoflurane	no	no	no	no
Meng (2012) [8]	14	elective non-neurosurgical	supine	propofol + remifentanil	yes (hypocapnia, normocapnia, hypercapnia)	yes (phenylephrine)	no	30–40

Blood Pressure Monitoring	Cardiac Output Monitoring	rSO$_2$ Monitoring	rSO2 Autoregulatory index	TCD Monitoring	TCD Autoregulatory Index	Conclusions
c-NIBP (Finapres®)	no	no	no	yes (2 mHz Neuroguard®)	yes (Mx, Sx and RoR with ICM+®)	Indices derived from the correlation between spontaneous fluctuations of blood flow velocity waveform and BP may be used for non-invasive and continous monitoring of cerebrovascular reactivity
Aline	no	no	no	yes (2 mHz Neuroguard®)	yes (ARI)	Under 1% sevoflurane PaCO$_2$ of 50 mmHg can impair autoregulation. Propofol maintains autoregulation at significantly higher PaCO$_2$ levels
Aline	no	no	no	yes (2 mHz Rimed®)	yes (THRR)	Cerebral autoregulation can be perioperatively impaired in up to 20% of neurosurgical patients. Large supratentorial tumours and midline shift of 5 mm were identified as risk factors
Aline	no	wave-NIRS (INVOS 5100® or FORE-SIGHT®)	no	yes (2 MHz DWL®)	yes (Mx with ICM+®)	During rewarming more than half of the patients had an Mx value that indicated impaired CBF autoregulation; with higher rate of postoperative strokes
Aline	no	cortical laser Doppler flowmetry + spectroscopy (O$_2$C-device®)	no	no	no	An increase in propofol dose (BIS 21) reduces cerebral metabolic demand in grey matter (2 mm) with altered CBF/CMRO$_2$ ratio. No changes in white matter (8 mm)
c-NIBP (Finapres®)	no	yes (NIRO200®)	yes (TOI)	yes (2 MHz DWL®)	yes (Mx with ICM+®)	Autoregulation is less efficient in patients > 65 y under sevoFlurane anaesthesia compared with patients between 18 and 40 y, but was not considered clinically relevant
Aline	no	wave-NIRS (INVOS 5100®)	yes (COX with ICM+®)	yes (2 MHz DWL®)	yes (Mx with ICM+®)	LLA MAP varies widely; rSO$_2$ derived index COX can provide real-time monitoring of AR
Aline (zeroed tragus)	yes (oesophageal Doppler)	FD-NIRS (Oxiplex®)	no	no	no	Hypocapnia intensifies and hypercapnia blunts the phenylephrine induced reduction in cerebral oxygenation

Table 12.1. (cont.)

	Subject Numbers	Surgery	Body Position	Anaesthetic Agents	$ETCO_2$ Changes	Vasoactive Drugs Test	Haemodynamic Challenges	Bispectral Monitoring Target
Jeong (2012)* [9]	42	shoulder	supine vs BCP	propofol + remifentanil vs sevoflurane/ N_2O	no ($ETCO_2$:35–40 mmHg)	no	no	40–50
Meng (2012) [10]	33	non-neurosurgical	30° HUT vs 30° HDT vs supine	propofol + remifentanil	yes ($ETCO_2$ 45 mmHg vs 25 mmHg)	no	no	30
Meng (2013) [11]	30	non-neurosurgical	supine	Induction with propofol + fentanyl	no (pre-induction vs post-intubation)	no	no	from 84 (pre-induction) to 24 (post-intubation)
Alexander (2013) [12]	26	non-neurosurgical	supine	propofol + remifentanil vs sevoflurane	yes ($ETCO_2$ 55 mmHg vs 25 mmHg)	no	no	30–50
Murphy (2014) [13]	70 (CT)	shoulder	BCP	sevoflurane	yes ($ETCO_2$ 30–32 mmHg vs 40–42 mmHg)	no	no	40–60
Tzeng (2014) [14]	18 healthy volunteers	no	sit to stand	no	yes (normocapnia and hypercapnia - $FiCO_2$ 5%-)	yes	yes (Aaslid's cuffs tests)	no
Ono (2014) [15]	450 (CT)	cardiac during CPB	supine	isoflurane	no	no	no	no
Moerman (215) [16]	34 (CT)	cardiac during CPB at 30 °C	supine	sevoflurane	no ($ETCO_2$ 40 mmHg)	yes (nitroprusside vs phenylephrine)	no	40–50

Blood Pressure Monitoring	Cardiac Output Monitoring	rSO$_2$ Monitoring	rSO2 Autoregulatory index	TCD Monitoring	TCD Autoregulatory Index	Conclusions
Aline (zeroed tragus)	no	wave-NIRS (INVOS 5100®)	no	no	no	In BCP sevoflurane/nitrous oxide provides a wider margin of safety against impaired cerebral oxygenation and better systemic haemodynamics than propofol/remifentanil
Aline (zeroed tragus)	yes (oesophageal Doppler + Vigileo®)	FD-NIRS (Oxiplex®)	no	no	no	Changes in rSO$_2$ and CBV correlate during 30° HUT and hyperventilation (25 mmHg). Changes in rSO$_2$ and CBV do not correlate with changes in MAP and CO during 30° HUT
Aline (zeroed tragus)	yes (Vigileo®)	FD-NIRS (Oxiplex®)	no	no	no	Cerebral tissue oxygenation remained stable during anaesthetic hypotension (MAP 84 to 53) during propofol induction (BIS 84 to 24)
Aline (zeroed tragus)	yes (oesophageal Doppler)	FD-NIRS (Oxiplex®)	no	no	no	Hyperventilation always significantly decreased rSO$_2$ values
arm NIBP	no	wave-NIRS (FORE-SIGHT®)	no	no	no	Cerebral oxygenation is significantly improved during BCP surgey when ventilation is adjusted to maintain EtCO$_2$ 40–42 compared with 30–32 mmHg
c-NIBP (Finapres®)	no	no	no	yes (2 MHz Spencer®)	yes (ARI)	Haemodynamic effects of hypercapnia during transient blood pressure challenges primarily reflects changes in Windkessel properties rather than pure CA impairment. There are many inter-individual differences
Aline	no	wave-NIRS (INVOS 5100®)	yes (COX with ICM+®)	no	no	19% patients had a disregulated pattern (COX≥0.3). A relationship was found between the duration and magnitude of MAP below the limits of CA and postop morbidity
Aline	no	wave-NIRS (INVOS 5100®)	yes (COX offline with Rugloop®)	no	no	65% of CPB surgery patients had functional autoregulation (COX 0.3). Paradoxical changes in rSO$_2$ after pharmacology induced pressure changes occurred exclusively in this patient group

Table 12.1. (cont.)

	Subject Numbers	Surgery	Body Position	Anaesthetic Agents	ETCO$_2$ Changes	Vasoactive Drugs Test	Haemodynamic Challenges	Bispectral Monitoring Target
Laflam (2015)[17]	218	shoulder	BCP vs LDP	sevoflurane or desflurane	no	no	no	40–55
Picton (2015) [18]	56 (CT)	shoulder	supine vs BCP	propofol vs desflurane	yes (ETCO$_2$ 30 mmHg +FiO$_2$ 0.5 vs 45 mmHg+FiO$_2$ 1)	no	no	no
Deschamps (2016) [19]	201 (CT)	cardiac	supine	Canadian Guidelines	control vs intervention when rSO$_2$ desaturation	control vs intervention when rSO$_2$ desaturation	no	no
Goettel (2016) [20]	136 (18–40 yo vs > 65 yo) (CT)	major surgery	supine	sevoflurane	no	no	no	no

vs= comparison between two groups

NIBP= non-invasive blood pressure monitoring

Aline= invasive blood pressure monitoring

c-NIBP= plethysmographic continuous non-invasive blood pressure monitoring

rSO$_2$= regional cerebral blood flow saturation

TCD= transcranial Doppler

COX = cerebral oximetry index (correlation between mean arterial pressure and rSO$_2$)

CT= clinical trial

NIRS= near infra-red spectroscopy

FD-NIRS = frequency domain-near infra-red spectroscopy

BCP = beach chair position

* the only study including jugular bulb venous saturation monitoring

TOI = tissue oxygenation index

HUT = head up tilt

HDT= Trendelenburg

THRR= transient hyperaemic response ratio (>1.1 defines normal autoregulation)

CBP= cardiopulmonary bypass

LDP = lateral decubitus position (Aaslid R, Lindegaard KF, Sorteberg W, Nornes H: Cerebral autoregulation dynamics in humans. Stroke. 1989; 20: 45–52)

ARI= Tieck's autoregulatory index (a value of 0 representants no cerebral autoregulation, a value of 9 represents perfect cerebral autoregulation). (Tiecks FP, Lam AM, Aaslid R, Newell SW: Comparison of static and dynamic cerebral autoregulation measurements. Stroke. 1995; 26: 1014–19)

SX= systolic index

RoR= rate of regulation

Blood Pressure Monitoring	Cardiac Output Monitoring	rSO$_2$ Monitoring	rSO2 Autoregulatory index	TCD Monitoring	TCD Autoregulatory Index	Conclusions
c-NIBP (Finapres®)	no	wave-NIRS (INVOS 5100®)	yes (COX with ICM+®)	no	no	BCP diminishes cerebral autoregulation (increases COX) compared with LDP in shoulder surgery patients
arm NIBP	no	wave-NIRS (INVOS 5100®)	no	no	no	rSO$_2$ decrease during BCP can be attenuated by normobaric hyperoxia and moderate hypercarbia, independent of the anaesthetic agent
Aline	no	wave-NIRS (INVOS 5100® or FORE-SIGHT® or EQUANOX®)	no	no	no	Cerebral desaturation was common during cardiac surgery. Episodes were reversed by applying an interventional algorithm in the study group; but no difference in adverse events
c-NIBP (Finapres®)	no	no	no	yes (2 MHz DWL®)	yes (Mx with ICM+®)	The autoregulatory plateau is shortened in both young and old patients receiving 1 MAC sevoflurane. Lower and upper limits of CBF autoregulation, as well as the range, are not influenced by the age of anaesthetized patients

Frequency-domain (FD) NIRS uses an amplitude modulated sinusoid signal [21]. The extra information contained in the reflected signals (both amplitude and phase changes) can distinguish light (photon) absorption from light scattering, making it possible to derive absolute changes in THC. Meng et al used this more quantitative approach [11].

The blood contained in brain tissue consists, on average, of 25% arterial and 75% capillary and venous blood. Normal values for SctSO$_2$ range between 60% and 80%. Most commercial devices consider a trend towards 20% below baseline a clinically relevant change. Many factors affect the NIRS: cardiac output, ABP, F_IO_2, temperature, PaCO$_2$ (both hypo- and hypercapnia), and extracranial blood [22].

Cerebral tissue oxygen saturation reflects the balance between O$_2$ supply and demand, while CBF only represents supply. While the reliability of SctO$_2$ as a surrogate measure of CBF is a matter of discussion, NIRS has been validated in numerous studies as a means to evaluate cerebral autoregulation [23, 24].

If autoregulation fails to maintain CBF, the brain will compensate for this by increasing O$_2$ extraction. NIRS thus becomes an indirect and non-invasive monitor of the vulnerability of cerebral perfusion. A decrease in NIRS can be attributed to any of the following, either alone or combined: (1) increased cerebral oxygen metabolic rate; (2) decreased oxygen delivery to the brain; and (3) decreased arterial and/or increased venous blood contribution(s).

A new concept derived from SctO$_2$ is the cerebral oxygen index (COx). The COx is obtained by calculating the correlation coefficient between 150 paired samples of 2-second recordings of mean arterial pressure (MAP) and 300-second epochs of SctO$_2$. A COx that approaches zero indicates that ABP is within the autoregulatory range. A COx approaching one indicates a pressure passive cerebral circulation, the situation where a decrease in cerebral perfusion pressure (CPP) causes a decrease in CBF. The COx threshold to discriminate between intact and impaired CA is arbitrary and varies between 0.25 and 0.50 [15].

Transcranial Doppler

Transcranial Doppler ultrasonography (TCD) provides relatively high-fidelity recordings of CBF velocity [25] and is one of the most commonly used methods to measure CBF in clinical studies [26]. TCD remains an indirect measure of CBF because blood velocity measurements accurately reflect volumetric blood flow only if the cross-sectional area of the insonated vessel remains constant. For this reason in some patients it might not reflect the actual CBF.

The rate of regulation (RoR) is an index calculated from TCD changes in response to a rapid, short-term decrease in ABP after, for example, sudden deflation of leg cuffs (dynamic) or after changing MAP itself by, for example, a phenylephrine bolus (static). The reaction of CBF velocity to different levels of perfusion pressure suggests that pressure-induced changes in cerebrovascular resistance (CVR) has two components, a 'rapid response component' (sensitive to pressure pulsations) followed by a 'slow response component' (sensitive to changes in MAP) [27].

One of the options to analyse data from haemodynamic or brain waveforms is ICM+® [28]. ICM+ collects data coming from the analogue output of the arterial blood pressure and TCD monitors. Using a method called time-wave integration, average values for MAP, intracranial pressure (ICP) and mean flow velocity (FVm) can be estimated. Mean Index (Mx) is a parameter extracted from those waveforms [29]. Mx reflects the moving linear correlation coefficient between values of CPP (see definition below) and FVm. Its strength is that it allows spontaneous fluctuations in MAP to be used to characterize autoregulation, eliminating the need for drugs or manoeuvres such as compression of the carotid artery or bilateral thigh cuffs to induce changes in MAP. Furthermore, it allows the efficiency of autoregulation to be quantified, with a higher Mx indicating a less efficient autoregulation.

While Mx and systolic (Sx) indices were originally calculated using CPP [29], Piechnik et al [1] found that MAP could be used as well. This modification does not invalidate the sensitivity of Mx and Sx to CO_2 induced changes of cerebral vasodilatory capacity. Although their reliability is not as good as RoR obtained with Aaslid's leg cuff tests [25], Mx and Sx have the advantage of being parameters that can be continuously measured and are considered particularly useful when continuous monitoring of cerebrovascular reactivity is needed.

The availability of new, non-invasive technologies that measure cerebral oxygen flow via image or signal analysis provides the clinician with reliable tools to assess the state of the brain almost in real time.

Cerebral Haemodynamics under Basal Conditions

Cerebral Perfusion Pressure

CPP is defined as the difference between MAP and ICP (or central venous pressure if it is higher than ICP). CPP represents the pressure gradient for CBF and thus is one of the key factors that determine oxygen and metabolite delivery. CPP must be kept within a very narrow range to avoid inadequate blood inflow to the brain.

Because the transmural pressure in distal cerebral veins is very close to zero, the ICP becomes the principal determinant of the postcapillary venous outflow pressure in a manner that is similar to a Starling resistor [30]. It has been suggested that the sum of ICP and the active tension produced by vascular smooth muscle contraction at the arteriolar level can be considered the pressure at which flow ceases. The arterial pressure at which cerebral flow ceases is called the zero flow pressure (ZFP). It is determined by arterial tone and represents the effective downstream pressure [31]. ZFP can be indirectly calculated from the instantaneous relationship between the blood flow velocity (FV) of the middle cerebral artery (MCA) and MAP during a cardiac cycle. The gradient between MAP and ZFP determines CPP. Because critical closing pressure can be as high as 30 mmHg in the supine position [32], the common practice of only considering MAP without taking effective downstream pressure into account can lead to marked overestimation of true CPP.

Maintaining an adequate CPP is fundamental when managing patients under anaesthesia or in critical condition. Abrupt changes in CPP may induce resistance changes in cerebral autoregulatory arterioles, i.e. arteriolar vasoconstriction when pressure increases and arteriolar vasodilation when pressure decreases. The resultant change in arterial to venous blood volume ratio can explain the observed change in $SctO_2$ [8, 16].

Cerebral Flow Autoregulation

A low MAP can cause inadequate cerebral perfusion, a situation where O_2 supply fails to meet O_2 demand.

However, whether or not this actually occurs in a given patient will depend on the autoregulatory response range (Fig. 12.1 [33]).

The classic teaching of cerebral autoregulation is that CBF is maintained at a constant level across a wide range (plateau) of MAPs, with a lower limit of autoregulation (LLA) of 50 mmHg and an upper limit (ULA) of 150 mmHg [34]. However, studies in awake healthy subjects indicate that the LLA usually is around 70 mmHg (higher than the 50 mmHg still reported in textbooks) and with a huge range (43–110 mmHg). It is therefore impossible to know the LLA in every patient at any given time [35]. In fact, 'preserved cerebral autoregulation' does not mean the position of the CBF–CPP plot remains unchanged; it only means that the link between the two remains intact. The LLA also depends on the cause of hypotension: in baboons, it is 65% of baseline MAP during experimental haemorrhagic hypotension but only 35% to 40% during drug-induced hypotension [36]. Meng et al [37] propose a framework that integrates the various CBF-regulating processes at the level of the cerebral arteries/arterioles. Depending on the mechanism, different segments of those vessels might be affected, e.g. sympathetic stimulation constricts large arteries, while an increase in MAP constricts the arterioles (Fig. 12.2 [37]).

Studies under various experimental settings have all demonstrated pressure–flow curves resembling Lassen's autoregulatory curve with the classic shape of a plateau and shoulders. However, most of these studies are inconsistent in that some report the plateau to be relatively wide (40 mmHg) [38] while others find it to be demonstrably narrow (i.e. 10–15 mmHg) [39]. Moerman et al [16] found substantial inter-subject variation in the response to pharmacology-induced pressure changes. This implies that the relation between MAP and $SctO_2$ may follow different patterns and that intact cerebral autoregulation may manifest itself not only as an autoregulatory plateau but also as a paradoxical response. Jones et al [40] demonstrated that the classic pattern is the result of averaging individual cerebral autoregulation curves, a finding confirmed by Moerman [16].

In patients with supratentorial tumours, preoperative cerebral autoregulation and autoregulation during the first 24 hours postoperatively was impaired in the 20% of patients (seven patients) that had a large tumour (average volume 100 cm³) and a midline shift of more than 5 mm, but not in those with smaller tumours (average volume 40 cm³) [3].

The Concepts of Static and Dynamic Autoregulation

An arterial blood pressure tracing recorded over several seconds is a complex pulsatile waveform with several characteristic features that are the result of

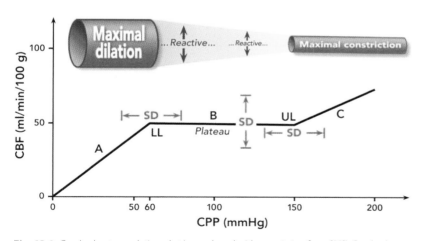

Fig. 12.1 Cerebral autoregulation plot (reproduced with permission from [33]). Cerebral autoregulation is visualized as a correlation plot between cerebral blood flow (CBF) and cerebral perfusion pressure (CPP). CBF remains stable between the lower limit (LL) and the upper limit (UL) (portion B, plateau). CBF is pressure passive at the CPP range below the lower limit (portion A) and above the upper limit (portion C). This illustration uses a CPP of 60 mmHg as the lower limit, a CPP of 150 mmHg as the upper limit, and a CBF of 50 mL/min per 100 g as the plateau. However, these regularly quoted numbers are not fixed; rather, they vary inter-individually and intra-individually depending on a variety of factors. Therefore, we take a note of SD to emphasize that these parameters have a wide range of distribution. The cerebrovascular reactivity is also illustrated. SD, standard deviation.

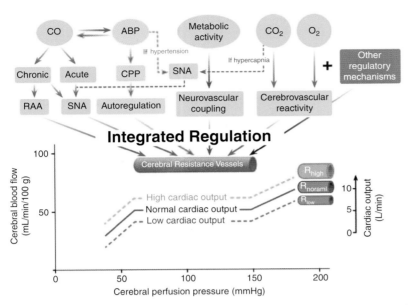

Fig. 12.2 Integrated regulation of brain perfusion. (Reproduced with permission from [37].) The conceptual framework of the integrated regulation of brain perfusion. The cerebrovascular resistance determined by the calibre of the cerebral resistance vessels is regulated by various physiological processes: (1) cardiac output (CO) likely via sympathetic nervous activity (SNA) and renin–angiotensin–aldosterone (RAA) system, depending on the chronicity of the change in CO, (2) arterial blood pressure (ABP) and cerebral perfusion pressure (CPP) via cerebral autoregulation, (3) cerebral metabolic activity via neurovascular coupling, and (4) arterial blood carbon dioxide (CO_2) and oxygen (O_2) via cerebrovascular reactivity. The SNA regulates cerebral blood flow and may play a prominent role during acute hypertension and hypercapnia as a protective mechanism preventing cerebral overperfusion (*dashed line*). These various regulatory mechanisms, together with other CBF-regulatory mechanisms that are not specified here such as anaesthetic effects, integrate at the level of the cerebral resistance vessels and, therefore, jointly regulate brain perfusion. The plateau of the autoregulation curve shifts downward when the CO is reduced and upward when augmented. The position of the plateau is determined by the calibre (R) of the cerebral resistance vessels at high (R_{high}), normal (R_{norm}), and low (R_{low}) CO. The scale of CO on the right side is smaller than that of CBF on the left side to reflect the lesser extent of change in CBF induced by an alteration of CO.

intrinsic cardiovascular properties (e.g. ventricular preload, vascular compliance, blood properties) and pulse wave reflection. But when recorded over a longer period (minutes, hours or days), the ABP exhibits different trends and oscillations. Superimposed, one can expect non-rhythmic blood pressure surges and dips that occur either spontaneously, or as a consequence of physical activities such as exercise, straining, coughing and changing body posture (see Fig. 12.3, and page 185). Thus, ABP is not a static variable, but rather represents a conglomerate of physiological changes that cannot be fully described in terms of simple numerical averages [30]. Clinical studies suggest that both short (minutes) and long-term (hours to days) episodes of high ABP variability increase the likelihood of adverse cerebrovascular outcomes.

Static cerebral autoregulation refers to the reflex adjustments in cerebral vascular resistance in response to steady-state alterations in ABP [30]. Static cerebral autoregulation can be evaluated by administering incremental doses of vasopressor drugs to reach a predetermined percentage increase or decrease of MAP while simultaneously monitoring the NIRS response ($SctO_2$ is used as a surrogate measure of the CBF response). The phenylephrine-induced increase in perfusion pressure induces vasoconstriction of the cerebral autoregulatory arterioles to prevent abrupt cerebral hyperperfusion, as occurs with increased sympathetic nerve activity. This causes a decreased arterial blood contribution to NIRS measurements resulting in a lower $SctO_2$. The $SctO_2$ increase with induced hypotension found by Moerman et al [16] could be explained by the same mechanism but in the opposite direction: to prevent cerebral hypoperfusion, cerebral arterioles dilate, increasing the arterial to venous blood volume ratio, which increases $SctO_2$. This phenomenon has been described as 'hyperautoregulation' [40].

Dynamic cerebral autoregulation refers to the vascular responses to higher frequency components of steady-state spontaneous ABP, or to dynamic changes in blood pressure such as those driven by altered body posture [30]; it is not affected by the acute change in CO [41]. Its integrity may be tested with the transient hyperaemic response (THR) of the middle cerebral artery after the release of a 10-second compression of the ipsilateral common carotid artery (monitored by TCD sonography). The transient hyperaemic response ratio (THRR) is calculated as the ratio of the mean systolic flow velocity from five heart cycles just prior to compression over the mean systolic value of two heart cycles after compression, with exception of the very first cycle. A value of THRR greater than 1.1 defines normal autoregulation. A valid THR test needs to meet some criteria [3]: (1) compression of the carotid artery leads to a sudden and maximum decrease in middle cerebral arterial blood velocity (Vmca); (2) heart rate and blood pressure remain stable during compression (within 10% of their respective pre-compression values); (3) no flow transients occur after release of compression; and (4) the power of the reflected Doppler signal does not change during the test.

Aaslid et al [25] tested cerebral autoregulation by using TCD to characterize the CBF velocity responses to abrupt release of inflated thigh occlusion cuffs. Cuff deflation induces sudden stepwise drops in ABP that remains depressed for approximately five to seven seconds before cardiac and vascular baroreflexes gradually restore it to baseline ABP over a 10–20 second period. The flow velocity (Vmca) response pattern is similar except for the fact that it recovered more rapidly.

The pressure and blood flow velocity recordings collected over prolonged periods (see above and Fig. 12.3) can be decomposed into their various oscillatory components. Transfer functions can be derived that define the relationships between blood pressure (input) and flow velocity (output) in terms of their linear statistical dependence (coherence), relative magnitudes (gain) and timing (phase) as a function of the frequency component of interest [30]. Between 0.07 and 0.20 Hz, there is a pattern of progressively increasing coherence and gain indicating that higher frequency blood pressure components are more linearly related to flow velocity than lower frequency components, and that the ratio between them increases. The transfer function characteristics within the 0.02–0.4 Hz range have been attributed to the capacity for cerebral arterioles to dilate and constrict dynamically in response to increases and decreases in the blood pressure. As yet, which of these metrics or combination of metrics one should use to assess dynamic cerebral autoregulation remains unknown.

Dynamic cerebral autoregulation can also be evaluated by using Mx, the moving linear correlation coefficient between values of cerebral perfusion pressure (CPP) and FVm [6].

Tiecks et al [42] demonstrated that in normal anaesthetized subjects measurement of dynamic cerebral autoregulation yields similar results to static testing of both the intact and pharmacologically impaired autoregulation.

Cerebrovascular Carbon Dioxide Reactivity

The interaction between the autoregulatory response and CO_2-induced dilation of cerebral vessels mainly involves the smaller arterial vessels [43]. Ito et al used positron emission tomography to demonstrate that changes in cerebral blood volume (CBV) during hypocapnia and hypercapnia are caused by changes in arterial blood volume without any changes in venous and capillary blood volume [44].

Carbon dioxide is a potent cerebral vasodilator, and a linear relationship exists between CBF and $PaCO_2$ within the range of 20 to 60 mmHg (2.5 and 8.0 kPa) [45]. The proposed mechanism for this effect is thought to be mediated via CO_2-related changes in extracellular pH [46]. Changes in CVR and CBF in response to changes in $PaCO_2$ are referred to as 'cerebrovascular reactivity to CO_2' or $CVR-CO_2$. Absolute $CVR-CO_2$ is defined as the change in CBF (mL/min or cm/s) per mmHg change in $PaCO_2$. Generally accepted values under anaesthesia are 1–2 mL/100g/min/mmHg (2.0 to 5.0 cm/s/mmHg). Relative $CVR-CO_2$ is defined as the percentage change relative to baseline: 2% to 4% change in mL/min/mmHg or 2.5% to 6% change in cm/s/mmHg from the baseline value. The relative reactivity value is by definition less dependent on baseline values than absolute reactivity and thus the better indicator of $CVR-CO_2$ for statistical analysis; it is also used as a measure of cerebrovascular integrity and cerebral autoregulation.

$CVR-CO_2$ can be influenced by disease states. A strong correlation has been reported between impaired $CVR-CO_2$ and high glycosylated haemoglobin (HBA1C) in insulin-dependent DM [47]. This impaired reactivity may be due to micro- and macro-angiopathic changes in cerebral arterioles associated with chronic hyperglycaemia. In patients with supratentorial tumours, however, CO_2 reactivity was normal preoperatively and remained so after tumour decompression [3].

Carbon dioxide is a modulator of cerebral vascular tone. Hancock et al [31] found that $EtCO_2$ changes

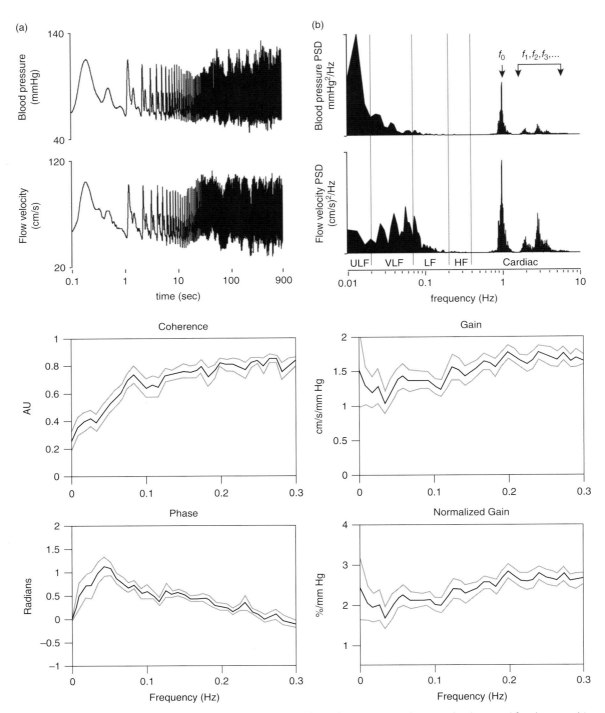

Fig. 12.3 Finger arterial blood pressure and middle cerebral blood flow velocity over 900 s (presented on long axes) for a human subject in the seated resting position (upper left). The corresponding power spectra, which decompose the time series signals into their various constituent component frequencies (upper right). Note that the fundamental frequency (f0) and its harmonics (f1, f2, f3) correspond to pulsations coincident with the pulse, whereas progressively lower frequency components reflect the longer term oscillations and trends in the time domain. ULF, ultra low frequency; VLF, very low frequency; LF, low frequency; HF, high frequency. Transfer function coherence, phase, gain and normalized gain for 105 healthy individuals (mean age 26±7 years) in the supine resting position. AU, arbitrary units. Values are mean ± SE (bottom) [30].

produce significant changes in estimated CPP (eCPP) and in ZFP in a group of healthy volunteers. Hypocapnia decreases eCPP and increases the pressure needed to perfuse the brain, while hypercapnia increases eCPP and decreases ZFP. The association of hypocapnia and hypotension decreases eCPP and increases ZFP, which implies that a higher MAP is needed to maintain adequate brain perfusion.

A common practice in neuroanaesthesia and neuro-critical care is to induce hypocapnia to reduce cerebral blood volume and intracranial pressure. Hypocapnia results in a shift of the plateau to lower cerebral blood flows, almost no change in LLA, and a poorly defined change of the ULA. Conversely, hypercapnia causes the CBF autoregulation plateau to progressively ascend as CO_2 rises, shifts the LLA to the right and the ULA to the left, thus narrowing the range over which CBF is maintained until it disappears, ultimately resulting in a pressure passive system [33] where CBF flow passively follows pressure.

Cardiac Output

The overall evidence shows that a change in cardiac output, either acute or chronic, can lead to a change in CBF that is independent of other CBF-regulating parameters including blood pressure and CO_2.

Meng et al [37] reviewed the studies that investigated the association between cardiac output and CBF in healthy volunteers and in patients with chronic heart failure. Even if blood pressure remains stable and within the autoregulatory range, a change in cardiac output, either acute or chronic, leads to a change in CBF. Disease states differently affect the association between cardiac output and CBF. Vasospasm, ischaemic stroke and sepsis are disease states where the association between cardiac output and CBF is evident. Head injury, neurological surgery, cardiac surgery and hepatic failure are diseases states where no association between cardiac output and CBF exists. The authors propose a conceptual framework that integrates the various CBF-regulating processes at the level of cerebral arteries/arterioles (also see Fig. 12.2). With acute cardiac output changes, each percentage change in cardiac output corresponds to a 0.35% change in CBF, meaning there is about a 10% CBF decrease for a 30% cardiac output reduction (based on eight datasets from five studies done in resting non-anaesthetized subjects). Physiologically, this is accomplished through the shunting of blood from the periphery to the brain by differential vasoconstriction in different vascular

beds. Physiologically it makes sense: brain perfusion is a priority during acute cardiac output reduction [37]. With chronically reduced cardiac output, CBF is reduced, for instance in patients with chronic heart failure. The extent of CBF reduction correlates with the severity of chronic heart failure. Cardiac transplantation, cardioversion or captopril treatment can reverse the situation [37]. Interestingly, there is an inappropriately high prevalence of cognitive dysfunction in patients diagnosed with chronic heart failure, but whether this is directly linked to a reduction in CBF is unclear [48].

Combined Effects of Haemodynamics and Carbon Dioxide Partial Pressure on Cerebral Blood Flow

CBF responses to transient blood pressure challenges are frequently attributed to cerebral autoregulation, but some evidence indicates that vascular properties like compliance ('windkessel effect') are also influential. The Windkessel effect is caused by distention of the elastic large arteries during systole and recoil during diastole. Since the rate of blood entering these elastic arteries exceeds that leaving them due to the peripheral resistance, there is a net storage of blood during systole which discharges during diastole. The distensibility of the large elastic arteries is therefore analogous to a capacitor: it dampens the fluctuation in blood pressure (pulse pressure) over the cardiac cycle and helps maintain organ perfusion during diastole when cardiac ejection ceases. Vascular compliance explained more than 50% of the MCA velocity variance during blood pressure manipulations such as bilateral thigh-cuff deflation and sit-to-stand manoeuvres under normocapnic and hypercapnic (5% CO_2) conditions in healthy volunteers [14]. The authors found that the response to acute transient systemic hypotension challenges was dominated by cerebrovascular elastance properties independent of cerebral autoregulation, that there was significant heterogeneity in these responses between individuals, and that the same principle applied to the cerebrovascular response to hypercapnia.

Effects of Body Position

In conscious subjects, the sitting position activates the sympathetic nervous system, resulting in an increase of systemic blood pressure (10–15%) along with increased systemic vascular resistance (30–40%) and reduced cardiac output (15–20%) [49]. In the upright position, cerebral hypoperfusion was more pronounced in patients with heart failure than in age- and sex-matched healthy controls, an effect that can be related to the neurohormonal activation by heart failure [50].

In the upright or semi-recumbent position (e.g. during shoulder surgery), the blood pressure measured at the level of the head (meatus acusticus externus) will be 1.35 mmHg (or 1 cm H_2O) lower per cm height difference relative to the site where MAP is measured (most often middle of the forearm). It is not clear whether this pressure gradient should be subtracted from the forearm MAP [51] when calculating CPP. It has been argued that according to the 'venous siphon model' venous pressure decreases as much as ABP, resulting in no net change in cerebral perfusion [52]. Other authors consider that collapsible veins prevent gravitational pressure gradients from being matched on the arterial and venous sides of the vascular loop above the heart, thus preventing the siphon from operating. According to the waterfall model they propose, CBF is independent of downstream resistance: the heart alone is responsible for pumping blood to the brain and overcoming viscous resistance to blood flow through the brain, and in the upright patient the descending limb does not 'aid' ascending flow. In this case, a pressure gradient from heart to brain will exist, and MAP in the brain will be lower than that in the arm according to the difference in height of the brain above the arm (and the heart) [52]. One approach to reconcile this debate is to view the cerebral circulation as a siphon in healthy patients, but as a waterfall in patients at risk of intracranial vascular disease or with intracranial disease and in those with reduced oxygen carrying capacity. In either case, a minimum effective cerebral perfusion pressure is needed [53].

What Do We Know about the Effects of Surgery and Anaesthesia on Perioperative Cerebral Haemodynamics?

Cerebral Metabolism, Effects of Anaesthesia on Neurovascular Coupling and Cerebral Autoregulation

The effect of an anaesthetic agent on CBF depends on the balance between its direct vasodilatory/vasoconstrictive properties and its indirect vasoconstrictive effect via flow–metabolism coupling [54]. Anaesthesia causes a decrease in neuronal activity, thus lowering metabolic demand, and a corresponding decrease in CBF (supply) if neurovascular coupling is preserved [55]. That is the case during propofol anaesthesia in healthy [56] and in head-injured patients [57]. Still, things may be slightly more complex. Klein et al studied the effect of propofol on human cerebral microcirculation with a device that used laser-Doppler flowmetry and photo-spectrometry to measure capillary venous blood flow (rvCBF), oxygen saturation (srvO$_2$), and haemoglobin amount (rvHb). The device was located on the surface of the cortex during craniotomy at 2 mm (grey matter) and 8 mm (white matter) of cerebral depth [5]. Increasing doses of propofol that decreased BIS from 40 to 21 increased SrvO$_2$ in grey matter without reducing rvCBF, indicating propofol did affect coupling of flow and metabolism. Because no changes were detected in white matter, the authors concluded that propofol may affect coupling of flow and metabolism differently in different areas of the brain [5].

Strebel et al tested dynamic and static autoregulation in anaesthetized patients. Both were preserved with propofol and 0.5MAC isoflurane and desflurane. At 1.5MAC both dynamic and static autoregulation were lost [27].

Burkhart et al [6] studied the effect of age on dynamic cerebral autoregulation (Mx) during sevoflurane anaesthesia and found that cerebral perfusion in older and younger patients may be more vulnerable to hypotension than in awake volunteers. Static cerebral autoregulation seems to be quite robust, even with high sevoflurane partial pressures [58].

The effective CBF autoregulation range appears to be shortened in both young and older patients receiving 1MAC sevoflurane [20]. This attenuation of autoregulation is likely due to the strong vasodilatory properties of volatiles. The brains of patients under general anaesthesia may be less well protected by the CBF autoregulation system and be more prone to ischaemia or oedema.

Anaesthesia and Systemic Haemodynamics

Even though the importance of preserving an adequate balance between cerebral oxygen supply and demand is well recognized, hypotension remains very common during induction of anaesthesia. The duration of hypotension, defined as a MAP ≤ 30% below baseline, is associated with postoperative stroke in patients undergoing non-cardiac, non-neurosurgical procedures (OR: 1.013/min of hypotension; 99.9% CI: 1.000–1.025). In the perioperative context, hypotension is best defined as a decrease in MAP relative to a preoperative baseline, rather than an absolute low blood pressure value [59].

Propofol causes hypotension by reducing stressed volume secondary to reduced venous and arterial resistance, with no changes in cardiac output [60]. Drugs that increase ABP, such as phenylephrine and noradrenaline may decrease cardiac output. In contrast, dobutamine and volume augmentation can increase cardiac output, but not necessarily ABP. The effect of a vasopressor on CBF likely depends on the choice of drug, the disease state and the functional status of the regulatory mechanisms of brain perfusion.

In a study by Meng et al, $SctO_2$ remained stable even though MAP decreased from a baseline 84.4 (SD 10.6) mmHg to 53.6 (SD 11.4) mmHg post-intubation after induction of anaesthesia with propofol and fentanyl [11]. This could be explained because neurovascular coupling was preserved (supported by many studies): the propofol-induced decrease in demand moves the plateau of the CPP–CBF curve downwards, allowing CBF to be maintained at a lower CPP value (Fig. 12.4, with permission). Whether there also is a leftward shift of the plateau of the CPP–CBF curve is unknown, but it is plausible due the neurovascular coupling mediated vasoconstriction (analogous to the effect of hypocapnia). This shift of the LLA curve to the left may help prevent the anaesthetic-induced hypotension from decreasing CBF and thus from disturbing the supply–demand balance. The leftward shift also implies that 'the same degree of hypotension that would have caused a passive decrease in CBF in an awake patient does not do so in a propofol-anaesthetized patient because the same CPP is still above the lower limit due the leftward shift of this lower limit' (i.e. the vessels still can vasodilate a bit more).

Anaesthesia and Cerebrovascular Carbon Dioxide Reactivity

Cerebrovascular reactivity to carbon dioxide (CVR-CO_2) is the change in CBF in response to a change in $PaCO_2$. Inhalational and intravenous anaesthetic agents have variable effects on CVR-CO_2, and their effects are further compounded by many physiological factors (age, body position), pathological conditions (diabetes, hypertension, stroke, other intracranial pathologic processes) (Table 12.2 [26]), or

the addition of nitrous oxide [61]. These are reviewed by Mariappan et al [26] based upon data from mostly non-neurosurgical patients in studies that had significant methodological heterogeneity. Changing minute ventilation was the most commonly used method to change $PaCO_2$. Because general anaesthesia alters the end-tidal to arterial CO_2 gradient, it is difficult to noninvasively (i.e. without arterial blood gas analysis) derive the 'true' slope of the CO_2 partial pressures–CBF response relationship. Only a limited number of studies have measured the CVR-CO_2 under both hypercapnic and hypocapnic conditions. At similar depths of anaesthesia, CO_2 reactivity was higher with isoflurane and lower with propofol. Hypocapnic responses were less apparent under propofol anaesthesia due to its vasoconstrictive effect. Hypercapnia-induced CBF responses were blunted with end-expired inhalational agents partial pressures > 1MAC due to their vasodilatory effects. CVR-CO_2 is impaired in elderly patients compared to young patients, during both sevoflurane and propofol anaesthesia. In patients with medical comorbidities, the CVR-CO_2 impairment under anaesthesia was associated with the severity of the underlying diseases and not the anaesthetic agent per se. Based upon their literature review, Mariappan et al [26] conclude that 'within the clinical anaesthesia concentrations, CVR-CO_2 is maintained under both propofol and inhalational agents'.

Combined Effects of Haemodynamic and Carbon Dioxide Partial Pressures during Anaesthesia

When CPP increases, cerebral resistance vessels constrict until the ULA is reached, the point of maximal vasoconstriction. However, if hypercapnia coexists, the ULA will be reached at a lower CPP than during normocapnia because the arteries are being dilated by CO_2 [33]. In humans, the average $PaCO_2$ threshold at which hypercapnia significantly impaired cerebral autoregulation was 56 mmHg and 61 mmHg during sevoflurane and propofol anaesthesia, respectively [2]. Autoregulation can already be impaired by the combination of a low sevoflurane partial pressure and a $PaCO_2$ of merely 50 mmHg, a $PaCO_2$ that is not uncommon under general anaesthesia and even in mechanically ventilated patients with severe lung pathology that are difficult ventilate.

Now let us consider what happens if CPP decreases in the presence of different $PaCO_2$ levels (Fig. 12.2

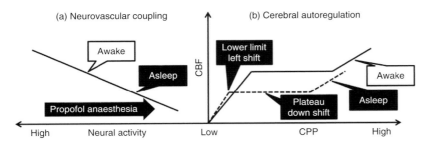

If neurovascular coupling and cerebral autoregulation are preserved
after propofol anaesthesia, then...

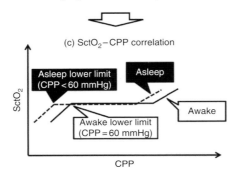

Fig. 12.4 Theoretical analysis of the mechanism responsible for the stable tissue oxygen saturation ($SctO_2$) following anaesthesia induction with propofol and fentanyl [11].

Table 12.2. Values of anaesthetic agents at which $CVR-CO_2$ is maintained (modified from Mariappan et al [26]).

Inhalation Agents	End-tidal Concentration	Minimum Alveolar Concentration
Sevoflurane	0.5–2.5%	0.3–1.5
Isoflurane	1.15–1.4%	Up to 1.3
Desflurane		Under 1 MAC
Intravenous agents	**Dose**	
Propofol	4–6 mg/kg/h (TCI concentration up to 6 µg/mL)	

TCI = target controlled infusion
MAC = minimum alveolar concentration

and Fig. 12.5). In the presence of hypotension under normocapnic conditions, autoregulation will cause cerebral resistance vessels to dilate, with maximum dilation – by definition – when the LLA is reached. If hypotension and hypercapnia induced vasodilation coexist, maximal vasodilation will already have occurred at a higher CPP than during normocapnia: the LLA is shifted rightward (based on the premise that the diameters of the maximally dilated cerebral resistance vessels during hypercapnia and normocapnia are the same) [33]. Finally, hypotension may also coexist with hypocapnia. There is evidence that the cerebrovascular reactivity to hypocapnia is significantly attenuated or even abolished during haemorrhage or anaesthesia-induced hypotension, and by a number of drugs. It is vital to understand that the effect of hypotension on cerebrovascular hypocapnia reactivity and effect of hypocapnia on cerebrovascular pressure reactivity (i.e. autoregulation), although related, are separate issues. During hypocapnia, the plateau of the autoregulation curve shifts downward, any change in LLA is unremarkable, and how ULA changes is not clear [33].

Not surprisingly, modifying $PaCO_2$ also affects $SctO_2$. Stepwise hyperventilation during both propofol–remifentanil and sevoflurane anaesthesia decreases $SctO_2$ [12]. During propofol–remifentanil anaesthesia in healthy patients, hypocapnia intensifies but hypercapnia blunts phenylephrine-induced decrease in $SctO_2$ [8]. In addition, phenylephrine also causes a significant decrease in CBV during hypocapnia, but not during normocapnia and hypercapnia.

Effects of Body Position, Systemic Haemodynamics and Carbon Dioxide Partial Pressure during Anaesthesia

The publication of a report of four middle-aged patients who suffered diverse catastrophic cerebral injuries after shoulder surgery in the (upright) beach chair position (BCP) opened the debate over the aetiology of their brain injury [62]. Systemic hypotension associated with head elevation and anaesthesia, more specifically the use of vasodilating agents and positive pressure ventilation, combined with the gravitational effects of head elevation may combine to cause cerebral hypoperfusion. Invasive blood pressure measurement with the transducer zeroed at the level of the circle of Willis (external ear canal) rather than at the level of the right atrium will obviate the need for the anaesthesiologist to mentally correct the CPP because of the height difference.

Laflam et al [17] reported that CBF was more pressure-passive (i.e. CBF decreased when MAP decreased) in patients undergoing surgery in 30° BCP than in lateral decubitus, supporting the hypothesis that failing to consider the abovementioned height difference may result in inadvertent cerebral hypotension. It is important to highlight that in Laflam's study head elevation was approximately 30°, while others have been reported to use head up tilt of 60° to even 90°, making the above gradient more pronounced. In addition, some patients undergoing shoulder surgery already experience episodes of MAP < LLA *regardless of position*. These patients may require elevated MAPs during surgery.

Some consider (partial) impairment of autoregulation during anaesthesia (e.g. by inhaled anaesthetics) to confer a margin of safety because CBF is bound to be higher at the same CPP.

During sevoflurane–nitrous oxide or propofol–remifentanil anaesthesia, Jeong et al found that changing the position of the patient from supine to BCP abruptly decreased MAP from baseline values, after which it restored over the course of seven to eight minutes [9]. The incidence of hypotension (MAP < 50 mmHg) and vasopressor use was lower in the sevoflurane–nitrous oxide group.

$SctO_2$ in 70 patients undergoing shoulder surgery in the BCP was higher with an $EtCO_2$ of 40–42 mmHg rather than the 30–32 mmHg range [13]. Most cerebral desaturation episodes occurred when MAP was more than 20% below baseline. Hypotension has to be avoided in patients undergoing surgery in BCP under general anaesthesia, and certainly so during concomitant hyperventilation.

In 56 patients undergoing shoulder surgery with desflurane or total intravenous (propofol) anaesthesia, F_IO_2 and $EtCO_2$ were initially maintained at 30% and 30 mmHg, respectively. Placing the patient in the BCP (80° to 90°) decreased regional cerebral oxygenation from an average 68% to 61% [18]. After being positioned in the BCP, increasing the F_IO_2 to 100% and the $EtCO_2$ to 45 mmHg increased regional cerebral oxygenation by 5% and 9%, respectively; both effects were independent of anaesthetic choice. The authors suggested that until LLA could be routinely monitored, blood pressure control alone cannot be assumed to be sufficient to protect patients from neurological injury during anaesthesia in the BCP.

Head up tilt and hyperventilation are the two most commonly used techniques to reduce brain bulk during neurosurgery. Of those two, common sense dictates we should preferentially use that intervention which causes the least decrease in $SctO_2$ and the greatest decrease in CBV. In normal healthy individuals under propofol anaesthesia, 30° head up tilt and hyperventilation to an $EtCO_2$ of 25 mmHg (from 45 mmHg) caused comparable small decreases in both $SctO_2$ and CBV [10]. During head up tilt, changes in $SctO_2$ and CBV did not correlate with changes in MAP and cardiac output but did correlate with changes in $EtCO_2$ during hyperventilation.

Head up tilt, hyperventilation and vasopressor administration all affect cerebral haemodynamics by different mechanisms, and it is hard to extrapolate findings from healthy patients to patients with intracranial pathology.

What Cerebral Perfusion Pressure to Maintain during Cardiopulmonary Bypass Surgery?

Cerebral oxygen desaturation during cardiac surgery has been associated with adverse perioperative outcomes. Deschamps et al [19] recently studied whether desaturation could be reversed by prompting the clinician to sequentially assess (and if needed correct) head and catheter position, MAP, SaO_2, $PaCO_2$,

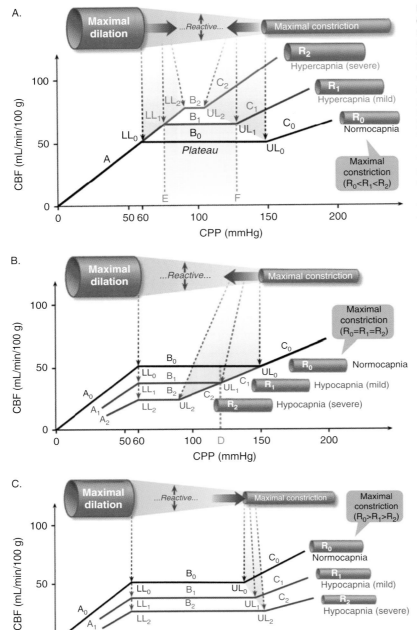

Fig. 12.5 Effect of hyper- and hypnocapnia on cerebral autoregulation. A. Hypercapnia moves the plateau upwards and shortens it (E-F), raises the LLA and lowers the ULA. B. If it is speculated that the diameters (R) of the maximally constricted cerebral resistance vessels at normocapnia and hypocapnia are the same (R0=R1=R2), hypocapnia will move the plateau downwards and shorten it, leave the lower limit unchanged (with few data to support this), and shift the ULA to the left. Note the slope of the curve above the ULA is unchanged. Data to support the effect on the LLA are scant, and none exist for the effect on the ULA. C. If it is speculated that the diameter of the maximally constricted cerebral resistance vessels during hypocapnia is smaller than during normocapnia due to the extra constriction imposed by hypocapnia (R0>R1>R2), the ULA may or may not shift rightward. As in scenario B, the plateau shifts downward, and any change in the lower limit is unremarkable. How the upper limit moves (i.e. whether pane B or C applies to real life) is not clear. Autoregulation curves during normocapnia, hypercapnia (upper pane), and hypocapnia (lower two panes) are black, red and blue, respectively. CBF = cerebral blood flow; CPP = cerebral perfusion pressure. The red cylinders depict cerebral resistance vessels with radius R, with the subscripts 0, 1 and 2 denoting whether $PaCO_2$ is normal, mildly aberrant or severely aberrant, respectively. In the middle pane it is speculated that the diameters of the maximally constricted cerebral resistance vessels at normocapnia and hypocapnia are the same (R0=R1=R2), while in the lower pane it is speculated that the calibre of the maximally constricted cerebral resistance vessels at hypocapnia is smaller than normocapnia (R0>R1>R2). The bold blue horizontal arrows on top of the graphs indicate the dynamic shift of the maximally dilated and constricted cerebral resistance vessels with the rise (upper pane) or decrease (lower two panes) of CO_2. The black vertical, dashed arrows left and right indicate the lower (LL0) and upper (UL0) autoregulation limits during normocapnia, respectively. The blue dashed arrows (vertical or slanted) indicate the lower (LL) and upper (UL) autoregulation limits with a mild (LL1 and UL1) or severely aberrant (LL2 and UL2) $PaCO_2$. Parts of the autoregulation curve labelled A, B and C refer to the part below the lower limit of autoregulation, the plateau and the part above the upper limit of autoregulation, with the subscripts 0, 1 and 2 again denoting whether $PaCO_2$ is normal, mildly aberrant or severely aberrant, respectively.

haemoglobin, mixed venous saturation and cerebral metabolic rate. Cerebral desaturation occurred in 56 (57%) of the 99 control group patients (no corrective action taken) and 71 (70%) of the 102 intervention group patients ($p = 0.04$). Reversal was successful in 69 (97%) of the intervention group patients. There were no differences in adverse events between the groups.

COx (see above) was used to study static cerebral autoregulation during moderately hypothermic cardiopulmonary bypass (CPB) by inducing 20% changes in MAP with sodium nitroprusside and phenylephrine. Patients received sevoflurane and fentanyl and $EtCO_2$ was maintained around 40 mmHg. COx was retrospectively calculated, and a value of 0.3 was chosen as the threshold to distinguish between intact and impaired cerebral autoregulation According to the effects of MAP changes on COx, four different patterns could be discerned:

1. **Pressure passive cerebral circulation:** in 35% of the patients MAP changed in parallel with $SctO_2$. These are the patients at high risk for neurological events. Higher $PaCO_2$ values, high sevoflurane partial pressures and hypothermic CPB are all associated with impaired autoregulation. The same percentage (35%) was reported by Joshi et al [4].

2. **Classic pattern of autoregulation:** in 18% of the patients COx approached zero at baseline and remained around zero after administration of vasoactive agents, indicating that CBF remained on the autoregulatory plateau.

3. **Paradoxical changes in $SctO_2$:** In 29% of the patients with intact baseline autoregulation COx became highly negative after administration of vasoactive drugs. A negative COx implies a paradoxical decrease in $SctO_2$ with a phenylephrine induced increase in MAP, and vice versa, a paradoxical increase in $SctO_2$ with a sodium nitroprusside induced decrease in MAP.

4. **Divergent effects of phenylephrine and sodium nitroprusside:** in 18% of the patients with intact baseline cerebral autoregulation, COx became negative after phenylephrine administration but increased above 0.3 after sodium nitroprusside administration. This paradoxical reaction ($SctO_2$ and blood pressure change in opposite directions) does not fit the classic concept of cerebral autoregulation, but the fact that they demonstrate paradoxical reactions only in

patients with intact cerebral autoregulation supports the hypothesis that it might be part of a normal physiological autoregulatory mechanism [16].

In a study of 232 patients undergoing coronary artery bypass grafting in which COx was determined during CPB, the MAP at the LLA was 66 mmHg (95% prediction interval, 43 to 90 mmHg) in the 225 patients in which it could be measured [7]. There was no relationship between preoperative MAP and the LLA after adjusting for age, gender, prior stroke, diabetes and hypertension, but a COx value of more than 0.5 was associated with the LLA.

Conclusion

The relationship between blood pressure and cerebral blood flow ('perfusion') is not passive or proportional, but is autoregulated. The autoregulatory curve that describes the relationship between MAP and CBF should be regarded as a dynamic process, with a huge range of thresholds in healthy awake individuals (43–110 mmHg) which makes it impossible to know the LLA in every individual patient at any given time [35]. The population LLA is not a fixed number but rather 'variable' because it can shift rightwards with chronic hypertension, return to a normal level when hypertension has been adequately treated, and because it can change with acute changes in $PaCO_2$ and sympathetic tone [63].

Because autoregulatory patterns differ so much amongst individuals, it becomes very difficult to define which MAP should be targeted in the individual. In healthy patients, a reasonable approach would be to maintain the MAP intraoperatively within 25–30% of the immediate preoperative values (i.e. measured in the preoperative holding area and the first MAP measured after entering the operating room) [59]. A MAP value below 30% of the basal values requires active intervention to restore it to baseline. Blood pressure should be kept closer to the baseline value in patients at increased risk of stroke, especially when there is a concomitant reduction in cardiac output and/or oxygen carrying capacity [53].

Cerebral autoregulation monitoring may provide a more effective means still, helping the clinician to define a target MAP in the individual patient, thus more effectively avoiding cerebral hyperperfusion and hypoperfusion than with the current standard of care. It seems reasonable to advocate intraoperative monitoring of cardiac output and CBF in patients with reduced cardiac function or cerebrovascular obstructive diseases, or during high-risk surgeries that have a greater chance of causing haemodynamic fluctuations [33].

The decision to use hypocapnia should be cautious because the resulting decrease in CBF renders the brain at risk of cerebral ischaemia, especially in the presence of hypotension and if cerebral metabolic rate remains unchanged.

Hypercapnia increases CBF and thus cerebral O_2 and substrate supply above demand (if cerebral metabolic rate remains unchanged). But even though this may be considered the safer situation in terms of maintaining supply of cerebral metabolic substrates, it needs to be noted that an acute increase in $PaCO_2$ not only *shifts* the plateau up but also *shortens* it. During general anaesthesia, a $PaCO_2 \geq 55$ mmHg should be considered to have eliminated cerebral autoregulation. Because under these conditions CBF will change passively with MAP, tighter CPP control is needed to avoid CBF fluctuations. Still, luxury perfusion might allow MAP and thus CPP to decrease more before ischaemia results (assuming a constant metabolic demand) [33].

References

1. Piechnik SK, Yang X, Czosnyka M, Smielewski P, Fletcher SH, Jones AL, Pickard JD: The continuous assessment of cerebrovascular reactivity: a validation of the method in healthy volunteers. Anesth.Analg. 1999; 89: 944–9.

2. McCulloch TJ, Visco E, Lam AM: Graded hypercapnia and cerebral autoregulation during sevoflurane or propofol anesthesia. Anesthesiology. 2000; 93: 1205–8.

3. Sharma D, Bithal PK, Dash HH, Chouhan RS, Sookplung P, Valivala MS: Cerebral autoregulation and CO_2 reactivity before and after supratentorial tumor resection. J.Neurosurg.Anesthesiol. 2010; 22: 132–7.

4. Joshi B, Brady K, Lee J, Easly B, Panigrahi R, Smielewski P, Czosnyka MM, Hogue CW: Impaired autoregulation of cerebral blood flow during rewarming from hypothermic cardiopulmonary bypass and its potential association with stroke. Anesth.Analg. 2010; 110: 321–8.

5. Klein KU, Fukui K, Schramm P, Stadie A, Fischer G, Werner C, Oertel J, Engelhard K: Human cerebral microcirculation and oxygen saturation during propofol-induced reduction of bispectral index. Br.J.Anaesth. 2011; 107 (5): 735–41.

6. Burkhart CS, Rossi A, Dell-Kuster S, Gamberini M, Möckli A, Siegemund M, Czosnyka M, Strebel SP, Steiner LA: Effect of age on intraoperative cerebrovascular autoregulation and near-infrared spectroscopy-derived cerebral oxygenation. Br.J.Anaesth. 2011; 107 (5): 742–8.

7. Joshi B, Ono M, Brown C, Brady K, Easley RB, Yenokyan G, Gottesman RF, Hogue CW: Predicting the limits of cerebral autoregulation during cardiopulmonary bypass. Anesth.Analg. 2012; 114: 503–10.

8. Meng L, Gelb AW, Alexander BS, Cerussi AE, Tromberg BJ, Yu Z, Mantulin MM: Impact of phenylephrine administration on cerebral tissue oxygen saturation and blood volume is modulated by carbon dioxide in anaesthetized patients. Br.J.Anaesth. 2012; 108 (5): 815–22.

9. Jeong H, Jeong S, Lim HJ, Lee J, Yoo KY: Cerebral oxygen saturation measured by near-infrared spectroscopy and jugular venous bulb oxygen saturation during arthroscopic shoulder surgery in beach chair position under sevoflurane-nitrous oxide or propofol-remifentanil anesthesia. Anesthesiology. 2012; 116: 1047–56.

10. Meng L, Mantulin WW, Cerussi AE, Tromberg BJ, Yu Z, Laning K, Kain ZN, Cannesson M, Gelb AW: Head-up tilt and hyperventilation produce similar changes in cerebral oxygenation and blood volume: an observational comparison study using frequency-domain near-infrared spectroscopy. Can.J.Anaesth. 2012; 59 (4): 357–65.

11. Meng L, Gelb AW, McDonagh DL: Changes in cerebral tissue oxygen saturation during anesthetic-induced hypotension: an interpretation based on neurovascular coupling and cerebral autoregulation. Anaesthesia. 2013; 68: 736–41.

12. Alexander BS, Gelb AW, Mantulin WW, Cerussi AE, Tromberg BJ, Yu Z, Lee C, Meng L: Impact of stepwise hyperventilation on cerebral tissue oxygen saturation in anesthetized patients: a mechanistic study. Acta. Anaesthesiol.Scand. 2013; 57 (5): 604–12.

13. Murphy GS, Szokol JW, Avram MJ, Greenberg SB, Shear TD, Vender JS, Levin SD, Koh JL, Parikh KN, Patel SS: Effect of ventilation on cerebral oxygenation in patients undergoing surgery in the beach chair position: a randomized controlled trial. Br.J.Anaesth. 2014; 113 (4): 618–27.

14. Tzeng YC, MacRae BA, Ainslie PN, Chan GSH. Fundamental relationships between blood pressure and cerebral blood flow in humans. J.Appl.Physiol. 2014; 117: 1037–48.

15. Ono M, Brady K, Easley RB Brown C, Kraut M, Gottesman RF, Hogue C: Duration and magnitude of blood pressure below cerebral autoregulation threshold during cardiopulmonary bypass is associated with major morbidity and operative mortality. J.Thorac. Cardiovasc.Surg. 2014; 147: 483–9.

16. Moerman AT, Vanbiervliet VM, Van Wesenmael A, Bouchez SM, Wouters PF, De Hert SG: Assessment of cerebral autoregulation patterns with near-infrared

spectroscopy during pharmacological-induced pressure changes. Anesthesiology. 2015; 123: 327–35.

17. Laflam A, Joshi B, Brady K, Yenokyan G, Brown C, Everett A, Selnes O, McFarland E, Hogue CW: Shoulder surgery in the beach chair position is associated with diminished cerebral autoregulation but no differences in postoperative cognition or brain injury biomarker levels compared with supine positioning: the anesthesia patient safety foundation beach chair study. Anesth.Analg. 2015; 120: 176–85.

18. Picton P, Dering A, Alexander A, Neff M, Miller BS, Shanks A, Housey M, Mashour GA: Influence of ventilation strategies and anesthetic techniques on regional cerebral oximetry in the beach chair position. A prospective interventional study with a randomized comparison of two anesthetics. Anesthesiology. 2015; 123: 765–74.

19. Deschamps A, Hall R, Grocott H, Mazer D, Choi PT, Turgeon AF, de Medicis E, Bussières JS, Hudson C, Syed S, Seal D, Herd S, Lambert J, Denault A: For the Canadian Perioperative Anesthesia Clinical Trials Group: Cerebral oximetry monitoring to maintain normal cerebral oxygen saturation during high-risk cardiac surgery. A randomized controlled feasibility trial. Anesthesiology. 2016; 124: 826–36.

20. Goettel N, Patet C, Rossi A, Burkhart CS, Czosnyka M, Strebel SP, Steiner LA: Monitoring of cerebral blood flow autoregulation in adults undergoing sevoflurane anesthesia: a prospective cohort study of two aged groups. J.Clin.Monitor.Comput. 2016; 30: 255–64.

21. Fantini S, Franceschini-Fantini MA, Maier JS, Walker SA, Barbieri B, Gratton E: Frequency-domain multichannel optical detector for non-invasive tissue spectroscopy and oximetry. Opt.Engineer. 1995; 34: 231–6.

22. Davie SN, Grocott HP: Impact of extracranial contamination on regional cerebral oxygen saturation: a comparison of three cerebral oximetry technologies. Anesthesiology. 2012; 116: 834–40.

23. Brady KM, Lee JK, Kliber KK, Easley RB, Koehler RC, Shaffner DH: Continuous time domain analysis of cerebrovascular autoregulation using near infrared spectroscopy. Stroke. 2007; 38: 2818–25.

24. Steiner LA, Pfister D, Strebel SP, Radolovich D, Smielewski P, Czosnyka M: Near-infrared spectroscopy can monitor dynamic cerebral autoregulation in adults. Neurocrit.Care. 2009; 10: 122–8.

25. Aaslid R, Lindegaard KF, Sorteberg W, Nornes H: Cerebral autoregulation dynamics in humans. Stroke. 1989; 20: 45–52.

26. Mariappan R, Mehta J, Chui J, Manninen P, Venkatraghavan L: Cerebrovascular reactivity to carbon dioxide under anaesthesia: a qualitative systematic review. J.Neurosurg.Anesthesiol. 2015; 27: 123–35.

27. Strebel A, Lam A, Matta B, Mayberg TS, Aaslid R, Newell DW: Dynamic and static cerebral autoregulation during isoflurane, desflurane and propofol anesthesia. Anesthesiology. 1995; 83: 66–76.

28. Smielewski P, Czosnyka M, Steiner L, Belestri M, Piechnik S, Pickard JD: ICM+: software for on-line analysis of bedside monitoring data after severe head trauma. Acta.Neurochir.Suppl. 2005; 95: 43–9.

29. Czosnyka M, Smielewski P, Kirkpatrick P, Menon DK, Pickard JD: Monitoring of cerebral autoregulation in head-injured patients. Stroke. 1996; 27: 1829–34.

30. Tzeng YCh, Ainsle PN: Blood pressure regulation IX: cerebral autoregulation under blood pressure challenges. Eur.J.Appl.Physiol. 2014; 114: 545–59.

31. Hancock SM, Mahajan RP, Athanassiou LA: Noninvasive estimation of cerebral perfusion pressure and zero flow pressure in healthy volunteers: the effects of changes in end-tidal carbon dioxide. Anesth.Analg. 2003; 96: 847–51.

32. Aaslid R, Lash SR, Bardy GH, Gild WH, Newell DW: Dynamic pressure–flow velocity relationships in the human cerebral circulation. Stroke. 2003; 34: 1645–9.

33. Meng L, Gelb AW: Regulation of cerebral autoregulation by carbon dioxide. Anesthesiology. 2015; 122: 196–205.

34. Lassen NA: Cerebral blood flow and oxygen consumption in man. Physiol.Rev. 1959; 39: 183–238.

35. Larsen FS, Olsen KS, Hansen BA, Paulson OB, Knudsen GM: Transcranial Doppler is valid for determination of the lower limit of cerebral blood flow autoregulation. Stroke. 1994; 25: 1985–8.

36. Fitch W, Ferguson GG, Sengupta D, Garibi J, Harper AM: Autoregulation of cerebral blood flow during controlled hypotension in baboons. J.Neurol. Neurosurg.Psychiatry. 1976; 39: 1014–22.

37. Meng L, Hou W, Chui J, Han R, Gelb AW: Cardiac output and cerebral blood flow. The integrated regulation of brain perfusion in adult humans. Anesthesiology. 2015; 123: 1198–208.

38. Brady KM, Easley RB, Kibler K, Kaczka DW, Andropoulos D, Fraser CD 3rd, Smielewski P, Czosnyka M, Adams GJ, Rhee CJ, Rusin CG: Positive end-expiratory pressure oscillation facilitates brain vascular reactivity monitoring. J.Appl.Physiol. 2012; 113: 1362–8.

39. Tan CO: Defining the characteristic relationship between arterial pressure and cerebral flow. J.Appl. Physiol. 2012; 113: 1194–200.

40. Jones SC, Radinsky CR, Furlan AJ, Chyatte D, Qu Y, Easley KA, Perez-Trepichio AD: Variability in the magnitude of the cerebral blood flow response and the shape of the cerebral blood flow-pressure autoregulation curve during hypotension in normal rats. Anesthesiology. 2002; 97: 488–96.

195

41. Deegan BM, Devine ER, Geraghty MC, Jones E, Ólaighin G, Serrador JM: The relationship between cardiac output and dynamic cerebral autoregulation in humans. J.Appl.Phsyiol. 2010; 109: 1424–31.

42. Tiecks FP, Lam M, Aaslid R, Newell DW: Comparison of static and dynamic cerebral autoregulation measurements. Stroke. 1995; 26 (6): 1014–19.

43. Harper M, Glass HI: Effect of alterations in the carbon dioxide tension on the blood flow through the cerebral cortex at normal and low blood pressures. J.Neurol. Neurosurg.Psychiatry. 1965; 28: 449–52.

44. Ito H, Ibaraki M, Kanno I, Fukuda H, Miura S: Changes in the arterial fraction of human cerebral blood volume during hypercapnia and hypocapnia measured by positron emission tomography. J.Cereb.Blood.Flow. Metab. 2005; 25: 852–7.

45. Ito H, Kanno IK, Ibaraki M, Hatazawa J, Miura S: Changes in human cerebral blood flow and cerebral blood volume during hypercapnia and hypocapnia measured by positron emission tomography. J.Cereb. Blood.Flow.Metab. 2003; 23: 665–70.

46. Low DA, Wingo JE, Keller DM, Davis SL, Zhang R, Crandall CG: Cerebrovascular responsiveness to steady-state changes in end-tidal CO_2 during passive heat stress. J.Appl.Physiol. 2008; 104: 976–81.

47. Kadoy Y, Himohara H, Kunimoto F, Saito S, Ide M, Hiraoka H, Kawahara F, Goto F: Diabetic patients have an impaired cerebral vasodilatory response to hypercapnia under propofol anaesthesia. Stroke. 2003; 34: 2399–403.

48. Vogels RL, Scheltens P, Schroeder-Tanka JM, Weinstein HC: Cognitive impairment in heart failure: a systematic review of the literature. Eur.J.Heart.Fail. 2007; 9: 440–9.

49. Smith JJ, Porth CM, Erickson M: Hemodynamic response to the upright posture. J.Clin.Pharmacol. 1994; 34: 375–86.

50. Fraser KS, Heckman GA, McKelvie RS, Harkness K, Middleton LE, Hughson RL: Cerebral hypoperfusion is exaggerated with an upright posture in heart failure: impact of depressed cardiac output. JACC Heart Fail. 2015; 3: 168–75.

51. Cullen DJ, Kirby RR: Beach chair position may decrease cerebral perfusion: catastrophic outcomes have occurred. APSF Newsletter. 2007; 22 (2): 25–7.

52. Lee L, Caplan R: APSF Workshop: Cerebral perfusion experts share views on management of head-up cases.

Anesthesia Patient Safety Foundation Newsletter. 2010; 24: 45–8.

53. Bijker JB, Gelb AW: The role of hypotension in perioperative stroke. Can.J.Anesth. 2013; 60: 159–67.

54. Lam A, Matta B, Mayberg T, Strebel S: Changes in cerebral blood flow velocity with onset of EEG silence during inhalational anesthesia in humans. Evidence of flow metabolism coupling. J.Cereb.Blood.Flow.Metab. 1994; 15: 714–17.

55. Attwell D, Buchasn AM, Charpak A, Macvicar BA, Newman EA: Glial and neuronal control of brain blood flow. Nature. 2010; 468: 232–43.

56. Oshima T, Karasawa F, Sato T: Effects of propofol on cerebral blood flow and the metabolic rate of oxygen in humans. Acta.Anaesth.Scand. 2002; 46: 232–43.

57. Steiner LA, Johnston AJ, Chatfield DA, Czosnyka M, Coleman MR, Coles JP, Gupta AK, Pickard JD, Menon DK: The effects of large-dose propofol on cerebrovascular pressure autoregulation in head-injured patients. Anesth.Analg. 2003; 97: 572–6.

58. Gupta S, Heath K, Matta BF: Effect of incremental doses of sevoflurane on cerebral pressure autoregulation in humans. Br.J.Anaesth. 1997; 79: 469–72.

59. Bijker JB, Persoon S, Peelen LM, Moons KGM, Kalkman CG, Kappelle LJ, van Klei WA: Intraoperative hypotension and perioperative ischemic stroke after general surgery. A nested case-control study. Anesthesiology. 2012; 116: 658–64.

60. De Wit F, van Vliet AL, de Wilde RB, Jansen JR, Vuyk J, Aarts LP, de Jonge E, Veelo DP, Geerts BF: The effect of propofol on haemodynamics: cardiac output, venous return, mean systemic filling pressure, and vascular resistance. Br.J.Anaesth. 2016; 116 (6): 784–9.

61. Aono MI, Sato J, Nishino T: Nitrous oxide increases normocapnic cerebral blood flow velocity but does not affect the dynamic cerebrovascular response to step changes in end-tidal $P(CO_2)$ in humans. Anesth. Analg. 1999; 89: 684–9.

62. Pohl A, Cullen DJ: Cerebral ischemia during shoulder surgery in the upright position: a case series. J.Clin. Anesth. 2005; 17: 463–9.

63. McCulloch TJ, Boesel TW, Lam AM: The effect of hypocapnia on the autoregulation of cerebral blood flow during administration of isoflurane. Anesth. Analg. 2005; 100: 1463–7.

Chapter 13

Targeted and Individualized Perioperative Medicine for Cognitive Dysfunction

Pauline Glasman, Alice Jacquens and Vincent Degos

Introduction

The ageing population in Western countries combined with advances in anaesthetic management and surgical techniques results in a growing number of frail patients presenting for surgery in the last 30 years. Increased age comes with reduced physiological reserves of major organs, and only worsens in the presence of concurrent disease. This fact undoubtedly contributes to an increase in perioperative complications.

Of all perioperative complications, cognitive impairment is a dreaded one. The association between perioperative changes and impaired cognitive status of elderly patients has been repeatedly confirmed since the first study of Bedford et al in 1955 [1–3]. However, contrary to common belief it seems that postoperative cognitive impairment is not caused by 'anaesthesia' and more specifically anaesthetic agents. Experimental and epidemiological evidence increasingly suggests that surgical stress is a key element in its genesis. Also, all cognitive dysfunction is not the same. The postoperative period is often followed by a short period of disrupted psychomotor performance and attention span. These phenomena are probably related to 'sickness behaviour' which is a normal behaviour in the aftermath of biological stress. However, cognitive dysfunction after the second postoperative day (on day three) should be considered pathological. Even though postoperative cognitive disorders remain poorly categorized, it is possible to discern two chronologically distinct pathologies: postoperative delirium (days three to seven), and postoperative cognitive dysfunction (POCD) (begins after the first week and can consolidate). More and more data suggest these two entities may have a common aetiological substratum and, for a subgroup of patients, there may be a continuum between the two pathologies.

Perioperative Cognitive Function and Dysfunction

Fragility in Brain Ageing

It is now well established that the brain, like any organ, goes through a normal ageing process.

Common sense dictates there should be a clinicopathological correlate to cognitive dysfunction, but it has proven difficult to find evidence for it. The normal ageing process is characterized by anatomical changes that have been visualized through standard imaging (atrophy or decreased fractional anisotropy in MRI-DTI), but it has no clinically detectable associated changes. Chronic diseases like hypertension and diabetes may accelerate these anatomical changes. Contrary to the normal ageing process, neurodegenerative disorders (e.g. Alzheimer's or Parkinson's diseases as well as vascular dementia) will directly affect cognitive skills. Acute brain diseases will inflict major brain damage and quickly degrade cognitive function.

The normal ageing process can be expressed as a loss of reserves relative to an initial cognitive potential evaluated through the Mini-Mental State Examination (MMSE) – see Fig. 13.1. Loss of reserves varies significantly between persons, and depends on socio-economic and environmental factors [4]. It is difficult to measure this loss without a proper neurocognitive measurement tool, and even in-depth neurocognitive assessment may not detect this loss. Nevertheless it seems crucial to detect preexisting loss of cognitive reserve (i.e. the frailty of the patient) early on during the perioperative phase [5]. It is challenging to identify and quantify loss of cognitive reserves, assess its different clinical presentations, and to track postoperative cognitive decay or recovery of postoperative cognitive function.

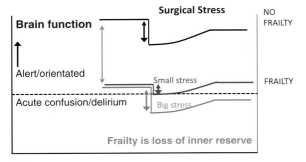

Fig. 13.1 Brain function over time. The normal ageing process can be expressed as a loss of reserves relative to an initial cognitive potential. When it decreases below a certain threshold, acute confusion/delirium results. Whether or not surgical stress results depends on (1) the frailty, which is the baseline position on the Y-axis at the time of stress and (2) the degree of stress (small versus big).

Early and Late Postoperative Cognitive Dysfunction

Early or Acute Postoperative Cognitive Dysfunction: Delirium

The American Psychiatry Association has recently defined delirium in the DSM-V Diagnostic and Statistical Manual of Mental Disorders 5th Edition. Postoperative delirium is a sudden event, usually occurring within 24 to 48 hours postoperatively [6]. It is characterized by disturbance of consciousness that fluctuates over time, reversal of sleep–wake rhythm, and cognitive impairment. The latter is global, with varied symptoms ranging from memory and behavioural disorders to temporo-spatial disorientation and anxiety. Three subtypes of delirium are discerned: hyperactive (25%), hypoactive (50%) and mixed (25%). This cerebral dysfunction is organic in origin and is in theory reversible [7].

Persistent Postoperative Cognitive Dysfunctions

The persistent form of POCD is less easily characterized than the acute one. While there is no formal definition in the DSM-V, it is conventionally accepted that a patient has 'persistent POCD' when one or more cognitive domains remain dysfunctional one week after a surgical procedure. The first reports on POCD in the 60s described how anterograde episodic memory and attention were affected after cardiac surgery [8], a finding later also described after non-cardiac surgery [9, 10]. Some authors have challenged this entity to be pathological, and argue these cognitive problems may represent normal age related decline of the cognitive

function of a subgroup of patients. During the perioperative period, the decline would only temporarily be accelerated; later, it would resume its preoperative rate of decline in such a manner that there would be no net change in decline relative to that to be expected had the patient not undergone surgery [11].

Epidemiology and Risk Factors

Delirium is one of the most common postoperative complications in patients over 60 years old, with an estimated incidence of 20% and 40% [12]. Risk factors associated with delirium in patients admitted for non-surgical (medical) reasons may also be involved in those admitted for surgery: age, chronic brain disease, depression, addiction, neurosensory deficit, chronic organ failure, endocrine disorders, iatrogenic factors and psychological factors. Certain types of surgery (orthopaedic, vascular or cardiac surgery) and emergency surgery, and a number of other perioperative factors have also been associated with an increased risk of postoperative confusion (Table 13.1). Delirium is associated with a deterioration of the patient's functional prognosis, reduced life expectancy [13, 14] and persistent POCD after cardiac surgery [15].

The incidence of persistent POCD in patients older than 60 undergoing non-cardiac surgery is between 10% and 54% [16]. After cardiac surgery, some studies show a higher incidence of POCD, regardless of whether or not extracorporeal circulation was used [17]. Because the diagnostic criteria are not clear yet, interpretation of the results of studies on POCD remains controversial [9]. Known risk factors include age, preoperative cognitive impairment, depression, perioperative sepsis and the metabolic syndrome. Individual and social consequences of POCD include an increase in mortality, and loss of ability to live autonomously and return to work [3].

Role of Neuroinflammation

Some pathophysiological mechanisms of delirium and persistent POCD seem to be similar. They appear to be related to the combination of preexisting vulnerability

Table 13.1. Limiting precipitating perioperative risk factors.

(a) Avoid anticholinergic drugs and benzodiazepines

(b) Improve cerebral perfusion

(c) Monitoring of the depth of anaesthesia

(d) Optimization of multimodal analgesia

(e) Limit the surgical stress

factors (cognitive impairment, addiction, age), the degree of operative stress (itself related to the type of surgery), and additional acute organic factors such as hydro-electrolytic disorders, sepsis and repeated episodes of low arterial blood pressure. In the past, these cognitive problems were often hypothesized to result (directly or indirectly) from general anaesthesia, i.e. from the pharmacological effect of the anaesthetic agents used, from haemodynamic instability, or from ventilation or oxygenation problems. However, epidemiological studies have found no causal link between low blood pressure, hypoxaemia and the occurrence of POCD. The type of anaesthesia (general versus locoregional) could not be correlated with persistent POCD [18].

The most likely cause is now hypothesized to be perioperative inflammatory stress, both in its initial phase and in its resolution. The immune response protects the body against pathogens by recognizing elements of 'non-self' pathogen associated molecular patterns (PAMPs). The same immune system is also involved in recognizing elements of 'self' named damage associated molecular patterns (DAMPs) in certain situations such as cancer and cell injury. Perioperative tissue damage releases DAMPs (both locally and into the bloodstream) that are recognized by PPRs (pattern recognition receptors), molecules expressed on the surface of leucocytes. Activation of these PPRs

causes nuclear translocation of transcription factors that serve to rapidly increase the release of proinflammatory cytokines such as IL-1β, TNF-α and IL-6. This response to PAMPs and DAMPS characterizes the initial phase of innate immunity (Fig. 13.2). It is hypothesized this is the manner by which surgery activates immune cells that can massively release proinflammatory agents.

The local and systemic effects of this immunological reaction are controlled by a mechanism called 'the resolution phase'. One of its local mechanisms is a vagal reflex [19] that inhibits macrophage activity via activation of the α-7 nicotinic acetylcholine receptor [20]. The brain and particularly the hippocampal region appear to be a particular target for these activated immunocytes. The cerebral response to surgical stress is characterized by local secretion of pro-inflammatory cytokines, recruitment of immune cells and activation of microglia (inflammatory brain cells), which combined generate a provisional neuroinflammatory profile. This can alter synaptic plasticity (disrupting hippocampal long-term potentiation, a neurobiological correlate of learning and memory) and has been associated with cognitive disorders in animals that clinically resemble perioperative cognitive impairment in humans [21] (Fig. 13.3). Age, systemic inflammation, infectious diseases and metabolic

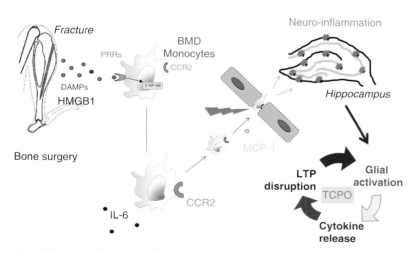

Fig. 13.2 Neuro-inflammation. The immune response protects the body against pathogens by recognizing elements of 'non-self' PAMPs (pathogen associated molecular patterns). The same immune system is also involved in recognizing elements of 'self' named DAMPs (damage associated molecular patterns) in certain situations such as cancer and cell injury. Perioperative tissue damage releases DAMPs (both locally and into the bloodstream) that are recognized by PPRs (pattern recognition receptors), molecules expressed on the surface of leucocytes. Activation of these PPRs causes nuclear translocation of transcription factors that serve to rapidly increase the release of proinflammatory cytokines such as IL-1β, TNF-α and IL-6. This response to PAMPs and DAMPS characterizes the initial phase of innate immunity. It is hypothesized this is the manner by which surgery activates immune cells that can massively release pro-inflammatory agents.

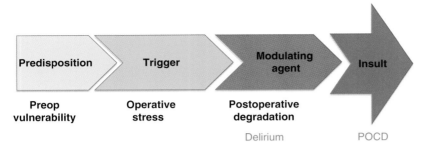

Fig. 13.3 Sequence of events leading to perioperative cognitive dysfunction.

syndrome can all modulate the inflammatory response by increasing the initial response and preventing the resolution phase.

While surgical stress appears to be the trigger of this inflammatory response, other perioperative events could also modulate the inflammatory response and thus play a role in the aetiology of cognitive disorders. These factors include (1) postoperative sleep disorders (especially in patients with sleep apnoea); (2) drugs used to provide anaesthesia and perioperative analgesia; (3) postoperative pain; and (4) perioperative infection. Finally, by reducing surgical stress, minimally invasive approaches (intraoperative techniques, avoiding cardiopulmonary bypass) are considered as an attractive therapeutic target to limit the incidence of POCD.

Early Postoperative Delirium: Causal Factor of Persistent Postoperative Cognitive Dysfunction?

Delirium after cardiac surgery is a risk factor for persistent pathology [16, 22]. Actually, because the risk factors for both diseases are so similar, more and more authors believe there to be a POCD continuum. Even though the issue is not yet completely resolved, two hypotheses exist that link delirium to POCD. A first hypothesis claims a causal link between delirium and POCD exists, and predicts that preventing delirium will have an impact on the incidence or severity of POCD. A second hypothesis claims delirium to be a marker associated with POCD, and therefore identifying delirium could enable us to determine which patients are at high risk of POCD and focus on this group to try to come up with both aetiological and symptomatic treatment.

With both hypotheses, it seems important to diagnose delirium early on, to establish when it started, and whether it is hyper- or hypo-active, and adopt

the necessary measures to treat it. The cornerstone of diagnosing POCD is a reliable, easy-to-use diagnostic tool to repeatedly assess the patient's cognitive state.

Is There a Marker of Cognitive Dysfunction?

One of the major challenges in the management of POCD is diagnosing it. There are currently no specific criteria to define persistent POCD. POCD screening tools reported in the literature are very heterogeneous, yet for optimal management and to facilitate comparisons between studies measurement of POCD ought to be standardized and able to be performed at the bedside. Better still, a specific brain marker should be identified.

Biomarkers

In post-traumatic or post-stroke patients, several brain injury biomarkers have been validated. Based upon these data, and assuming that POCD also involves some degree of brain injury, several authors have studied the link between the dynamic changes in the levels of these biomarkers and the changes in cognitive function. Besides allowing POCD to be diagnosed per se, a specific biomarker would allow us to diagnose POCD before the appearance of the first clinical symptoms, opening the possibility for individualized prophylactic measures. However, a blood test to diagnose POCD remains elusive at this time. In one study that followed 150 patients after non-cardiac surgery [23], increased plasma GFAP (an astrocyte protein) measured immediately after surgery could be correlated with POCD one month later, yet two other biomarkers, PS100 and NSE, could not. In another study [24], the same biomarkers and the APOE4 genotype (involved in the aetiology of Alzheimer's disease) again could not predict POCD.

Brain Imaging

MRI has been studied as a tool to predict or diagnose POCD. Preoperative temporal lobe abnormalities on MRI correlated with the risk of POCD. In a prospective study in elderly subjects undergoing gastrointestinal surgery, a small hippocampal volume predicted the occurrence of early POCD well [25]. This was expected since it is known that one of the main risk factors for POCD is preexisting cognitive impairment, which has been associated with changes in hippocampal volume [26, 27]. Because temporal MRI abnormalities may occur several years before the onset of clinical signs, MRI could detect patients at risk of POCD even at a very early stage.

But some investigators also reported negative results when exploring the use of imaging techniques such as brain MRI in diagnosing POCD. Acute MRI lesions after cardiac (CABG) [28] and non-cardiac surgery did not correlate with delirium or persistent POCD. Summarized, brain imaging is currently not a completely effective tool to detect or predict early persistent POCD at every point during the surgical process, but it can help to preoperatively define patients at risk for POCD. Therapeutic implications remain, however, limited.

Neuropsychological Tests

The 'Troponin like biomarker' that diagnoses POCD will probably result from neuropsychological tests. POCD is widely underdiagnosed, especially in the elderly population. Indeed, a postoperative delirium in an elderly patient it is often trivialized and put on the account of preexisting dementia. Delirium can present in several forms clinically, as previously described. In more than 50% of patients symptoms are not recognized because of the high percentage of patients that have a 'hypoactive' presentation without any associated agitation. That is why it is essential to come up with a reliable tool to screen for POCD: standardized, repeatable, fast, simple and easily performed at the bedside by a nurse or physician.

Early POCD, delirium, can be diagnosed with the CAM (Confusion Assessment Method), which is the only validated and reliable clinical tool that can detect the symptoms of delirium. The CAM can be performed by health professionals without neuropsychiatric training [29], takes less than 5 minutes, can be done at the bedside, and has a high sensitivity and specificity [30]. CAM assesses the acute nature of POCD, and whether any of

the following are present: inattention or lack of focus, disorganized thinking, psychomotor agitation or apathy, and fluctuations and changes in the sleep–wake cycle. The CAM has been adapted for use in the ICU patient (CAM-ICU).

Diagnosing persistent POCD is more complex. In the absence of well-defined criteria, it is generally considered that a patient presents with late POCD if there is a deterioration of cognitive tests *compared to the preoperative or immediate postoperative period*. Different clinical studies have used a battery of neuropsychological tests with variable diagnostic thresholds [5, 31]. But a standardized, simple and reliable screening test that would allow us to routinely diagnose and grade cognitive function throughout the perioperative course has not yet been developed.

Perioperative Global Care
Primary Prevention: Identify Groups at Risk

The patient's preoperative cognitive trajectory [32] has to be known because it is predictive of the postoperative course. A history of any neurodegenerative or neurovascular disorder could be an important risk factor for postoperative delirium. The preoperative baseline cognitive level may provide the clinician with relevant information regarding possible cognitive postoperative complications and provides a reference against which postoperative cognition can be compared.

Cognitive reserve is affected by somatic or psychological diseases, as well as by cardiovascular risk factors. Amnesic or cognitive complaints, even in their early stage, should be actively searched for. The patient should undergo a complete physical and psychological assessment to identify at an early stage memory or cognitive problems, loss of temporospatial orientation, etc. But such in depth evaluation cannot be performed by the anaesthesiologist during a single preoperative interview. What is needed is a reliable and easy to perform cognitive test or tests that can be used by an anaesthesiologist during preoperative consultation.

The most widely used test to assess cognition is the MMSE. It explores overall cognition, including time and space orientation, anterograde memory, calculation and attentional abilities, and language and visual-praxis abilities. However, because it takes 10–15 minutes to take the test and does not detect early cognitive disorders, a shorter test that is still able to detect early symptoms is warranted. Of these, the so called 'test of the five categorical words' allows the clinician to better explore memory deficits. Two other tests have proven to be practical during pre-anaesthesia consultation to detect preoperative cognitive impairment and to predict the risk of POCD: the Mini-Cog and Codex (cognitive disorder examination). These two tests consist of two tasks. The first one is 'the test of the three words' which consists of memorizing three words and then recalling them. The second one is asking the patient to draw a clock. The Codex is slightly different from the Mini-Cog: depending on how the patient performs in both tasks, five questions will be asked to evaluate orientation in space. The test takes only a few minutes, is well accepted by patients, and has a specificity of 93% and a sensitivity of 99% to detect cognitive disorders [33, 34].

The IQCODE-R (Informant Questionnaire on Cognitive Decline in the Elderly) can be completed by the caregiver in the waiting room; the short version is faster than the full version because it contains 16 instead of 26 questions [35].

More sensitive cognitive tests that diagnose cognitive disorders in an early phase are being evaluated in the perioperative context. The Isaac Test Set for example is a short (two-minute) test of verbal fluency that spots symptoms several years before the actual dementia diagnosis is made.

What do we do with these tests after identifying the patient at risk of POCD? First, the risk is explained to the patient. One can consider admitting the patient preoperatively to a geriatric service for a global and more detailed assessment of cognitive function, optimize any existing treatment and involve the support of the family.

Secondary Prevention: Reducing the Incidence of Postoperative Cognitive Dysfunction

Limit Precipitating Perioperative Risk Factors

As mentioned before, contrary to popular belief, anaesthesia-related factors like anaesthetic drugs, maintenance of physiological homeostasis, or choice of anaesthetic technique contribute little or not at all to POCD. Still, it might be possible to decrease the incidence of POCD (particularly early postoperative delirium) by avoiding or limiting factors known to affect CNS function in more general terms. Anticholinergic

drugs (including glycopyrrolate) and benzodiazepines should be avoided because they have been implicated in the onset, worsening and persistence of cognitive impairment in the elderly. Cerebral hypoperfusion can lead to brain damage and POCD, especially in hypertensive patients with vascular disease, who have an impaired cerebral autoregulation. Even though the results of the different studies are contradictory, one can consider the use of aesthetic depth monitoring in these patients, and maintain arterial blood pressure optimally to ensure cerebral perfusion (also see Chapter 12) [36, 37]. Pain is a factor known to cause agitation and must be optimally treated postoperatively. Although occurring simultaneously, the effects of pain and inflammation appear to affect cognitive function separately. Some studies have shown that surgical management of chronic pain (such as hip/knee surgery for severe and disabling osteoarthritis) can improve the quality of life of patients.

Finally, because surgical stress induced neuroinflammation may be the main culprit in POCD, any surgical technique that minimizes tissue damage might be expected to minimize the inflammation, shorten its resolution and reduce the risk of POCD.

Non-pharmacological Prevention

Because the aetiology of POCD is multifactorial, a multi-pronged approach may be more effective than just acting on a single risk factor: the more risk factors identified and targeted, the more effective preventive therapy is likely to be. Care protocols should be developed that address those factors that have a proven impact on the incidence and duration of delirium. Prevention programmes focus on optimizing analgesia, making sure the patient is wearing her or his glasses or hearing aids, early rehabilitation, ensuring sleep quality and close monitoring of hydration status.

Because there currently is no clearly defined treatment for POCD, we remain limited to implementing multiple, non-specific measures to optimize the overall care of the patient.

Pharmacological Prevention

There is no pharmacological approach known to reliably prevent POCD. Pharmacological prevention has been attempted with neuroleptics, acetylcholinesterase inhibitors and drugs with anti-inflammatory action. Although some studies show antipsychotics to have a (small) effect on the incidence of delirium, their side effects outweigh their benefits and thus they should not be used. Similarly, the potential effectiveness of acetylcholinesterase inhibitors is largely offset by their adverse events. The most promising studies may be those that focus on limiting intraoperative neuro-inflammation. Ketamine's effects are contradictory [38]. Statins may have a beneficial effect on the incidence of POCD [39, 40]. Finally, the highly selective alpha-2 adrenergic agonist dexmedetomidine decreased the incidence of early POCD after cardiac and non-cardiac surgery [41]. This drug, which has analgesic and hypnotic effects, has been studied primarily as a sedative in the intensive care setting where it has the advantage of keeping the patient sedated yet arousable without affecting ventilation. A limited number of animal and clinical studies seem to support a neuroprotective mechanism of action of dexmedetomidine that involves a reduction of the surgical stress response and decreased hippocampal apoptosis via inhibition of neuronal hyperexcitability.

Tertiary Prevention: How to Treat Delirium?

Delirium is a real emergency that requires rapid aetiological and symptomatic treatment. The first step is to look for and treat any possible organic causes: hypoxaemia, hypercarbia, hypotension, stroke, metabolic disorders, sepsis, pain (including an undetected full bladder), drug and ethanol withdrawal.

At the same time, symptoms should be treated, first by non-pharmacological means. The care provider should help the patient refocus and reconnect with reality. The non-pharmacological measures mentioned above have to be applied. The patient should not be isolated, and the use of physical restraints should be the exception and, if used, be limited in time because they reduce mobility and increase agitation. Pharmacological treatment is reserved for patients whose clinical symptoms could compromise their own safety. As first-line drugs, antipsychotics such as haloperidol are often recommended (although rigorous scientific support for this recommendation is lacking). The lowest dose should be used for the shortest time possible. Benzodiazepines are reserved for withdrawal syndromes and delirium tremens. Finally, dexmedetomidine warrants further study in this setting.

Whatever the short-term evolution of any episode of POCD, it is advised to schedule a neurology or geriatric consultation to assess if the delirium persists, and to identify the patients at risk for persistent cognitive impairment.

Conclusion

The different clinical presentations of postoperative cognitive dysfunction have become a public health burden, as shown by the increasing number of studies in this domain. The physiopathology of this clinical entity remains poorly understood and likely is multifactorial. Surgical stress seems to play a central role and likely is the triggering factor. Some authors suggest that a combination of preoperative risk factors and cognitive tests might be predictive of POC. A postoperative hypo- or hyperactive delirium is a risk factor for the development of late (persistent) POCD. Monitoring of cognition throughout the perioperative phase will be a key point to individualize the treatment of the patient.

References

1. Moller JT, Cluitmans P, Rasmussen LS, Houx P, Rasmussen H, Canet J, et al: Long-term postoperative cognitive dysfunction in the elderly ISPOCD1 study. ISPOCD investigators. International Study of Post-Operative Cognitive Dysfunction. Lancet.Lond.Engl. 1998; 351 (9106): 857–61.

2. Bedford PD: Adverse cerebral effects of anaesthesia on old people. Lancet.Lond.Engl. 1955; 269 (6884): 259–63.

3. Monk TG, Weldon BC, Garvan CW, Dede DE, van der Aa MT, Heilman KM, et al: Predictors of cognitive dysfunction after major noncardiac surgery. Anesthesiology. 2008; 108 (1): 18–30.

4. Clegg A, Young J, Iliffe S, Rikkert MO, Rockwood K: Frailty in older people. Lancet. 2013; 381 (9868): 752–62.

5. Evered L, Silbert B, Scott DA, Ames D, Maruff P, Blennow K: Cerebrospinal fluid biomarker for Alzheimer disease predicts postoperative cognitive dysfunction. Anesthesiology. 2016; 124 (2): 353–61.

6. Duppils GS, Wikblad K: Acute confusional states in patients undergoing hip surgery. A prospective observation study. Gerontology. 2000; 46 (1): 36–43.

7. Parikh SS, Chung F: Postoperative delirium in the elderly. Anesth.Analg. 1995; 80 (6): 1223–32.

8. Lewis MC, Barnett SR: Postoperative delirium: the tryptophan dyregulation model. Med. Hypotheses. 2004; 63 (3): 402–6.

9. Whitlock EL, Vannucci A, Avidan MS: Postoperative delirium. Minerva.Anestesiol. 2011; 77 (4): 448–56.

10. van Harten AE, Scheeren TWL, Absalom AR: A review of postoperative cognitive dysfunction and

neuroinflammation associated with cardiac surgery and anaesthesia. Anaesthesia. 2012; 67 (3): 280–93.

11. Avidan MS, Evers AS: The fallacy of persistent postoperative cognitive decline. Anesthesiol.J.Am.Soc. Anesthesiol. 2016; 124 (2): 255–8.

12. Dyer CB, Ashton CM, Teasdale TA: Postoperative delirium. A review of 80 primary data-collection studies. Arch.Intern.Med. 1995; 155 (5): 461–5.

13. Gustafson Y, Berggren D, Brännström B, Bucht G, Norberg A, Hansson LI, et al: Acute confusional states in elderly patients treated for femoral neck fracture. J. Am.Geriatr.Soc. 1988; 36 (6): 525–30.

14. Marcantonio ER, Flacker JM, Michaels M, Resnick NM: Delirium is independently associated with poor functional recovery after hip fracture. J.Am.Geriatr. Soc. 2000; 48 (6): 618–24.

15. Newman MF, Kirchner JL, Phillips-Bute B, Gaver V, Grocott H, Jones RH, et al: Longitudinal assessment of neurocognitive function after coronary-artery bypass surgery. N.Engl.J.Med. 2001; 344 (6): 395–402.

16. Androsova G, Krause R, Winterer G, Schneider R: Biomarkers of postoperative delirium and cognitive dysfunction. Front.Aging.Neurosci. 2015; 7.

17. Hueb W, Lopes NH, Pereira AC, Hueb AC, Soares PR, Favarato D, et al: Five-year follow-up of a randomized comparison between off-pump and on-pump stable multivessel coronary artery bypass grafting. The MASS III Trial. Circulation. 2010; 122 (11 Suppl): S48–52.

18. Ghoneim MM, Hinrichs JV, O'Hara MW, Mehta MP, Pathak D, Kumar V, et al: Comparison of psychologic and cognitive functions after general or regional anesthesia. Anesthesiology. 1988; 69 (4): 507–15.

19. Pavlov VA, Parrish WR, Rosas-Ballina M, Ochani M, Puerta M, Ochani K, et al: Brain acetylcholinesterase activity controls systemic cytokine levels through the cholinergic anti-inflammatory pathway. Brain Behav. Immun. 2009; 23 (1): 41–5.

20. Czura CJ, Tracey KJ: Autonomic neural regulation of immunity. J.Intern.Med. 2005; 257 (2): 156–66.

21. Degos V, Vacas S, Han Z, van Rooijen N, Gressens P, Su H, et al: Depletion of bone marrow-derived macrophages perturbs the innate immune response to surgery and reduces postoperative memory dysfunction. Anesthesiology. 2013; 118 (3): 527–36.

22. Rudolph JL, Marcantonio ER, Culley DJ, Silverstein JH, Rasmussen LS, Crosby GJ, et al: Delirium is associated with early postoperative cognitive dysfunction. Anaesthesia. 2008; 63 (9): 941–7.

23. Rappold T, Laflam A, Hori D, Brown C, Brandt J, Mintz CD, et al: Evidence of an association between brain cellular injury and cognitive decline after non-cardiac surgery. BJA.Br.J.Anaesth. 2016; 116 (1): 83–9.

24. McDonagh DL, Mathew JP, White WD, Phillips-Bute B, Laskowitz DT, Podgoreanu MV, et al: Cognitive function after major noncardiac surgery, apolipoprotein E4 genotype, and biomarkers of brain injury. Anesthesiology. 2010; 112 (4): 852–9.

25. Chen M, Liao Y, Rong P, Hu R, Lin G, Ouyang W: Hippocampal volume reduction in elderly patients at risk for postoperative cognitive dysfunction. J.Anesth. 2013; 27 (4): 487–92.

26. Brown CH, Faigle R, Klinker L, Bahouth M, Max L, LaFlam A, et al: The association of brain MRI characteristics and postoperative delirium in cardiac surgery patients. Clin.Ther. 2015; 37 (12): 2686–99.e9.

27. Cavallari M, Hshieh TT, Guttmann CRG, Ngo LH, Meier DS, Schmitt EM, et al: Brain atrophy and white-matter hyperintensities are not significantly associated with incidence and severity of postoperative delirium in older persons without dementia. Neurobiol.Aging. 2015; 36 (6): 2122–9.

28. Gerriets T, Schwarz N, Bachmann G, Kaps M, Kloevekorn W-P, Sammer G, et al: Evaluation of methods to predict early long-term neurobehavioral outcome after coronary artery bypass grafting. Am.J.Cardiol. 2010; 105 (8): 1095–101.

29. Inouye SK, van Dyck CH, Alessi CA, Balkin S, Siegal AP, Horwitz RI: Clarifying confusion: the confusion assessment method. A new method for detection of delirium. Ann.Intern.Med. 1990; 113 (12): 941–8.

30. Cole MG, Dendukuri N, McCusker J, Han L: An empirical study of different diagnostic criteria for delirium among elderly medical inpatients. J. Neuropsychiatry.Clin.Neurosci. 2003; 15 (2): 200–7.

31. Dokkedal U, Hansen TG, Rasmussen LS, Mengel-From J, Christensen K: Cognitive functioning after surgery in middle-aged and elderly Danish twins. J.Neurosurg. Anesthesiol. 2016; 28 (3): 275.

32. Nadelson MR, Sanders RD, Avidan MS: Perioperative cognitive trajectory in adults. Br.J.Anaesth. 2014; 112 (3): 440–51.

33. Robinson TN, Wu DS, Pointer LF, Dunn CL, Moss M: Preoperative cognitive dysfunction is related to adverse postoperative outcomes in the elderly. J.Am.Coll.Surg. 2012; 215 (1): 12–17; discussion 17–18.

34. Mézière A, Paillaud E, Belmin J, Pariel S, Herbaud S, Canouï-Poitrine F, et al: Delirium in older people after proximal femoral fracture repair: role of a preoperative screening cognitive test. Ann.Fr.Anesth.Reanim. 2013; 32 (9): e91–96.

35. Priner M, Jourdain M, Bouche G, Merlet-Chicoine I, Chaumier JA, Paccalin M: Usefulness of the Short IQCODE for predicting postoperative delirium in elderly patients undergoing hip and knee replacement surgery. Gerontology. 2008; 54 (2): 116–19.

36. Chan MTV, Cheng BCP, Lee TMC, Gin T, CODA Trial Group. BIS-guided anesthesia decreases postoperative delirium and cognitive decline. J.Neurosurg. Anesthesiol. 2013; 25 (1): 33–42.

37. Ballard C, Jones E, Gauge N, Aarsland D, Nilsen OB, Saxby BK, et al: Optimised anaesthesia to reduce post operative cognitive decline (POCD) in older patients undergoing elective surgery, a randomised controlled trial. PloS.One. 2012; 7 (6): e37410.

38. Bilotta F, Gelb AW, Stazi E, Titi L, Paoloni FP, Rosa G: Pharmacological perioperative brain neuroprotection: a qualitative review of randomized clinical trials. Br.J.Anaesth. 2013; 110 (Suppl 1): i113–20.

39. Vallabhajosyula S, Kanmanthareddy A, Erwin PJ, Esterbrooks DJ, Morrow LE: Role of statins in delirium prevention in critical ill and cardiac surgery patients: A systematic review and meta-analysis. J. Crit. Care. 2017; 37: 189–96.

40. Mariscalco G, Mariani S, Biancari F, Banach M: Effects of statins on delirium following cardiac surgery – evidence from literature. Psychiatr.Pol. 2015; 49 (6): 1359–70.

41. Li B, Wang H, Wu H, Gao C: Neurocognitive dysfunction risk alleviation with the use of dexmedetomidine in perioperative conditions or as ICU sedation: a meta-analysis. Medicine. (Baltimore). 2015; 94 (14): e597.

Cardiac and Haemodynamic Function

Kai Kuck, Natalie Silverton and Michael K. Cahalan

Introduction

In Europe, approximately 30% of surgeries are performed in patients with cardiovascular comorbidities and up to 42% of intraoperative complications are cardiac related [4]. Often, the anaesthesiologist needs to intervene to maintain haemodynamic function and prevent perioperative complications.

Cardiac and Haemodynamic Function

The haemodynamic system has a large reserve capacity, redundancy, closed-control loops and compensatory mechanisms. Critical failures that overwhelm these mechanisms lead to catastrophic physiological sequelae very quickly. Part of the quantitative assessment of

the cardiac and haemodynamic system is to ascertain the degree to which these compensatory mechanisms are active, and how much reserve capacity the system still has available. An important end-point of cardiac and haemodynamic performance is the maintenance of adequate tissue perfusion and tissue oxygen delivery. Figure 14.1 illustrates the physiological mechanisms and relationships affecting tissue oxygen delivery.

Anaesthetic Medications

Volatile anaesthetic agents depress myocardial contractility and reduce SVR leading to a decrease in MAP. Nitrous oxide alone, for example, in sedative concentrations, has only slight systemic haemodynamic

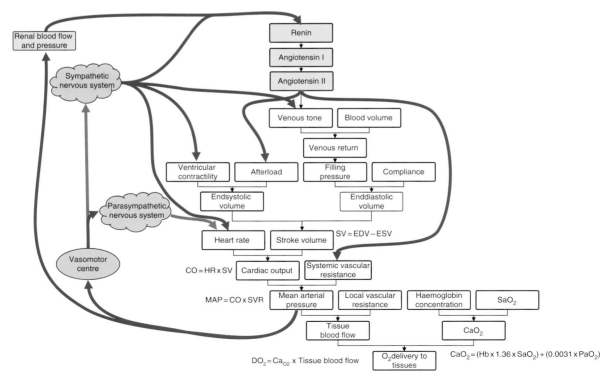

Fig. 14.1 Cardiac and haemodynamic quantitative factors and their hormonal and autonomic feedback control loops that determine tissue blood flow and oxygen delivery to the tissues [1, 2].

Table 14.1. Cardiovascular effects of intravenous anaesthetic drugs, including propofol [95], ketamine [95, 96], etomidate [95], and opioids [97].

	BP	CO	SVR	HR
Propofol bolus induction	25–40% decrease	15% decrease	15–25% decrease	unchanged
Propofol infusion maintenance	20–30% decrease	unaltered	30% decrease	variable
Ketamine	increase	increase		increase
Etomidate				almost no effect on cardiovascular system
Opioids	(decrease)		(decrease)	(decrease, especially fentanyl)	milder than other IV anaesthetics

effects [5]. However, when combined with volatile anaesthetic agents, vascular resistance and blood pressure are increased, when compared to using the volatile anaesthetic without nitrous oxide but adjusted to achieve the same level of anaesthesia [6, 7]. Many anaesthetic agents also alter autonomic reflexes, e.g. avoiding or counteracting the increases in HR and blood pressure from surgical stimulation or from the irritating airway effects of some volatile anaesthetics. Among the intravenous anaesthetic agents, propofol has the most profound effects on the cardiovascular system (Table 14.1), including negative inotropy and vasodilation, resulting in marked hypotension. Ketamine, etomidate and opioids have considerably less impact (Table 14.1).

Therapeutic Intervention Options for Haemodynamic Management

A recent survey revealed that only 5.4% of North American anaesthesiologists and 30.4% of European anaesthesiologists indicate that their institution or group have a written haemodynamic management protocol [3].

Table 14.2 lists pharmaceutical agents used in intraoperative haemodynamic management, their pharmacokinetic characteristics and their haemodynamic effect.

Fluid shifts, haemorrhage, evaporation and changes in vascular capacity necessitate the administration of fluids. Outcome is affected by the volume, the type of fluid and timing of administration. Goal-directed therapy (GDT) aims to provide protocol-based guidance about fluid administration but there is no agreement on which if any of the published GDT approaches is best. Some have suggested that the variability in the preoperative and intraoperative conditions, patient

comorbidities and anaesthetic management require marked individualizations of fluid management [8]. Moreover, determining the adequacy of fluid therapy is very difficult and frequently unreliable. Cannesson and Gan summarize the philosophy of GDT as providing fluids only, if the patient responds to the fluid [9]. Myburgh et al provide a thorough review of the different types of resuscitation fluids, but conclude that there is currently no ideal resuscitation fluid [10].

Haemodynamic Variables and Their Target Ranges

In a meta-analysis, a proactive haemodynamic monitoring strategy combined with targeted haemodynamic interventions has been shown to reduce surgical mortality and complications [11]. The ideal variables for haemodynamic management reflect end-organ perfusion and can be measured easily, accurately, reproducibly and continuously, or at least rapidly. Tissue hypoperfusion was one of the three strongest intraoperative predictors of postoperative complications in a study of 438 patients undergoing moderate-risk elective surgeries [12]. Tissue hypoxia has been found to play a central role in organ dysfunction [13], which in turn can compromise perioperative patient outcome [14]. However, tissue perfusion and tissue oxygenation are difficult to measure. Often, surrogate variables are used instead.

Even though most organs require blood flow rather than blood pressure [15], the most commonly used variable for managing haemodynamics is blood pressure. Blood pressure values vary with age [16]. USA data indicate that hypertension (>= 140–159/90–99 mmHg systolic/diastolic blood pressure) is prevalent in approximately 30% of the population, making it one of the most common chronic medical conditions [17, 18]. A meta-analysis of 30 observational studies associates

Table 14.2. Pharmaceutical options for haemodynamic management [17, 23, 98–105].

Drug	Onset of action (min)	Duration of action (min)	α	β	CO	HR	SVR	MAP	PuVR	PerVR
Adrenaline	Immediate	5–15	+	+	↑	↑	↑	↑	0	
Isoproterenol	1–5	15–30	0	+	↑	↑	↓	↓	0	
Noradrenaline	Immediate	5–15	+	+	0	0	↑	↑	↑	
Dopamine	2–4	10–15	+	+	↑	↑	↑	↑	0	
Dobutamine	1–2 (peak at 10)	10–15	0	+	↑	↑	↓	↓	↓	
Milrinone	1	45–60	0	0	↑	0	↓	↓	↓	
Phenylephrine	1–3	10–20	+	0	0	↓	↑	↑	↑	
Vasopressin	1–3	5–10	0	0	0	0	↑	↑	0	
Ephedrine	1–3	15–20	+	+	↑	↑	↑	↑	0	
Levosimendan	5	1–2 h	0	0	↑	0	↓	↓	↓	
Esmolol	1	10–20	0	-	↓	↓	0	↓	0	
Labetalol	2–5	6h	-	-	0	(↓)	↓	↓		
Clevidipine	2–4	5–15	0	0	↑	0		↓	↓	
Nicardipine	2 (5–15 for infusion)	2–4 h (4–6 h for infusion)	0	0	↑		↓*	↓		
Nitroprusside	Immediate	1–2	0	0	0		↓	↓		↓
Nitroglycerin	2–5	3–5	0	0	↓	↑	↓	↓		↓
Clonidine	30	4-6 h	+**		(↓)	↓	↓	↓		↑
Urapidil	2	4-5 h	-		0	0	↓	↓		↓
Enalaprilat	15	6h	0	0	(↑)	0	↓	↓	↓	
Fenoldopam	5	30–60	0	0	↑	↑	↓	↓		↓
Hydralazine	5–15	6–12 h			↑	↑	↓	↓		↓

PuVR … Pulmonary Vascular Resistance, PerVR … Peripheral Vascular Resistance
* coronary, ** cerebral

preoperative hypertension with a 35% increase in risk of intraoperative cardiovascular complications [19].

However, evidence for optimal perioperative blood pressure targets is lacking [4, 20]. A systematic literature review found 140 different definitions of intraoperative hypotension in 130 articles, where the most frequent definition was a systolic blood pressure below 80 mmHg, a systolic blood pressure decrease of more than 20%, or a combination of absolute and relative thresholds (100 mmHg and 30% decrease) [21]. Patients presenting with chronic hypertension may have a shifted or impaired cerebral or renal autoregulation. Population-based blood pressure targets will likely not be adequate in these patients. Instead an individualized approach is needed, supported by monitoring of indicators that reflect end-organ perfusion [20].

A transient increase in blood pressure (by 20–30 mmHg) and heart rate (by 15–20 bpm) can be seen after laryngoscopy and intubation [22]. The blood pressure increase may be blunted by using opioids during induction. Anaesthetic agents can trigger a decrease in blood pressure and heart rate. Low blood pressure has also been observed in about a third of patients after spinal anaesthesia, one of the most common spinal anaesthesia complications [23]. Another frequent cause of perioperative hypotension is hypovolaemia due to dehydration or haemorrhage. A retrospective study in 33,330 non-cardiac surgeries found an increase in the risk of acute kidney injury or myocardial injury dependent on the duration of intraoperative MAP below 55 mmHg [24]. Surgical technique (e.g. laparoscopic insufflation), patient positioning and positive pressure ventilation can lower blood pressure by decreasing venous return and cardiac output.

Perioperative goal-directed therapy (PGDT) provides a rational, protocol-driven approach to haemodynamic optimization, often using IV fluids and vasoactive medications. A 2013 Cochrane review of 31 studies of PGDT in 5292 patients found that PGDT did not have an impact on mortality but that it did reduce postoperative renal failure, respiratory failure and wound infections [25]. Studies of GDT show a wide variety of protocols, endpoints and haemodynamic monitoring techniques [9]. The Surviving Sepsis campaign guideline recommends CVP 8–12 mmHg, MAP >= 65 mmHg, urine output >= 0.5 mL/kg/h, and central venous oxygen saturation (Scv_{O2}) or mixed venous oxygen saturation (Sv_{O2}) 70% or 65%, respectively, and suggests using lactate levels as an indicator of tissue hypoperfusion [26]. Some studies have found HR's association with outcome not to be consistent and to be confounded with other variables, such as patient presentation, beta-blocker medications and operative variables – raising doubts about the value of HR as a good variable for haemodynamic management [27, 28].

In their meta-analysis of proactive perioperative haemodynamic management trials, Hamilton et al [11] found in 29 studies target values similar to those recommended by the Surviving Sepsis campaign. These were CVP 6–15 mmHg, MAP of a minimum of 60–110 mmHg (average 74 mmHg) and maximum of 100–110 mmHg (average of 105 mmHg), urine output

at least 0.5–1 mL/kg/h, and Sv_{O2} minimally 65–70%. Only five of the reviewed studies used heart rate using a target of a maximum heart rate of between 100 to 120 beats per minute.

Of note, these surrogate variables, with the exception of Sv_{O2} and Scv_{O2}, may be normal, even when tissue hypoperfusion is present [29, 30]. In high-risk patients undergoing major surgery, 65% [31] and 73% [32] were found to be the optimal cut-off Scv_{O2} values to predictively discriminate complications. However, using Scv_{O2} to guide goal-directed therapy failed to improve mortality [30].

Indicators of the patient's need for intravenous fluids include positive pressure variations (PPV) and stroke volume variations (SVV) with typical thresholds for indicating fluid responsiveness of 10–15% during closed chest positive pressure ventilation of at least 7 mL/kg [33–36].

Intraoperative events result in haemodynamic variable deviations from their normal range, as detailed in Table 14.3.

Monitoring

Invasive and non-invasive arterial blood pressure, central venous pressure, cardiac output and pulmonary capillary wedge pressure are the top five modalities used in North America and Europe during high risk surgery (Fig. 14.2) [3].

Invasive arterial blood pressure monitors display the continuous blood pressure waveform and calculate systolic (SYS), diastolic (DIA) and mean arterial (MAP) blood pressure as well as heart rate. Similar set-ups with catheters connected to an external pressure sensor are used to measure pressures other than arterial, e.g. central venous pressure and pulmonary artery pressures.

Non-invasive arterial blood pressure monitors most commonly use an oscillometric cuff wrapped around an extremity, typically the upper arm. Measurements are intermittent, and should be limited in frequency to help avoid peripheral nerve injury from inflation of the cuff. Oscillometry is known to have limited accuracy, especially in patients with stiff arteries [37–39]. In a comparison of non-invasive and invasive arterial blood pressures in more than 24,000 cases, Wax et al found that non-invasive blood pressure was underestimated during hypertension and overestimated during hypotension [40].

Table 14.3. Haemodynamic changes during various intraoperative events [106, 107].

	ECG	Pulse				PA				SpO$_2$	Sv$_{O2}$	TEE
		HR	CO	BP	Pressure	CVP	Pressure	PCWP	PPV			
Acute haemorrhage		↑		↓				–	–		↓	Hypovolaemia
Cardiac arrest	Arrhythmias (VT, VF, asystole)			absent	absent					absent		Lack of ventricular contraction
Sepsis		>90		(↓)						>70		
Acute coronary syndrome	ST segment elevation	↑/↓		↓		–		–				Wall motion abnormalities
Anaphylactic and anaphylactoid reactions	Arrhythmias	↓		↓↓						↓		
Cardiac tamponade	Low-amplitude ST changes	↑	↓	↓	↓							Pericardial fluid visible atrial and/or ventricular collapse abnormal ventricular septal motion with respiration IVC plethora
Non-lethal ventricular arrhythmias	PVC, VT, torsades des points											
Pulmonary oedema	Arrhythmias	↑		↑/↓						↓		
Pulmonary oedema (cardiogenic)	Arrhythmias	↑		↑/↓		↑		↑				
Pulmonary embolism (patient conscious)		↑		↓		↑						
Pulmonary embolism (anaesthesia)	ST-T changes, PEA, asystole, RBBB	↑		↓		↑		↑		↓		
Sinus bradycardia	Junctional or idioventricular escape beats	↓		↓								
Supraventricular arrhythmias	Abnormal Syncope or presyncope	↑		↓								
Venous air embolism	Tachyarrhythmias ST-T changes		↓	↓		–	–			↓		Air in cardiac chambers

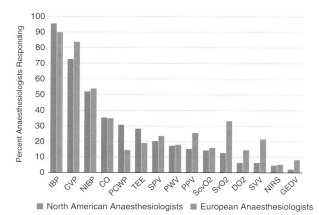

Fig. 14.2 Haemodynamic monitoring modalities used by North American and European anaesthesiologists for managing patients during high-risk surgery [3]. Legend: IBP (Invasive arterial pressure), CVP (Central venous pressure), NIBP (Non-invasive arterial pressure), CO (Cardiac output), PCWP (Pulmonary capillary wedge pressure), TEE (Transesophageal echocardiography), SPV (Systolic pressure variation), PWV (Plethysmographic waveform variation), PPV (Pulse pressure variation), ScvO$_2$ (Central venous saturation), SvO$_2$ (Mixed venous saturation), DO2 (Oxygen delivery), SVV (Stroke volume variation), NIRS (Near-infrared spectroscopy), GEDV (Global end diastolic volume).

Arterial tonometry and volume clamping allows continuous non-invasive blood pressure monitoring as well as display and derivation of the same or similar variables as invasive blood pressure monitoring. Cannesson et al systematically reviewed and analysed 29 studies of commercially available devices and found that their accuracy and precision did not meet the Association for the Advancement of Medical Instrumentation's performance requirements (accuracy <= 5 mmHg and precision <= 8 mmHg) for non-invasive blood pressure monitors [41]. It might be that the requirements that target intermittent non-invasive blood pressure monitors are not appropriate for continuous non-invasive blood pressure monitors.

Most anaesthesiologists indicated in a recent survey [3] that they monitor central venous pressure (CVP) in high risk surgery cases. CVP is used as an indicator for volume expansion in these cases, together with blood pressure, urine output and clinical experience. This is in spite of the fact that more than 95% of anaesthesiologists acknowledge that CVP is not the best predictor for fluid responsiveness, and that there are 'no data to support the widespread practice of using central venous pressure to guide fluid therapy' [42].

The development of the Swann–Ganz pulmonary artery catheter (PAC) in the 1970s led to the widespread adoption of thermodilution cardiac output measurement – and eventually GDT. The PAC-based thermodilution method can be performed either intermittently by injecting room temperature or iced saline into the right atrium, or continuously, using a PAC with integrated heating filaments. The resulting change in temperature is measured downstream, in the pulmonary artery, and used to calculate cardiac output, assuming the indicator mixed completely with the blood and no indicator was lost. Accuracy is better the colder the indicator solution is and the lower the cardiac output is, because of a better signal to noise ratio. The PAC also allows measurement of pulmonary artery pressure, pulmonary artery wedge pressure and, with some PAC catheters, continuous monitoring of mixed venous oxygen saturation (SvO$_2$). Evidence has amassed that data provided through use of the PAC, including thermodilution, is not accurate, that the PAC is associated with significant risk and poor outcome, that many clinicians are not able to correctly interpret information obtained through the PAC and that information may not help in the management of critically ill patients and in fact may result in overtreatment [43–46].

Less invasive and non-invasive cardiac output approaches have become available as alternatives to PAC-based thermodilution. Oesophageal Doppler cardiac output measures flow velocity in the descending aorta using a small-diameter dedicated ultrasonic probe inserted through the mouth or nose. Oesophageal Doppler can show beat-to-beat stroke volume, cardiac output, heart rate and a number of parameters derived from the flow velocity waveform. It assumes a homogeneous (or known) velocity profile across the aortic cross-section, a known cross-sectional area that stays constant over a heartbeat, a fixed and known ratio of cardiac output distribution between ascending and descending aorta and a correct positioning of the Doppler probe to make sure the ultrasonic beam is directed towards the descending aorta. Oesophageal Doppler cardiac output has been found in human and animal studies to be just slightly less accurate than thermodilution and associated with improved patient outcome [47].

Thoracic bioimpedance cardiac output measures the voltage drop across thoracic electrodes resulting from the injection of a small high-frequency electrical current across the thorax using two additional electrodes and measuring the resulting voltage drop. Assuming a certain bioimpedance model of the thorax and assuming that changes in impedance are related to changes in blood volume within the thorax, aortic flow rate and stroke volume are calculated. The approach is sensitive to the appropriateness of the thorax model, the placement of the electrodes, non-cardiac output related fluid shifts in the thorax and electrical noise. Variations of bioimpedance such as electrical velocimetry (relates impedance changes not to aortic flow but to aortic blood velocity) and bioreactance (considers the phase shift between electrical current and voltage drop) aim to ameliorate the sensitivity to electrode placement and thorax model. Studies of bioimpedance cardiac output agree that it lacks interchangeability with thermodilution but some indicate that bioimpedance might be successfully employed as a trend monitor and to judge fluid responsiveness [48].

In partial CO_2 rebreathing cardiac output the volume of CO_2 excreted through the lungs per breath is related to cardiac output. This method assumes that cardiac output, venous CO_2 concentration and the slope of the CO_2 dissociation curve stay constant during the measurement period and that end-tidal CO_2 can be measured reliably and reflects alveolar CO_2. Human and animal studies report mixed results. A meta-analysis by Peyton et al [49] found partial CO_2 rebreathing to perform similarly to other non-invasive cardiac output approaches (oesophageal Doppler, bioimpedance and pulse contour). However, just like other non-invasive methods, it did not meet Critchley and Critchley's postulated criteria of 30% or better agreement [50].

Pulse contour cardiac output analyses the continuous arterial blood pressure waveform and estimates cardiac output from vascular impedance and the area under the blood pressure curve during systole. Pulse contour cardiac output may become inaccurate if vascular impedance changes. Some of the commercially available pulse contour cardiac output monitors require occasional calibration, usually with less invasive methods, e.g. transpulmonary thermodilution or lithium dilution. A recent literature review of five commercially available pulse contour cardiac output monitors that use invasive blood pressure measurement found a total pooled underestimation bias of 40% and a standard deviation of the error of 1.25 L/min and only limited agreement with thermodilution during haemodynamically unstable periods. Frequent recalibration with thermodilution improved the accuracy of cardiac output estimations [51]. Another review showed that cardiac output estimated using non-invasive continuous blood pressure provides reasonable estimates of cardiac output, but does not reach the threshold for interchangeability with invasive thermodilution cardiac output [52].

Less invasive cardiac output indicator dilution approaches do not require a PAC. Instead, the indicator is injected through a central venous catheter and the thermodilution temperature curve is then measured in a large peripheral artery, e.g. the femoral or axillary artery. The shape of this transpulmonary indicator dilution waveform can then also be used to derive other variables of interest, such as extravascular lung water (EVLW), a measure of pulmonary oedema, and global end-diastolic volume (GEDV), an indicator of preload. EVLW estimation by transpulmonary thermodilution has been well validated and its ability to predict mortality in critically ill patients demonstrated in a number of studies [53]. In order to determine the need for fluid administration or fluid responsiveness, static preload indicators, such as central venous pressure, are inadequate. Static preload indicators do not consider where on the Frank Starling curve the heart is operating: preload is not the same as preload-responsiveness. In contrast, dynamic indicators involve changing the preload, and assessing the impact on stroke volume. Preload is changed as a matter of course by positive pressure ventilation and its impact on venous return. A mix of spontaneous and mechanically provided breaths will compromise the performance of this approach. This method assumes that the transmission of airway pressure to the thorax is not impeded, e.g. through low lung compliance or open chest or laparoscopic surgery. SVV might be assessed directly using continuous cardiac output approaches, through changes in pulse pressure measured from a continuous invasive or non-invasive blood pressure waveform (PPV), or through changes of the plethysmographic waveform, for example from a pulse oximeter. For these approaches, a trend monitor is sufficient; they do not require an absolute measurement. A systematic review encompassing 29 studies of mechanically ventilated patients demonstrated high sensitivity and specificity for predicting fluid responsiveness using respiratory variations of pulse pressure or stroke volume [54].

Oxygen saturation of haemoglobin helps determine the blood's oxygen carrying capacity of arterial blood, tissue oxygenation. The utility of pulse oximeters that measure arterial oxygen saturation have been expanded by adding an indicator of peripheral perfusion, measurement of carbon monoxide and methaemoglobine saturation, absolute haemoglobin, and respiratory rate.

Venous oxygen saturation can be measured optically and continuously in mixed venous blood (Sv_{O_2}) of the pulmonary artery by some of the modern PACs. It can be used to gauge, at constant SpO_2, how much oxygen the body has extracted. As an alternative, if PAC use is not indicated, central venous oxygen saturation (Scv_{O_2}) can be measured, instead, at the tip of the central venous catheter. Because the relationship between Scv_{O_2} and Sv_{O_2} is not constant they cannot always be interchanged with each other [55].

Near-infrared spectroscopy (NIRS) approaches have been developed that allow non-invasive monitoring of cerebral oxygenation. Cerebral oximetry measures non-pulsatile average tissue oxygenation, with a majority signal contribution from venous blood (approximately 70%) and the balance from arterial blood. Factors that might affect accuracy include changes in haemoglobin, haematoma, skull thickness and cerebrospinal fluid area, deviation from the assumed 70/30% ratio of venous to arterial signal contribution and jaundice.

Because of wide ranges of normal cerebral tissue oxygenation (60–75%), a coefficient of variation of the absolute baseline of 9.4% [56], and the large variability of algorithmic differences, cerebral oximetry is best used as a trend monitor. Thresholds between 12% and 20% decrease from baseline have been reported to be able to predict clinical symptoms of cerebral ischaemia during carotid surgeries. In an intervention algorithm based on cerebral oxygenation monitoring proposed by Denault et al [57] a decrease of cerebral oxygenation of 20% or more triggered an in-depth inspection of other haemodynamic parameters. The evidence for improved outcome from use of cerebral oximetry is still elusive, however [58].

Left Ventricular Echocardiography

Perioperative physicians use transthoracic (TTE) and transoesophageal echocardiography (TEE) in the operating room, emergency room and critical care settings. Evaluation of global LV systolic function is a universal requirement. No other bedside diagnostic technique offers the immediacy or comprehensiveness that echocardiography provides for this evaluation.

The most common and clinically useful LV echocardiographic modalities are fractional area change, fractional shortening and myocardial velocity assessment. In urgent clinical situations, experienced practitioners estimate LV systolic function qualitatively recognizing that only very marked abnormalities produce life-threatening consequences.

Fractional area change: the fractional area change (FAC) of the LV may be obtained with any of a number of different cross-sections, but the transgastric (TG) mid-ventricular short-axis (SAX) is usually the best choice because foreshortening of the left ventricle is a common problem with the TEE long-axis cross-sections. The simple formula for this calculation is:

$$FCA = \frac{EDA - ESA}{EDA} \tag{1}$$

where EDA is the end-diastolic area and ESA is the end-systolic area. Usually, the result is expressed as a percentage. Software packages provide an easy way to make these measurements by tracing the endocardial borders in both systole and diastole. By convention, the papillary muscles are included within the area measurements. Although this measurement is obtained easily, its interpretation has inherent limitations. For example, when FAC is measured using the TG mid-ventricular cross-section, segmental wall motion abnormalities (SWMA) in the ventricular base or apex will lead to overestimation of global LV function. Also, FAC is dependent on ventricular preload and afterload. Thus, changes in FAC may not reflect changes in LV global function unless loading conditions remain constant.

Fractional shortening (FS) is analogous to FAC in that it measures the change in dimension (instead of cross-sectional area as used in FAC) occurring during systole. The equation for this measurement is:

$$FS = \frac{(LVED - LVES)}{LVED} \tag{2}$$

where LVED is the LV end-diastolic diameter and LVES is LV end-systolic diameter. FS was the principal measure of LV function in the early days of echocardiography when only M-mode technology was available. However, it is still a commonly cited measurement in reports and studies. The TG mid-ventricular cross-section is the most useful for this measurement with

Table 14.4. Normal LV function values.

TG Short Axis Cross-Section	Men	Women
Fractional area change	59% ± 8%	62% ± 6%
Fractional shortening	34% ± 9%	37% ± 7%
Systolic wall thickening	30% ± 7%	28% ± 8%

the M-mode cursor placed across the myocardium of interest. FS has the same limitations as FAC when used for the assessment of global LV function. In fact, given the one-dimensional nature of M-mode, FS is less likely than FAC to reflect global ventricular function in the presence of any SWMA. Unlike the textbook values, Table 14.4 provides normal values for anaesthetized patients [59]. Wall thickening is included for completeness.

Three-dimensional (3-D) systems capture real-time end-diastolic and end-systolic volumes and allow measurement of ejection fraction and stroke volume. However, these systems are expensive and complicated to operate. Like the parameters in Table 14.4, ejection fraction and stroke volume measurements are impacted substantially by changes in LV preload and afterload.

Doppler tissue imaging: Doppler tissue imaging (DTI) uses pulsed-wave Doppler technology adapted to measure myocardial velocities instead of blood flow velocities [60]. Typically, myocardial velocities range between +20 and –20 cm/s. During normal LV contraction, the mitral annulus descends toward the apex of the heart. DTI measures the velocity of this descent (S'). S' correlates with traditional measures of LV function including ejection fraction and the rate of rise of LV systolic pressure (dP/dt) [60, 61]. In addition, S' decreases in the presence of myocardial ischaemia and responds to changes in inotropy [62, 63]. The four chamber cross-section is best for measuring S': the sampling volume is placed at the lateral insertion point of the mitral valve into the left ventricle and the cross section is aligned so that the sampling cursor is directly parallel with the motion of the annulus. The resulting Doppler tracing shows the downward S' systolic wave caused by the descent of the base of the LV as well as two upward diastolic waves E' and A'. These waves are caused by the upward motion of the base of the LV associated with the early and late phases of left atrial filling. S' is an easy and reproducible measurement. However, Ama et al tested its load dependence in 42 haemodynamically stable patients with normal

segmental LV function after coronary surgery. S' did not change significantly in response to a 20% increase or decrease in MAP induced by phenylephrine or nitroglycerine [64]. However, it increased significantly when preload was augmented by rapid infusion of colloid [63]. In summary, S' is less dependent on afterload than FAC and FS, but like these other two measures, it remains critically dependent on preload. However, DTI provides a quick and easy way to estimate LV ejection fraction: an S' greater that 7 cm/s usually correlates with an LV ejection fraction ≥ 50% [65]. This correlation was established using TTE. TTE estimates of S' may be somewhat greater than TEE measurements because with TTE the Doppler beam and annular motion may be better aligned. However, Sevimli et al estimated that difference to be less than 2% [66]. Clearly, in an individual patient, if the TEE Doppler beam and annular motion are off parallel alignment by more than 30°, you should expect significant underestimation. Likewise, if a segmental wall motion abnormality affects annular motion, the S' may not reflect global LV systolic function.

Right Ventricular Echocardiography

Traditionally, echocardiography has focused more on the evaluation of LV function and the RV has often been termed 'the forgotten ventricle'. Barring significant intra-cardiac shunt, however, these two pumps in series must provide the same cardiac output and therefore the function of the right ventricle is equally important as the function of the left.

Classic teaching about RV failure in the setting of myocardial infarction (MI) has been to give the patient IV fluids, elevate their CVP and turn the RV into a 'conduit' for passive blood flow. Outcome studies, however, showed that patients with right-sided MI had significantly greater morbidity and mortality than those with left-sided MI [67] and, recently, the importance of RV dysfunction has been demonstrated in patients with systolic heart failure [68], in right-sided MI [69] and in those undergoing cardiac surgery [70–72]. Objective measures of RV function are therefore becoming a more essential component of the echocardiographic exam.

The biggest challenge to the echocardiographic assessment of RV function is its complex geometric shape. The LV has a simple bullet shape that is amenable to two-dimensional (2-D) modelling and allows relatively accurate approximations of ejection fraction (EF) from 2-D images. The RV, on the other hand, has a relatively complex crescentic shape and 2-D approximations of RV volumes and EF are not valid [73]. The objective evaluation of the RV, therefore, has relied on surrogate measures of function such as tricuspid annular plane motion and cross-sectional area change.

The most widely used measure of RV function in echocardiography is the tricuspid annular plane systolic excursion (TAPSE), which is a measure of the distance the tricuspid valve annulus is displaced during systole. A four-chamber view of the heart is obtained and the motion of the tricuspid annulus is tracked over time using M mode echocardiography. The vigorous contraction of a normal healthy RV results in a tricuspid annular excursion of around 2–3 cm. A TAPSE < 1.7 cm suggests RV dysfunction [74]. Another common measure of RV function is the peak velocity of the tricuspid annulus as it descends from the base of the heart during systole (S'). This velocity is measured using TDI and an S' < 9.5 cm/s suggests RV dysfunction [74].

These two measures of tricuspid annular motion are the most commonly reported objective measures of RV function with transthoracic echocardiography (TTE). When compared to the 3-D assessment of the RV using MRI, however, these surrogate measures of RV function show poor correlation with RV EF [75], most likely because they assess the function of only a single segment of only one of the four walls of the RV. In addition, geometric changes that occur with the heart after pericardiotomy appear to result in a decrease in TAPSE that persists for greater than 12 months after cardiac surgery even though 3-D measures of RV ejection fraction are unchanged [76], suggesting that TAPSE may not be a valid measure of RV function after cardiac surgery. Finally, measurements of systolic excursion and tissue Doppler based velocity are highly angle dependent. Whereas the angle of the ultrasound beam aligns well with tricuspid annular motion in a four-chamber view using TTE, this is not true of the corresponding measurement in TEE. These measures of RV function, therefore, should probably not be used for the intraoperative assessment of RV function.

Two additional echocardiographic measures of RV function are fractional area change (FAC) and myocardial performance index (MPI). The FAC is percentage change in the cross-sectional area of the RV through the cardiac cycle. Analogous to EF, FAC is calculated by subtracting the end-systolic area of the RV in a four-chamber view from the end-diastolic area and then normalizing it by the end-diastolic area. RV

dysfunction is suggested by an RV FAC < 35% [74]. Despite being a 2-D estimation of 3-D EF, RV FAC has been shown to correlate better with RV 3-D EF than either TAPSE or S' [75], can be used intraoperatively with TEE and is a significant predictor of outcome after cardiac surgery [71].

Myocardial performance index (MPI) is a measure of the ratio of duration of the isovolumic phases of ventricular contraction and relaxation to the duration of the systolic ejection period. A healthy RV will have relatively short isovolumic times and a relatively long ejection period making this ratio a small number. In RV dysfunction, the isovolumic times are prolonged and the ejection period shortens. MPI can be measured using spectral Doppler of a tricuspid regurgitation jet and the right ventricular outflow tract ejection. Alternatively, simultaneous measurements of MPI can be made using TDI. RV dysfunction is suggested by a pulsed wave Doppler MPI > 0.43 or a tissue Doppler MPI > 0.54 [74]. MPI has also been shown to predict outcome after cardiac surgery [70] and is applicable to both TTE and TEE.

Two relatively new measures of RV function are speckle-tracking strain and 3-D RV EF measured with echocardiography. Both of these methods require specialized software that was initially only offered offline on a separate computer. Recently, however, major manufacturers have started making these software applications available on the echo machine itself such that these calculations can now be made during image acquisition or in the operating room.

Speckle-tracking strain echocardiography uses echogenic 'speckles' in the myocardium to track movement of the myocardium over time [77, 78]. RV strain is calculated as the percentage of myocardial shortening during systole. RV *global longitudinal* strain is the average strain of the three segments of the lateral wall in a four-chamber view and the three segments of the inter-ventricular septum. The septum is included because of the contribution it is thought to make to RV ejection and cardiac output. RV *free wall* strain (RV FWS) is the same measurement; only the inter-ventricular septum values are removed and thus it is the average strain of the three segments of the lateral wall of the RV. This measure is analogous to TAPSE except that speckle-tracking echocardiography is relatively angle independent and instead of only measuring the excursion of the tricuspid annulus, it measures myocardial shortening of the entire lateral wall of the RV. RV FWS is a promising new technology that is the best predictor of RV dysfunction when compared to more traditional echocardiographic measures of RV function [75]. RV strain has also been shown to predict outcome in patients with systolic heart failure [68] and right-sided MI [69], and those undergoing cardiac surgery [72].

Three-dimensional echocardiography is not a new technology. However, only in the last decade has computer processing on echo machines been fast enough to incorporate this technology into day-to-day practice. Most new echo machines have the capability of acquiring 3-D images of the heart and when applied to the RV, volumetric data can be obtained and then used to calculate 3-D EF. TTE measurements of 3-D RV EF have been shown to correlate well with the gold standard of cardiac MRI [79]. 3-D RV EF has also been shown to be feasible to measure with TEE in the operating room [80], although the software to make these calculations is expensive and not available on most echo machines.

To summarize, despite its reputation as 'the forgotten ventricle', multiple studies now demonstrate the importance of RV function in patients with cardiovascular disease. The assessment of RV function is difficult because the complex shape of the RV precludes accurate estimations of ejection fraction using 2-D echocardiography. Surrogate measures of RV function such as TAPSE and S' are often used, but these have limitations, particularly when used with TEE in the operating room. Newer measures such as RV strain and 3-D RV EF show promise in terms of their diagnostic accuracy but require specialized software. Hopefully over time, this new software will become less expensive and more available to end-users in the operating room.

Closed Loop

As discussed, it is hard to set and justify specific absolute haemodynamic target values for the individual patient based on population statistics. When appropriate target values have been determined by the clinician, closed-loop systems might help reaching and maintaining these values automatically. Academic research going back decades [81] has shown systems that have demonstrated lower inter-patient variability for fluid management [82], more consistent and stable control of blood pressure [83] and good performance of a number of other haemodynamic closed-loop systems [84]. However, hardly any device has taken the requisite regulatory and safety engineering steps to make it to the market, with one of the notable and rare exceptions being the GenESA closed-loop system for the

control of a synthetic beta agonist for cardiac stress test applications [85]. Closed-loop and autonomous systems are rapidly emerging even in areas in which safety is a top priority. It may be expected that such systems will find their way into anaesthesia and perioperative haemodynamic management eventually [86].

Models and Displays

Pilots, operators of complex industrial plants and professionals in similar occupations have decreased cognitive workload and improved performance if they use integrated graphical data displays rather than single variable indicators [87]. These findings were confirmed with anaesthesiologists [88, 89]. Physiological haemodynamic models may provide a framework for creating graphic displays that relate measured haemodynamic variables to each other. The landmark model described by Guyton [90] contains 500 variables, constants and parameters. A simpler model developed by Smith et al [91] shows reactions to simulated haemodynamic events, such as hypovolaemic shock, septic shock, tamponade, etc., that are consistent with clinical observations. Still, even this relatively simple model has more than 20 parameters.

Advanced ecological haemodynamic displays use very simple models. For example, Blike et al [92] visualize the relationship:

$$CO = SV \times HR \qquad (3)$$

with a rectangle in which the sides represent HR and SV and the area CO. In their graphical display design, Agutter et al represented cardiovascular relationships that conform to the anaesthesiologist's mental model [89]. Anaesthesiologists using the Blike or the Agutter display showed modest performance improvement compared to use of traditional displays.

Pharmacokinetic (PK) and pharmacodynamic (PD) models have been the basis for displays supporting anaesthesiologists administering anaesthetic drugs [93]. The inter-patient variability in sensitivity to vasoactive drugs makes the use of PK/PD models for haemodynamic management particularly challenging. Gorges et al used models for dobutamine, dopamine and nitroprusside to create a display that supports the titration of these drugs. The system uses slight variations in infusion rate to determine the particular patient's drug model parameters. In a study in which nine nurses used this system, accuracy, time to titrate, and number of rate adjustments improved significantly [94].

In conclusion, the large number of confounding factors limits the ability to manage haemodynamic variables, and makes it very difficult to define exact quantitative haemodynamic targets or protocols for each individual patient and circumstance. Successful haemodynamic management involves a comprehensive assessment of the patient and the pathophysiological context, often the testing of hypotheses, and then the selection and careful titration of haemodynamic interventions. More direct measurements of tissue perfusion and oxygenation are emerging, which will help guide haemodynamic management in the individual patient.

References

1. Katzung BG: *Basic and Clinical Pharmacology*, 5th ed. Norwalk, Conn.: Appleton and Lange, 1992, xiii, 1017.

2. Crystal GJ, Heerdt PM: Cardiovascular physiology: integrative function. In: Hemmings HC, Egan TD, eds. *Pharmacology and Physiology for Anesthesia: Foundations and Clinical Application*. London: Elsevier Health Sciences: 2013, 253–71.

3. Cannesson M, Pestel G, Ricks C, Hoeft A, Perel A: Hemodynamic monitoring and management in patients undergoing high risk surgery: a survey among North American and European anesthesiologists. Crit. Care. 2011; 15 (4): R197.

4. Longrois D, Hoeft A, De Hert S: European Society of Cardiology/European Society of Anaesthesiology guidelines on non-cardiac surgery: cardiovascular assessment and management: A short explanatory statement from the European Society of Anaesthesiology members who participated in the European Task Force. Eur.J.Anaesthesiol. 2014; 31 (10): 513–16.

5. Wynne J, Mann T, Alpert JS, Green LH, Grossman W: Hemodynamic effects of nitrous oxide administered during cardiac catheterization. JAMA. 1980; 243 (14): 1440–2.

6. Malan TP, Jr., DiNardo JA, Isner RJ, Frink EJ, Jr., Goldberg M, Fenster PE, et al: Cardiovascular effects of sevoflurane compared with those of isoflurane in volunteers. Anesthesiology. 1995; 83 (5): 918–28.

7. Cahalan MK, Weiskopf RB, Eger EI, 2nd, Yasuda N, Ionescu P, Rampil IJ, et al: Hemodynamic effects of desflurane/nitrous oxide anesthesia in volunteers. Anesth.Analg. 1991; 73 (2): 157–64.

8. Tatara T: Context-sensitive fluid therapy in critical illness. J. Intens.Care. 2016; 4: 20.

9. Cannesson M, Gan TJ. PRO: Perioperative goal-directed fluid therapy is an essential element of an enhanced recovery protocol. Anesth.Analg. 2016; 122 (5): 1258–60.

10. Myburgh JA, Mythen MG: Resuscitation fluids. N. Engl.J.Med. 2013; 369 (13): 1243–51.

11. Hamilton MA, Cecconi M, Rhodes A: A systematic review and meta-analysis on the use of preemptive hemodynamic intervention to improve postoperative outcomes in moderate and high-risk surgical patients. Anesth.Analg. 2011; 112 (6): 1392–402.

12. Bennett-Guerrero E, Welsby I, Dunn TJ, Young LR, Wahl TA, Diers TL, et al: The use of a postoperative morbidity survey to evaluate patients with prolonged hospitalization after routine, moderate-risk, elective surgery. Anesth.Analg. 1999; 89 (2): 514–19.

13. Lobo SM, Rezende E, Knibel MF, Silva NB, Paramo JA, Nacul FE, et al: Early determinants of death due to multiple organ failure after noncardiac surgery in high-risk patients. Anesth.Analg. 2011; 112 (4): 877–83.

14. Grocott MP, Mythen MG, Gan TJ: Perioperative fluid management and clinical outcomes in adults. Anesth. Analg. 2005; 100 (4): 1093–106.

15. Jarisch A: Kreislauffragen. Deutsche Med Wochenschr. 1928; 29: 1211–13.

16. Lewington S, Clarke R, Qizilbash N, Peto R, Collins R: Age-specific relevance of usual blood pressure to vascular mortality: a meta-analysis of individual data for one million adults in 61 prospective studies. Lancet. 2002; 360 (9349): 1903–13.

17. Varon J, Marik PE: Perioperative hypertension management. Vasc.Health.Risk.Manag. 2008; 4 (3): 615–27.

18. Chobanian AV, Bakris GL, Black HR, Cushman WC, Green LA, Izzo JL, Jr., et al: Seventh report of the Joint National Committee on Prevention, Detection, Evaluation, and Treatment of High Blood Pressure. Hypertension. 2003; 42 (6): 1206–52.

19. Howell SJ, Sear JW, Foex P: Hypertension, hypertensive heart disease and perioperative cardiac risk. Br.J.Anaesth. 2004; 92 (4): 570–83.

20. Sanders RD: How important is peri-operative hypertension? Anaesthesia. 2014; 69 (9): 948–53.

21. Bijker JB, van Klei WA, Kappen TH, van Wolfswinkel L, Moons KG, Kalkman CJ: Incidence of intraoperative hypotension as a function of the chosen definition: literature definitions applied to a retrospective cohort using automated data collection. Anesthesiology. 2007; 107 (2): 213–20.

22. Kristensen SD, Knuuti J, Saraste A, Anker S, Botker HE, De Hert S, et al: ESC/ESA Guidelines on non-cardiac surgery: cardiovascular assessment and management: The Joint Task Force on non-cardiac surgery: cardiovascular assessment and management of the European Society of Cardiology (ESC) and

217

the European Society of Anaesthesiology (ESA). Eur.J.Anaesthesiol. 2014; 31 (10): 517–73.

23. Lonjaret L, Lairez O, Minville V, Geeraerts T: Optimal perioperative management of arterial blood pressure. Integr. Blood Press.Control. 2014; 7: 49–59.

24. Walsh M, Devereaux PJ, Garg AX, Kurz A, Turan A, Rodseth RN, et al: Relationship between intraoperative mean arterial pressure and clinical outcomes after noncardiac surgery: toward an empirical definition of hypotension. Anesthesiology. 2013; 119 (3): 507–15.

25. Grocott MP, Dushianthan A, Hamilton MA, Mythen MG, Harrison D, Rowan K, et al: Perioperative increase in global blood flow to explicit defined goals and outcomes after surgery: a Cochrane Systematic Review. Br.J.Anaesth. 2013; 111 (4): 535–48.

26. Dellinger RP, Levy MM, Rhodes A, Annane D, Gerlach H, Opal SM, et al: Surviving sepsis campaign: international guidelines for management of severe sepsis and septic shock: 2012. Crit.Care.Med. 2013; 41 (2): 580–637.

27. Scali S, Bertges D, Neal D, Patel V, Eldrup-Jorgensen J, Cronenwett J, et al: Heart rate variables in the Vascular Quality Initiative are not reliable predictors of adverse cardiac outcomes or mortality after major elective vascular surgery. J.Vasc.Surg. 2015; 62 (3): 710–20.e9.

28. Waldron N, Miller T, Gan T: Endpoints of goal-directed therapy in the OR and in the ICU. In: Cannesson M, Pearse R, eds. *Perioperative Hemodynamic Monitoring and Goal Directed Therapy: From Theory to Practice.* Cambridge: Cambridge University Press, 2014, 372–90.

29. Shoemaker WC, Montgomery ES, Kaplan E, Elwyn DH: Physiologic patterns in surviving and nonsurviving shock patients. Use of sequential cardiorespiratory variables in defining criteria for therapeutic goals and early warning of death.Arch. Surg. (Chicago, Ill: 1960). 1973; 106 (5): 630–6.

30. Lobo SM, de Oliveira NE: Clinical review: what are the best hemodynamic targets for noncardiac surgical patients? Crit.Care. 2013; 17 (2): 210.

31. Pearse R, Dawson D, Fawcett J, Rhodes A, Grounds RM, Bennett ED: Changes in central venous saturation after major surgery, and association with outcome. Crit.Care. 2005; 9 (6): R694–9.

32. Collaborative Study Group on Perioperative Scv OM. Multicentre study on peri- and postoperative central venous oxygen saturation in high-risk surgical patients. Crit.Care. 2006; 10 (6): R158.

33. Tseng GS, Wall MH: Endpoints of resuscitation: what are they anyway? Semin.Cardiothorac.Vasc.Anesth. 2014; 18 (4): 352–62.

34. Vallet B, Blanloeil Y, Cholley B, Orliaguet G, Pierre S, Tavernier B, et al: Guidelines for perioperative haemodynamic optimization. Ann.Fr.Anesth.Reanim. 2013; 32 (10): e151–8.

35. Cannesson M: Arterial pressure variation and goal-directed fluid therapy. J.Cardiothorac.Vasc.Anesth. 2010; 24 (3): 487–97.

36. Monnet X, Dres M, Ferre A, Le Teuff G, Jozwiak M, Bleibtreu A, et al: Prediction of fluid responsiveness by a continuous non-invasive assessment of arterial pressure in critically ill patients: comparison with four other dynamic indices. Br.J.Anaesth. 2012; 109 (3): 330–8.

37. Mireles SA, Jaffe RA, Drover DR, Brock-Utne JG: A poor correlation exists between oscillometric and radial arterial blood pressure as measured by the Philips MP90 monitor. J.Clin.Monit.Comput. 2009; 23 (3): 169–74.

38. Ribezzo S, Spina E, Di Bartolomeo S, Sanson G: Noninvasive techniques for blood pressure measurement are not a reliable alternative to direct measurement: a randomized crossover trial in ICU. Scient.World.J. 2014: 353628.

39. Meng X, Zang G, Fan L, Zheng L, Dai J, Wang X, et al: Non-invasive monitoring of blood pressure using the Philips Intellivue MP50 monitor cannot replace invasive blood pressure techniques in surgery patients under general anesthesia. Exp.Ther.Med. 2013; 6 (1): 9–14.

40. Wax DB, Lin HM, Leibowitz AB: Invasive and concomitant noninvasive intraoperative blood pressure monitoring: observed differences in measurements and associated therapeutic interventions. Anesthesiology. 2011; 115 (5): 973–8.

41. Kim SH, Lilot M, Sidhu KS, Rinehart J, Yu Z, Canales C, et al: Accuracy and precision of continuous noninvasive arterial pressure monitoring compared with invasive arterial pressure: a systematic review and meta-analysis. Anesthesiology. 2014; 120 (5): 1080–97.

42. Marik PE, Cavallazzi R: Does the central venous pressure predict fluid responsiveness? An updated meta-analysis and a plea for some common sense. Crit. Care.Med. 2013; 41 (7): 1774–81.

43. Harvey S, Stevens K, Harrison D, Young D, Brampton W, McCabe C, et al: An evaluation of the clinical and cost-effectiveness of pulmonary artery catheters in patient management in intensive care: a systematic review and a randomised controlled trial. Health. Technol.Assess. 2006; 10 (29): iii–iv, ix–xi, 1–133.

44. Rajaram SS, Desai NK, Kalra A, Gajera M, Cavanaugh SK, Brampton W, et al: Pulmonary artery catheters for adult patients in intensive care. Cochrane.Database. Syst.Rev. 2013; 2: CD003408.

45. Marik PE: Obituary: pulmonary artery catheter 1970 to 2013. Ann.Intensive Care. 2013; 3 (1): 38.

46. Schwann NM, Hillel Z, Hoeft A, Barash P, Mohnle P, Miao Y, et al: Lack of effectiveness of the pulmonary artery catheter in cardiac surgery. Anesth.Analg. 2011; 113 (5): 994–1002.

47. Kuper M, Gold SJ, Callow C, Quraishi T, King S, Mulreany A, et al: Intraoperative fluid management guided by oesophageal Doppler monitoring. BMJ. 2011; 342: d3016.

48. Fellahi JL, Fischer MO: Electrical bioimpedance cardiography: an old technology with new hopes for the future. J.Cardiothorac.Vasc.Anesth. 2014; 28 (3): 755–60.

49. Peyton PJ, Chong SW: Minimally invasive measurement of cardiac output during surgery and critical care: a meta-analysis of accuracy and precision. Anesthesiology. 2010; 113 (5): 1220–35.

50. Critchley LA, Critchley JA: A meta-analysis of studies using bias and precision statistics to compare cardiac output measurement techniques. J.Clin.Monit. Comput. 1999; 15 (2): 85–91.

51. Schloglhofer T, Gilly H, Schima H: Semi-invasive measurement of cardiac output based on pulse contour: a review and analysis. Can.J.Anaesth. 2014; 61 (5): 452–79.

52. Ameloot K, Palmers PJ, Malbrain ML: The accuracy of noninvasive cardiac output and pressure measurements with finger cuff: a concise review. Curr. Opin.Crit.Care. 2015; 21 (3): 232–9.

53. Jozwiak M, Teboul JL, Monnet X. Extravascular lung water in critical care: recent advances and clinical applications. Ann.Intens.Care. 2015; 5 (1): 38.

54. Marik PE, Cavallazzi R, Vasu T, Hirani A: Dynamic changes in arterial waveform derived variables and fluid responsiveness in mechanically ventilated patients: a systematic review of the literature. Crit.Care. Med. 2009; 37 (9): 2642–7.

55. Dueck MH, Klimek M, Appenrodt S, Weigand C, Boerner U: Trends but not individual values of central venous oxygen saturation agree with mixed venous oxygen saturation during varying hemodynamic conditions. Anesthesiology. 2005; 103 (2): 249–57.

56. Thavasothy M, Broadhead M, Elwell C, Peters M, Smith M: A comparison of cerebral oxygenation as measured by the NIRO 300 and the INVOS 5100 Near-Infrared Spectrophotometers. Anaesthesia. 2002; 57 (10): 999–1006.

57. Denault A, Deschamps A, Murkin JM: A proposed algorithm for the intraoperative use of cerebral near-infrared spectroscopy. Semin.Cardiothorac.Vasc. Anesth. 2007; 11 (4): 274–81.

58. Ghosh A, Elwell C, Smith M: Review article: cerebral near-infrared spectroscopy in adults: a work in progress. Anesth.Analg. 2012; 115 (6): 1373–83.

59. Skarvan K, Lambert A, Filipovic M, Seeberger M: Reference values for left ventricular function in subjects under general anaesthesia and controlled ventilation assessed by two-dimensional transoesophageal echocardiography. Eur.J.Anaesthesiol. 2001; 18 (11): 713–22.

60. Pai RG, Bodenheimer MM, Pai SM, Koss JH, Adamick RD: Usefulness of systolic excursion of the mitral anulus as an index of left ventricular systolic function. Am.J.Cardiol. 1991; 67 (2): 222–4.

61. Yamada H, Oki T, Mishiro Y, Tabata T, Abe M, Onose Y, et al: Effect of aging on diastolic left ventricular myocardial velocities measured by pulsed tissue Doppler imaging in healthy subjects. J.Am.Soc. Echocardiogr. 1999; 12 (7): 574–81.

62. Alam M, Wardell J, Andersson E, Samad BA, Nordlander R: Effects of first myocardial infarction on left ventricular systolic and diastolic function with the use of mitral annular velocity determined by pulsed wave doppler tissue imaging. J.Am.Soc.Echocardiogr. 2000; 13 (5): 343–52.

63. Gorcsan J, 3rd, Strum DP, Mandarino WA, Gulati VK, Pinsky MR: Quantitative assessment of alterations in regional left ventricular contractility with color-coded tissue Doppler echocardiography. Comparison with sonomicrometry and pressure-volume relations. Circulation. 1997; 95 (10): 2423–33.

64. Ama R, Segers P, Roosens C, Claessens T, Verdonck P, Poelaert J: The effects of load on systolic mitral annular velocity by tissue Doppler imaging. Anesth.Analg. 2004; 99 (2): 332–8.

65. Vinereanu D, Khokhar A, Tweddel AC, Cinteza M, Fraser AG: Estimation of global left ventricular function from the velocity of longitudinal shortening. Echocardiogr. 2002; 19 (3): 177–85.

66. Sevimli S, Arslan S, Gundogdu F, Aksakal E, Buyukkaya E, Tas H, et al: Can transesophageal pulse-wave tissue Doppler imaging be used to evaluate left ventricular function? Echocardiogr. 2007; 24 (9): 946–54.

67. Zehender M, Kasper W, Kauder E, Schonthaler M, Geibel A, Olschewski M, et al: Right ventricular infarction as an independent predictor of prognosis after acute inferior myocardial infarction. N. Engl.J.Med. 1993; 328 (14): 981–8.

68. Cameli M, Righini FM, Lisi M, Bennati E, Navarri R, Lunghetti S, et al: Comparison of right versus left ventricular strain analysis as a predictor of outcome in patients with systolic heart failure referred for heart transplantation. Am.J.Cardiol. 2013; 112 (11): 1778–84.

69. Park SJ, Park JH, Lee HS, Kim MS, Park YK, Park Y, et al: Impaired RV global longitudinal strain is associated with poor long-term clinical outcomes in patients with acute inferior STEMI. JACC.Cardiovasc.Imaging. 2015; 8 (2): 161–9.

70. Haddad F, Denault AY, Couture P, Cartier R, Pellerin M, Levesque S, et al: Right ventricular myocardial performance index predicts perioperative mortality

219

or circulatory failure in high-risk valvular surgery. J. Am.Soc.Echocardiogr. 2007; 20 (9): 1065–72.

71. Maslow AD, Regan MM, Panzica P, Heindel S, Mashikian J, Comunale ME: Precardiopulmonary bypass right ventricular function is associated with poor outcome after coronary artery bypass grafting in patients with severe left ventricular systolic dysfunction. Anesth.Analg. 2002; 95 (6): 1507–18.

72. Ternacle J, Berry M, Cognet T, Kloeckner M, Damy T, Monin JL, et al: Prognostic value of right ventricular two-dimensional global strain in patients referred for cardiac surgery. J.Am.Soc.Echocardiogr. 2013; 26 (7): 721–6.

73. Rudski LG, Lai WW, Afilalo J, Hua L, Handschumacher MD, Chandrasekaran K, et al: Guidelines for the echocardiographic assessment of the right heart in adults: a report from the American Society of Echocardiography endorsed by the European Association of Echocardiography, a registered branch of the European Society of Cardiology, and the Canadian Society of Echocardiography. J.Am.Soc. Echocardiogr. 2010; 23 (7): 685–713; quiz 86–8.

74. Lang RM, Badano LP, Mor-Avi V, Afilalo J, Armstrong A, Ernande L, et al: Recommendations for cardiac chamber quantification by echocardiography in adults: an update from the American Society of Echocardiography and the European Association of Cardiovascular Imaging. J.Am.Soc.Echocardiogr. 2015; 28 (1): 1–39.e14.

75. Focardi M, Cameli M, Carbone SF, Massoni A, De Vito R, Lisi M, et al: Traditional and innovative echocardiographic parameters for the analysis of right ventricular performance in comparison with cardiac magnetic resonance. Eur.Heart.Cardiovasc.Imaging. 2015; 16 (1): 47–52.

76. Tamborini G, Muratori M, Brusoni D, Celeste F, Maffessanti F, Caiani EG, et al: Is right ventricular systolic function reduced after cardiac surgery? A two- and three-dimensional echocardiographic study. Eur.J.Echocardiogr. 2009; 10 (5): 630–4.

77. Blessberger H, Binder T: Two dimensional speckle tracking echocardiography: clinical applications. Heart. 2010; 96 (24): 2032–40.

78. Blessberger H, Binder T: Non-invasive imaging: Two dimensional speckle tracking echocardiography: basic principles. Heart. 2010; 96 (9): 716–22.

79. Leibundgut G, Rohner A, Grize L, Bernheim A, Kessel-Schaefer A, Bremerich J, et al: Dynamic assessment of right ventricular volumes and function by real-time three-dimensional echocardiography: a comparison study with magnetic resonance imaging in 100 adult patients. J.Am.Soc.Echocardiogr. 2010; 23 (2): 116–26.

80. Fusini L, Tamborini G, Gripari P, Maffessanti F, Mazzanti V, Muratori M, et al: Feasibility of intraoperative three-dimensional transesophageal echocardiography in the evaluation of right ventricular volumes and function in patients undergoing cardiac surgery. J.Am.Soc.Echocardiogr. 2011; 24 (8): 868–77.

81. Bowman RJ, Westenskow DR: A microcomputer-based fluid infusion system for the resuscitation of burn patients. IEEE.Trans.Biomed.Eng. 1981; 28 (6): 475–9.

82. Rinehart J, Alexander B, Le Manach Y, Hofer C, Tavernier B, Kain ZN, et al: Evaluation of a novel closed-loop fluid-administration system based on dynamic predictors of fluid responsiveness: an in silico simulation study. Crit.Care. 2011; 15 (6): R278.

83. Keogh BE, Jacobs J, Royston D, Taylor KM: Microprocessor-controlled hemodynamics: a step towards improved efficiency and safety. J.Cardiothorac. Anesth. 1989; 3 (1): 4–9.

84. Rinehart J, Liu N, Alexander B, Cannesson M: Review article: closed-loop systems in anesthesia: is there a potential for closed-loop fluid management and hemodynamic optimization? Anesth.Analg. 2012; 114 (1): 130–43.

85. Ketteler T, Krahwinkel W, Wolfertz J, Godke J, Hoffmeister T, Scheuble L, et al: Arbutamine stress echocardiography. Eur.Heart.J. 1997; 18 Suppl D: D24–30.

86. Kuck K, Johnson KB: The three laws of autonomous and closed-loop systems in anesthesia. Anesth.Analg. 2017; 124 (2): 377–80.

87. Drews FA, Westenskow DR: The right picture is worth a thousand numbers: data displays in anesthesia. Hum. Factors. 2006; 48 (1): 59–71.

88. Blike GT, Surgenor SD, Whalen K, Jensen J: Specific elements of a new hemodynamics display improves the performance of anesthesiologists. J.Clin.Monit. Comput. 2000; 16 (7): 485–91.

89. Agutter J, Drews F, Syroid N, Westenskow D, Albert R, Strayer D, et al: Evaluation of graphic cardiovascular display in a high-fidelity simulator. Anesth.Analg. 2003; 97 (5): 1403–13.

90. Guyton AC, Coleman TG, Granger HJ: Circulation: overall regulation. Annu.Rev.Physiol. 1972; 34: 13–46.

91. Smith BW, Andreassen S, Shaw GM, Jensen PL, Rees SE, Chase JG: Simulation of cardiovascular system diseases by including the autonomic nervous system into a minimal model. Comput.Methods.Programs. Biomed. 2007; 86 (2): 153–60.

92. Blike GT, Surgenor SD, Whalen K: A graphical object display improves anesthesiologists' performance on a simulated diagnostic task. J.Clin.Monit.Comput. 1999; 15 (1): 37–44.

93. Billard V: Pharmacokinetic-pharmacodynamic relationship of anesthetic drugs: from modeling to clinical use. F1000Res. 2015; 4.

94. Gorges M, Westenskow DR, Kuck K, Orr JA: A tool predicting future mean arterial blood pressure values improves the titration of vasoactive drugs. J.Clin. Monit.Comput. 2010; 24 (3): 223–35.

95. Patel S: Cardiovascular effects of intravenous anesthetics. Int.Anesthesiol.Clin. 2002; 40 (1): 15–33.

96. Doenicke A, Angster R, Mayer M, Adams HA, Grillenberger G, Nebauer AE: The action of S-(+)-ketamine on serum catecholamine and cortisol. A comparison with ketamine racemate. Der. Anästhesist. 1992; 41 (10): 597–603.

97. Ogura T, Egan TD: Opioid agonists and anagonists. In: Hemmings HC, Egan TD, eds. *Pharmacology and Physiology for Anesthesia : Foundations and Clinical Application*. London: Elsevier Health Sciences, 2013, 253–71.

98. Zimmerman J, Cahalan M: Vasopressors and inotropes. In: Hemmings HC, Egan TD, eds. *Pharmacology and Physiology for Anesthesia : Foundations and Clinical Application*. London: Elsevier Health Sciences, 2013, 390–404.

99. Shipley JB, Tolman D, Hastillo A, Hess ML: Milrinone: basic and clinical pharmacology and acute and chronic management. Am.J.Med.Sci. 1996; 311 (6): 286–91.

100. Figgitt DP, Gillies PS, Goa KL: Levosimendan. Drugs. 2001; 61 (5): 613–27; discussion 28–9.

101. Sear JW: Antihypertensive drugs and vasodilators. In: Hemmings HC, Egan TD, eds. *Pharmacology and Physiology for Anesthesia : Foundations and Clinical Application*. London: Elsevier Health Sciences, 2013, 405–25.

102. Mitchell A, Buhrmann S, Opazo Saez A, Rushentsova U, Schafers RF, Philipp T, et al: Clonidine lowers blood pressure by reducing vascular resistance and cardiac output in young, healthy males. Cardiovasc. Drugs.Ther. 2005; 19 (1): 49–55.

103. Fontana F, Allaria B, Brunetti B, Arienta R, Favaro M, Trivellato A, et al: Cardiac and circulatory response to the intravenous administration of urapidil during general anaesthesia. Drugs.Exp.Clin.Res. 1990; 16 (6): 315–18.

104. Boldt J, Schindler E, Wollbruck M, Gorlach G, Hempelmann G: Cardiorespiratory response of intravenous angiotensin-converting enzyme inhibitor enalaprilat in hypertensive cardiac surgery patients. J.Cardiothorac.Vasc.Anesth. 1995; 9(1): 44–9.

105. Wagner F, Yeter R, Bisson S, Siniawski H, Hetzer R: Beneficial hemodynamic and renal effects of intravenous enalaprilat following coronary artery bypass surgery complicated by left ventricular dysfunction. Crit.Care.Med. 2003; 31 (5): 1421–8.

106. Harrison TK, Goldhaber-Fiebert S: Generic events. In: Gaba DM, Fish KJ, Howard SK, Burden A, eds. *Crisis Management in Anesthesiology*. 2nd ed. London: Elsevier Health Sciences, 2014, 88–136.

107. Steyn J, Dorfling J: Cardiovascular events. In: Gaba DM, Fish KJ, Howard SK, Burden A, eds. *Crisis Management in Anesthesiology*. 2nd ed. London: Elsevier Health Sciences, 2014, 137–72.

Chapter 15

Effects of Anaesthesia on Thermoregulation

Oliver Kimberger

Introduction

The ability of the human body to maintain normothermia via physiological reactions or behavioural changes to vastly different climatic circumstances is an evolutionarily well preserved mechanism. It is a key feature that has allowed humans to adapt to changing environmental conditions, enabling *Homo sapiens* worldwide evolutionary success and distribution. Humans possess a *homeothermic* thermoregulatory system, and all enzymatic processes in the human body are optimized to work within a tightly regulated so-called 'normothermic' temperature range [1].

The non-anaesthetized human body reacts very aggressively to even minor changes of its core temperature. The importance of core temperature regulation and how it is affected by anaesthesia only started to receive the attention it deserves in the 1990s (see Fig. 15.1). The importance of maintaining normothermia and the consequences of accidental perioperative hypothermia have been studied extensively since. More recently, the therapeutic effects of deliberately altering core temperatures are being explored, such as therapeutic hypothermia in the setting of cardiac arrest, myocardial infarction and neuropathologies, fever management (permissive, restrictive or therapeutic) and therapeutic hyperthermia as part of oncological therapies.

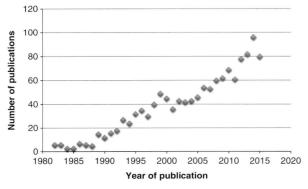

Despite these new insights, core temperature measurement is often still considered an optional parameter or 'vital sign of minor importance' in many hospitals and operating rooms [2, 3]. However, methods of core temperature manipulation (warming, cooling) and methods of core temperature monitoring should be considered inseparable twins.

A Definition of Core Temperature, Thermoregulatory Compartments and Heat Distribution

Heat distribution can be modelled with a two-compartment model consisting of a core and a peripheral compartment. It suffices to demonstrate the main thermoregulatory functions.

The core compartment consists of all deep body tissues that maintain the organism's normothermic operating temperature, i.e. the organs in the trunk plus the central nervous system. The peripheral compartment consists of the limbs, the skin and peripheral tissues covering the trunk and the head. The contribution of the latter though is very small.

In a moderate climate (i.e. room temperature of 23°C) the temperature of the peripheral compartment is 2–4°C lower than that of the core compartment. This (radial) gradient depends on the vasoconstrictive or vasodilatatory state of the organism: in a colder environment, a distinct radial temperature gradient is observed, while in a warmer environment vasodilation increases blood flow to the peripheral compartment, decreasing the gradient. Adults produce around 100 Watts of heat while resting, with substantially higher rates during strenuous activity. This heat flows from the core to the peripheral compartment via two mechanisms: convection (i.e. via blood flow, a fast longitudinal heat transfer) and conduction (i.e. via adjacent tissues, a slow radial heat transfer).

To *maintain* a thermal steady state where heat production matches heat losses, the heat generated by the body must be able to leave and dissipate to the

Fig. 15.1 Pubmed entries for the search terms 'perioperative' and 'hypothermia'.

environment. This heat is dissipated mostly via skin, with only 5% of heat being lost via respiration. The most efficient way to lose heat via the skin is by sweating: sweating can dissipate ten times the heat generated by the basal metabolism [4].

Numerous formulas and models with more or less elaborate assumptions and simplifications have been developed to calculate heat content, heat production and heat transfer rates of the human body. These models could be used in clinical practice to predict which patients are prone to develop hypothermia (see below), or to individualize patient warming options.

Since there are (at least, simplistically) two compartments present in human thermoregulation, measuring core temperature alone is not sufficient to assess the full thermal state of the human body. The concept of 'mean body temperature' recognizes this. Mean body temperature is the mass-weighted average of tissue temperatures throughout the body. While core temperature is relatively easy to measure (as demonstrated in the next sections), the exact measurement of temperatures of the peripheral compartment requires the insertion of multiple needle thermometers into the limbs at different depths, and both proximally and distally. However, sufficiently accurate estimates of mean body temperature can also be obtained in a much simpler and less invasive manner by using core temperature and non-invasive skin temperatures [5].

The Physiology of Core Temperature

While the body's core temperature set point itself can vary by approximately 1°C individually due to circadian variation or hormonal changes (menstrual cycle), temperature deviations from this set point as small as ± 0.1°C activate regulatory processes (physiological and behavioural reactions) to counteract the temperature change [6]. This makes sense from an evolutionary point of view, because the enzymes of the body optimally function within the normothermic temperature range (usually defined as a range from 36.5 to 37.5°C).

Physiological thermoregulatory control consists of the three elements: temperature measurement, temperature regulation, and the reactions that core temperature changes trigger. Temperature measurement integrates the input of sensors located in the skin (C-fibres and Aδ-fibres), in deep tissues (i.e. the organs in the trunk and the brain) and in the spinal cord and various regions in the brain (hypothalamus). Most input comes from the skin (50% of all temperature information input) and the hypothalamus [7]. Temperature

regulation mostly occurs in the hypothalamus. The third component is the sum of the reactions that core temperature changes trigger. Autonomic responses include vasoconstriction and vasodilation, shivering and sweating; in the non-anaesthetized patient, these reactions also include behavioural changes (e.g. putting on clothes, moving into the sunlight, etc.).

Non-shivering thermogenesis by brown fat occurs to a relevant degree in infants only [8].

The aforementioned autonomic responses (vasoconstriction and vasodilation, shivering and sweating) are very tightly regulated. From a physiological standpoint the properties of these responses can be described by the thresholds at which they are activated, their gain (relationship between the degree of core temperature change and the intensity of autonomic reaction) and their maximum response.

While vasodilation and sweating share the same threshold temperature, shivering occurs up to 1°C below the vasoconstriction threshold. The interval between the sweating and the vasoconstriction threshold includes the so called 'normothermic range', also known as the 'interthreshold range' (see Fig. 15.2). This interthreshold range is increased by many anaesthetic drugs used and altered by several other medications [9].

There is no general consensus on what exactly constitutes the normal normothermic core temperature range, but most authors agree this is 36.5°C to 37.5°C. Most physicians agree that a core temperature below 36°C definitely constitutes hypothermia, but a grey area remains between 36.0°C and 36.5°C. Reported 'fever' thresholds range from 37.2°C to 38.0°C, below which some authors define a 'subfebrile' range to describe moderately elevated core temperatures or 'low-grade fever'.

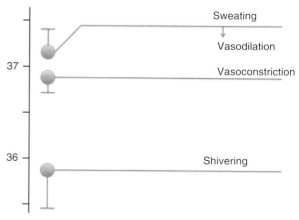

Fig. 15.2 Thermoregulatory thresholds in non-anaesthetized humans: sweating, vasodilation, vasoconstriction and shivering.

How Anaesthetic Drugs Affect Core Temperature

General Anaesthesia

Almost all anaesthetic drugs alter thermoregulatory homeostasis in numerous ways. This phenomenon applies to both intravenous drugs (propofol [10], opioids [11]) and inhaled anaesthetics (desflurane [12], isoflurane [13], N_2O) [14]. Their effects are mostly comparable: increased sweating threshold, decreased vasoconstriction and shivering thresholds, and near-abolition of non-shivering thermogenesis in infants. The reductions of the thermoregulatory thresholds for shivering and vasoconstriction are typically linearly dose dependent for intravenous drugs, while for volatile anaesthetics the vasoconstriction and shivering thresholds are typically nonlinearly decreased with higher volatile gas concentrations (see Fig. 15.3). Also the gain of vasoconstriction is reduced by volatile anaesthetics, as is maximum shivering intensity. Interestingly, opioids and particularly midazolam have no clinically relevant impact on thermoregulatory

thresholds, gain and maximum intensity of shivering [15]. Even though vasoconstriction and shivering thresholds are lowered during general anaesthesia, these compensatory mechanisms are still active beyond these (altered) thresholds. Despite numerous advances in the basic understanding of the mechanisms of anaesthesia, the exact mechanism why and how anaesthetics change thermoregulatory thresholds remains mostly unclear. A potential hypothesis for the understanding of the mechanism is the effect of volatile anaesthetics on the TRPV1 receptor, possibly contributing to both the analgesic effect of volatile anaesthetics and their modification of thermoregulatory input [16].

Different anaesthetic drugs have different effects on the thermoregulatory thresholds of the three key thermoregulatory mechanisms, as displayed in Table 15.1.

Neuraxial Anaesthesia (Spinal or Epidural Anaesthesia)

The effect of neuraxial anaesthesia on thermoregulation is remarkably similar to that of anaesthetic drugs, i.e. an increased interthreshold range and linear decrease of the vasoconstriction and shivering thresholds (dependent on the number of dermatomes

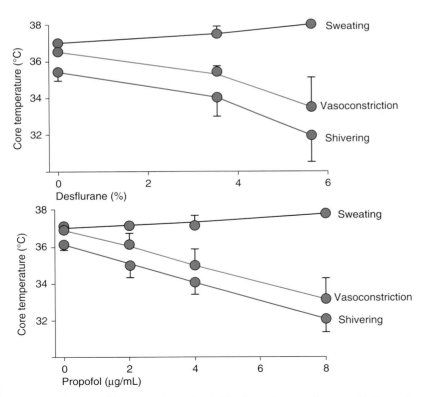

Fig. 15.3 Changes of thermoregulatory thresholds – linear decrease of vasoconstriction and sweating threshold with increased propofol concentration [10], nonlinear decrease with increased concentration of volatile anaesthetic (desflurane) [12].

Table 15.1. Effect of different anaesthetic drugs on thermoregulatory thresholds.

Medication	Vasoconstriction	Shivering	Sweating
Desflurane [12]	pronounced, nonlinear decrease	pronounced, nonlinear decrease	minor linear increase
Isoflurane [13]	pronounced, nonlinear decrease	pronounced, nonlinear decrease	minor linear increase
Propofol [10]	pronounced, linear decrease	pronounced, linear decrease	slight linear increase
Midazolam [15]	minimal, linear decrease	minimal, linear decrease	minimal linear increase
Meperidine [17]	pronounced, linear decrease	marked effect on vasoconstriction, linear decrease	slight linear increase
Alfentanil [18]	pronounced, linear decrease	pronounced, linear decrease	slight linear increase

blocked) [19]. Gain and maximum intensity of shivering are also decreased [20]. An accepted hypothesis for this phenomenon is that the thermometric 'input signal' is being modified by blocking of the cold sensation from the blocked dermatomes [21]. Blocking the vasomotor nerves causes the vessels in the blocked dermatomes to vasodilate, which accelerates heat loss. After neuraxial anaesthesia, patients have a sensation of warmth, even if they become hypothermic [22, 23, 24]. The effect of epidural and general anaesthesia on thermoregulatory thresholds is additive, causing these patients to be at particular risk of perioperative hypothermia [21].

How Core Temperature Affects Anaesthetic Drugs

If core temperature is lowered, enzymatic activity decreases and the half-life (elimination half-life) of almost all drugs used perioperatively is consequently prolonged. Plasma clearance of vecuronium is decreased by 11% for every 1°C [25]. In the recovery room, propofol plasma concentrations are 28% higher in hypothermic individuals ($\approx 34°C$) [26]. These factors cause emergence from anaesthesia and recovery room stay of accidentally hypothermic patients to be prolonged [27](also see below).

Complications of Accidental Hypothermia

Thermal Discomfort

Patients experience thermal discomfort if they are hypothermic after anaesthesia [28]. This can be readily alleviated by active skin warming: because the brain integrates the thermometric input of both the skin and the core into a single input to the hypothalamus, active skin warming will trick the hypothalamus into calculating a higher overall mean body temperature [29] closer to the normothermic 'comfort-zone'.

Impairment of Coagulation

The effects of hypothermia on coagulation are well documented. Impairment of platelet aggregation and reduced clot formation (due to impairment of the enzymatic coagulation cascades) may increase perioperative blood losses: a temperature difference of just 1°C increases the relative risk of transfusion by 22% [30].

Wound Infection and Length of Stay in the Postoperative Care Unit and in the Hospital

Hypothermia can increase the incidence of wound infection in several ways. First, hypothermia-induced vasoconstriction decreases wound perfusion and thus oxygen delivery. The resulting lower tissue O_2 partial pressures negatively affect oxidative killing, which typically acts as a first barrier against bacteria [31]. Second, the motility of immune cells vital for bacterial defence is decreased [32]. Finally, impaired formation of collagen fibres compromises wound healing, facilitating wound dehiscence [33]. The clinical relevance for surgical wound healing has been documented in two studies; one in patients undergoing colorectal surgery [34], and one in patients undergoing 'clean' surgery after prewarming [35].

Cardiac Complications

Hypothermia causes a stress response, with increased catecholamine levels and increased oxygen consumption [36]. While common sense dictates this might increase cardiac morbidity in patients at risk for cardiac ischaemia, clinical evidence for this complication relies on only a single study with rather coarse methods for the detection of cardiac complications [37].

Shivering

Postoperative shivering can be a response of the autonomic nervous system to accidental perioperative hypothermia. But not all postoperative shivering is caused by hypothermia – the differential diagnosis

Table 15.2. Quantification of shivering, scale by Crossley and Mahajan [39].

0	No shivering
1	No visible muscle activity, but one or more of the following: piloerection, peripheral vasoconstriction, or peripheral cyanosis (after exclusion of other causes).
2	Muscular activity in one muscle group
3	Moderate muscular activity in more than one muscle group but no generalized shaking
4	Violent muscular activity involving the whole body

Table 15.3. Treatment of hypothermia-induced shivering.

Drug	Dose (in Respective Study)	Effect on Shivering
Pethidine [42]	25 mg	Very strong; can be used in combination with other drugs
Clonidine [43]	75 µg	Good
Dexmedetomidine [44]	0.5 µg/kg	Stronger than clonidine but with more sedation
Ketamine [45]	0.5 mg/kg	Low dose effective
Nefopam [46]	20 mg	Moderate; only on shivering *threshold*
Magnesium [47]	80 mg/kg + 2 g/h	No clinically relevant effect
Doxapram [48]	Titrated to 2.5 µg/ml plasma level	No clinically relevant effect
Odansetron [49, 50]	4–8 mg	Effect controversial
Buspirone [51]	60 mg	Synergistic effect with pethidine
Dantrolene [52]	2.5 mg/kg	Primary effect on *gain* of shivering
Other methods		
Counterwarming/Skin warming [53]	n/a	Reduces shivering threshold; additive effect with pethidine

should include pain, stress, over-activity of the sympathetic nervous system, and unknown causes [38].

Shivering can be quantified by one of several scales, the most widely used being that by Crossley and Mahajan [39].

Shivering has to be treated rapidly and effectively because it is very uncomfortable for the patient and increases the patient's oxygen consumption and metabolic rate [40, 41]. There are several drugs with potent anti-shivering properties, which share one common feature: they lower the thermoregulatory threshold for shivering. A potent non-pharmacological therapy is 'counter'-warming, i.e. actively warming the hypothermic patient's skin, the mechanism of which has been explained above.

In summary, over the last decades scientific evidence has led perioperative normothermia to become a standard-of-care in anaesthesia. Even though many of the studies were published almost 20 years ago, and even though some of them are considered to provide only 'low to moderate' evidence by today's scientific standards, they are unlikely to be repeated using a 'no-active-warming' control group because *not* actively warming perioperatively can no longer be accepted and would be considered unethical [54, 55].

How to Measure Core Temperature

While properly measuring the temperature of a patient might seem a pretty straightforward task, it is not, because there is no consensus on where exactly the patient's core temperature is actually 'located' (in which tissue or body cavity). The problem of definition becomes even more difficult when a patient is undergoing surgery: while cerebral tissue temperature and pulmonary artery temperature are both supposed to be gold standards of core thermometry, they will become invalid e.g. during brain surgery or cardiac/thoracic surgery, respectively. And even though pulmonary artery temperature and intracerebral temperature are both considered 'gold standards' of core temperature measurement, even these 'core temperatures' are not always in agreement, e.g. after brain injury, with higher temperatures in the cerebral tissue [56–58]. In addition, intracerebral temperature probes and pulmonary artery catheters are too invasive to be used just for core temperature measurement. Thus less invasive surrogate measurements are needed. These surrogate core temperature measurement methods are presented below, from most invasive to least invasive method.

Distal Oesophageal Temperature

During general anaesthesia, distal oesophageal temperature measurement is one of the best substitutes according to numerous studies. Furthermore it is highly resistant to artefacts [59] and dislocation [60]. The text-book recommended placement of the probe is the region of the oesophagus bounded by the left ventricle and aorta, corresponding to the level of the eighth and ninth thoracic vertebrae, but exactly positioning it there can be difficult (particularly in paediatric patients) [61, 62] (see Fig. 15.4a).

Contact Tympanic Temperature

A contact tympanic thermometer very accurately measures brain temperature via a specialized cotton swab probe placed in direct contact with the eardrum (tympanic membrane). The probe may be poorly tolerated by the awake patient, with the sensation ranging from negligible to uncomfortable and even painful. Perforation of the tympanic membrane is a possible complication [63] (see Fig. 15.4b).

Nasopharyngeal Temperature

Nasopharyngeal measurement of core temperature is also often used in the patient undergoing general anaesthesia. Measurements can be affected by airflow over the nasopharyngeal airways and by failing to insert the probe deep enough (10–20 cm) [64]. Care has to be taken so as not to provoke epistaxis during insertion [65] (see Fig. 15.4).

Sublingual Temperature

To measure sublingual temperature accurately, the thermometer has to remain in the 'sublingual pocket' during the entire measurement period, which makes continuous measurement difficult and dependent on patient compliance. Oral temperature fluctuates with mouth opening, oral food or fluid intake, and mucosal inflammation [66]. Nevertheless, if used correctly, the sublingual measurement method is a good trade-off between noninvasiveness and accuracy [67] (see Fig. 15.4c).

Bladder Temperature

Bladder temperature is an adequate substitute for core temperature (if the surgical field does not involve the lower abdomen). Complications do not differ from those of regular bladder catheters (i.e perforation, infection, urethral lesions, etc.), since there is no clinically significant difference in size between bladder catheters with and without built-in thermometers [68]. Urine flow may have some influence on the accuracy of the measurement [69] (see Fig. 15.4d).

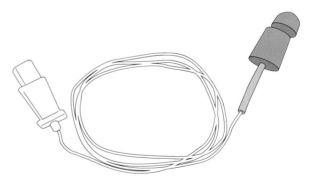

Fig. 15.4b Contact tympanic thermometer.
© Fa. Drägerwerk AG &Co.KGaA, Lübeck, Germany

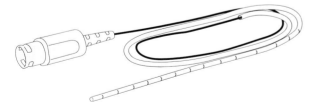

Fig. 15.4 Thermometry methods: a. Distal oesophageal temperature. © Fa. Drägerwerk AG &Co.KGaA, Lübeck, Germany

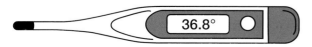

Fig. 15.4c Standard thermometer for oral, axillary, rectal use.
© Fa. Drägerwerk AG &Co.KGaA, Lübeck, Germany

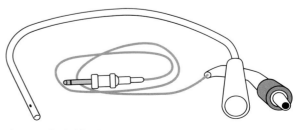

Fig. 15.4d Bladder thermometer.
© Fa. Drägerwerk AG &Co.KGaA, Lübeck, Germany

Rectal Temperature

While some authors claim rectal temperature to be an accurate and relatively noninvasive substitute for core temperature, its time lag of up to one hour prevents it from detecting the rapid onset of fever and hypothermia [70, 71]. Intestinal perforation has been described after the probe has been introduced too deeply or vigorously, which is a particular risk in paediatric patients [72] (see Fig. 15.4c for spot measurements or 15.4d for continuous rectal thermometry).

Temporal Artery Thermometer

Temporal artery thermometers (TATs) – theoretically – measure the temperature above the temporal artery. The actual measurement involves moving the thermometer in a slow, continuous and sweeping motion from the centre of the forehead to the retroauricular area. TATs are less accurate than the aforementioned more invasive measurements and are more affected by environmental factors (cold or heat exposure) and patient factors (vasoconstriction, sweating) [73]. Measurements cannot be made continuously (see Fig. 15.4e).

Axillary Temperature

Despite ample evidence of its low accuracy and poor precision, axillary temperature measurement is still one of the most widely used thermometry methods. Axillary temperature is typically 1–2°C lower than actual core temperature [74, 75]. Accuracy may be decreased even further if the measurement period is too short – at least 4 minutes are required if a mercury-in-glass thermometer is used) [76] or if the probe is not adjacent to the axillary artery (see Fig. 15.4c).

Skin Temperature

Another popular method of thermometry is the measurement of skin temperature, typically on the forehead (via a liquid crystal thermometer or via the human hand). To derive an estimation of core temperature, 2°C have to be added to the measurement. Still, the resulting estimate of core temperature is so inaccurate [77] as to render electronic and liquid crystal forehead thermometers unsuitable for clinical use [78]. Surprisingly, the human hand performs as well as less accurate, yet more high-tech methods in detecting fever, such as liquid crystal forehead thermometers [79] (see Fig. 15.4f).

Infra-red Tympanic

Another very common core thermometry method is infra-red (IR) tympanic thermometry via the external aural canal. However, the method typically measures the temperature of the external ear canal rather than that of the tympanic membrane. This is a result of its shape, designed to prevent deep insertion to minimize the likelihood of tympanic membrane perforation. Cerumen may deteriorate its accuracy. The method is not accurate enough to obtain a reasonable estimate of core temperature in clinical practice [80, 81].

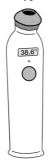

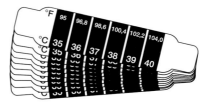

Fig. 15.4e Temporal artery thermometer.
© Fa. Drägerwerk AG &Co.KGaA, Lübeck, Germany

Fig. 15.4f Forehead liquid crystal thermometer.
© Fa. Drägerwerk AG &Co.KGaA, Lübeck, Germany

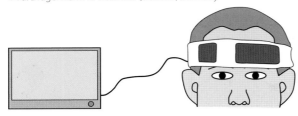

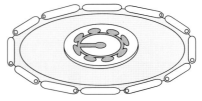

Fig. 15.4g Zero heat flux thermometer.
© Fa. Drägerwerk AG &Co.KGaA, Lübeck, Germany

Fig. 15.4h Double sensor thermometer.
© Fa. Drägerwerk AG &Co.KGaA, Lübeck, Germany

Zero Heat Flux

Zero heat flux technology combines thermal isolation of a skin area (most often the forehead) with a heating element above this area. A thermal equilibrium is established between the heating element and the patient's core. This allows the core temperature to be derived from the measured skin temperature in the isolated area. This technology is noninvasive, continuous and well tolerated in awake patients. Due to its high accuracy, the technology can provide an alternative to more invasive thermometry [82–84] (see Fig. 15.4g).

Heat Flux/Double Sensor Technology

While heat flux/double sensor technology does not need an active warming element, the double-sensor technology similarly relies on an isolated skin area on the forehead where the effluent heat flow is measured between two thermistors with a standardized insulator in between. Again, the sensor has a high accuracy and can be used as an alternative to more invasive thermometry [85–88] (see Fig. 15.4h).

Experimental Temperature Measurement Methods

Experimental methods used to measure or estimate core temperature include ultrasound [89], MRI [90], measurement via the inner canthus of the eye [91] and simulation (see further) [92–95]. Thermography can be used for fever screening, but is not accurate enough to derive core temperature [96].

How to Model Core Temperature

Modelling and simulation of human core temperature have been facilitated by modern computer technology. Several programmes are available to simulate perioperative patient temperature curves, which can be used as a teaching aid on physiology and thermoregulation or to predict perioperative hypothermia risk and the need for active warming.

Mechanical Models

The most basic mechanical model for human thermoregulation is a simple, passive cylinder.

However, one cylinder alone cannot adequately simulate heat loss because it cannot account for the different shapes of the head, arms, legs and torso that all differ in their surface/mass-ratio. More elaborate models thus do include multiple cylinders [97], and more elaborate models also simulate the effect of sweating and heat distribution between the core and periphery via circulation. Despite several simplifications, some of these models have been successfully used to test patient warming devices [98, 99], and to address other clinical questions that cannot be addressed by clinical studies for practical and/or ethical reasons [100].

Numerical Models

The complexity of numerical models is only limited by the ingenuity of the researcher and computing power. Numerical models divide the human body into several segments that each have their individual thermal capacity, heat production and heat balance. The different segments are connected via blood flow. The most basic model consists of a peripheral and a central compartment, which is able to simulate the main mechanisms of thermoregulation and to predict core and peripheral temperature trends under different ambient and physiological conditions.

Vasoconstriction, Blood Flow and Metabolism in a Basic Two Compartment Model

Blood, circulating in the central compartment, has a high thermal conductivity. A resistor models vasomotion: the resistance changes depending on the difference between the core temperature's set point and the 'actual' core temperature. If the core is too warm, the resistance is decreased and blood flow from the central to peripheral compartment rises to a certain maximum; if the core is too cold, the resistance increases and blood flow from the peripheral to central compartment decreases to a certain minimum.

Heat production generated by metabolism is modelled in an analogue manner, i.e. it will adjust itself depending on the difference between core temperature set point and actual core temperature. When the core temperature is close to its set point, the metabolic rate is typically at its baseline value. When core temperature drops 2°C below the set point temperature, metabolic rate becomes maximal. If core temperature decreases even more, metabolic rate decreases as well.

Example of Model-based Simulation of Thermoregulation

In the following section, the Bussman model is used [101].

This two compartment model incorporates heat losses to the environment by convection, radiation and evaporation and simulates blood flow between the core and peripheral compartment as described above. Body surface area is calculated by an empirical equation [102].

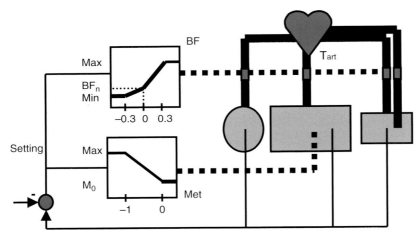

Fig. 15.5 Simple block model of thermoregulation with two compartments (head with torso representing the core, and peripheral tissues), metabolic rate (Met) and the blood flow (BF) between the compartments, which are controlled by the difference between the temperature setpoint and the body temperature input.
© Fa. Drägerwerk AG &Co.KGaA, Lübeck, Germany

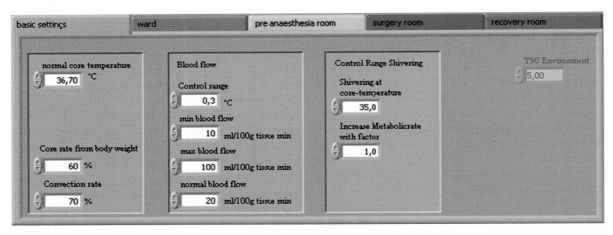

Fig. 15.6 Basic settings.
© Fa. Drägerwerk AG &Co.KGaA, Lübeck, Germany

The equation for *convection* includes ambient air temperature and humidity as well as air velocity between patient and environment or active warming therapy device. Heat exchange via *radiation* is calculated via skin temperature of the patient and wall temperature of the room. For *conduction*, heat transfer to or from the insulated blanket or the actively heated device are added to the calculation. The *evaporation* rate is described by an empirical equation [103]. The core and peripheral temperatures represent the mean temperatures of these body compartments that are considered homogeneously mixed. Blood flows freely between the central organs, but blood flow to the periphery is regulated by vasoconstriction and vasodilation. When the patient's core temperature and set point differ, vasoconstriction decreases the core-to-peripheral blood flow from approximately 20 mL/kg tissue/min to 1 mL/kg/min if the core temperature is too low or vasodilation increases the core-to-peripheral blood flow up to 50 mL/kg/min if the core temperature is too high.

Covariates of metabolic rate are gender, age and weight. Anaesthesia reduces metabolic rate. The heat conductivity of the tissue (bone, fat tissue and skin) is estimated. The model also takes into account the effect of BMI and body fat (fat is a good insulator), heat loss by respiration, heat loss by unwarmed IV fluids, and the effect of areas of the body that cannot be warmed due to surgical access.

Figures 15.6–15.8 show three of the many dialogue pages, overall > 50 parameters can be entered into the

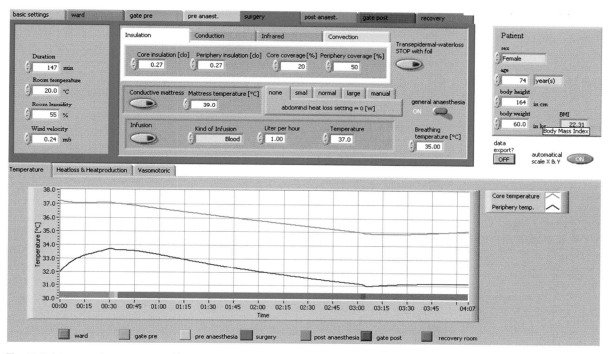

Fig. 15.7 Intraoperative parameters with temperature curve output.

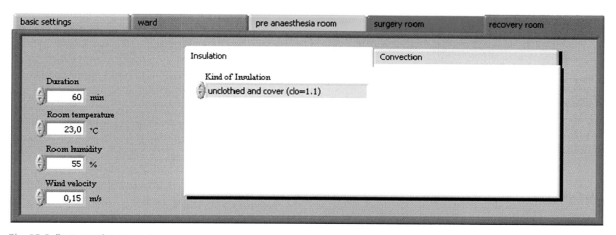

Fig. 15.8 Postoperative parameters.

simulation (see Table 15.4 for an abbreviated list of input parameters).

The model was validated by comparing it with core temperature measurements of 40 patients. Bland Altman analysis indicated that a simple two compartment model suffices to predict core temperatures perioperatively (see Fig. 15.9).

More detailed models have been developed with special emphasis on different climatic conditions [104], on garments [105], on physical activities [106], etc. These models can be very complex with multi-segmental, multi-layered representations of the human body, including spatial subdivisions and with additional calculations on the basis of computational fluid dynamics [107]. However, for real-time predictions of a patient's likelihood to become hypothermic the more basic model described above suffices.

Table 15.4. Abbreviated list of input parameters.

Patient

Sex	Age
Height	Weight

Basic physiological parameters

Baseline temperature	Body fat content
Metabolic rate	

Environment (ward, preoperative, intraoperative, postoperative)

Duration of stay in environment	Room temperature
Room humidity	Wind velocity
Insulation type of patient	

Additional preoperative parameters

Warming by conduction/convection/infra-red	Warming matress yes/no with temperature
Intravenous fluid temperature and rate	

Additional intraoperative parameters

General anaesthesia	Ventilator temperature

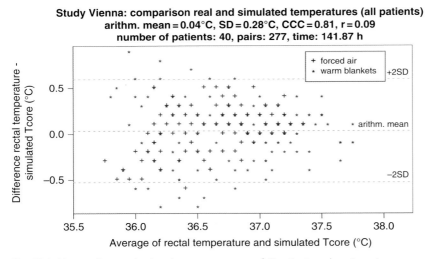

Fig. 15.9 Measured versus simulated core temperatures of 40 patients undergoing minor surgery. Bias 0.04°C; standard deviation 0.28°C; Lin's concordance correlation coefficient: 0.81

How to Avoid and Manage Accidental Perioperative Hypothermia

After induction of anaesthesia, core temperature drops over the first 60 minutes in almost all patients due to the core-to-peripheral redistribution of heat caused by drug induced vasodilation [108]. This 'redistribution hypo-thermia' occurs even if active warming is immediately initiated, but can (at least partly) be prevented by pre-induction warming [109]. After this initial drop, core temperature gradually decreases further until a plateau temperature is reached where heat production and heat loss are equal. Active warming during this phase can prevent this, and can even increase core temperature.

Of the many factors that determine the likelihood of accidental hypothermia, the following are particularly important: ambient temperature, location and extent of surgery, patient characteristics (age, weight, height), open versus laparoscopic surgery, and type of (active) warming technology [110, 111].

Insulation alone with special coated blankets covering the patient does not prevent hypothermia in the majority of patients [112], in contrast to *active* warming, which has become the *de facto* standard method to preserve normothermia. Heat is transferred to the patient's skin via active warming devices. Heat transfer to the skin can be achieved with any of the following technologies: forced air, water mattresses [113], resistive-electric warming [114], and chemical warming (using an exothermic chemical reaction, when a vacuum-sealed blanket is exposed to air) [115]. Of these, forced air warming is the method most commonly used. One crucial technical advantage of forced air warming is that the convection it uses can easily dissipate heat over a larger skin surface area than actually covered with the blanket. In contrast the efficiency of conductive warming systems (resistive heating, chemical heating, water mattresses) depends on actual direct contact between the patient's skin and the respective device, which is not always so easy to achieve (the most efficient conductive methods rely on pads 'glued' to the patient's skin).

It is not possible to warm patients perioperatively solely with fluids because this would require either very high, poorly tolerated fluid temperatures or very large amounts of fluid. Fluid warming may thus only serve to avoid further cooling by preventing the administration of unwarmed fluids. Cooling patients with fluids on the other hand can be done rapidly and is fairly easy, and is used to induce therapeutic hypothermia with relatively small amounts (up to two litres of cold crystalloid i.v. fluids) given in a short period of time [116].

Other warming methods are semi-invasive (e.g. oesophageal heat exchange catheter) or invasive (intravenous heat exchange catheters) and are only used for very specific indications, e.g. in patients where skin warming is not possible due to the extent of surgery (such as in burn victims undergoing plastic surgery) [117, 118].

Most warming technologies use open-loop feedback, i.e. they rely on a manual control of the warming device to maintain normothermia. However, more efficient technologies (e.g. intravenous warming, conductive warming systems with water infused pads attached to the patient) demand mandatory core temperature feedback as a safety precaution.

Conclusion

Research over the last decades in the fields of therapeutic hypothermia, accidental perioperative hypothermia, and thermometry has positioned core temperature as a truly *vital* parameter, that must be routinely monitored and managed perioperatively. Perioperative core temperature management and preservation of normothermia affect not only short-, but also mid- and long-term outcome of a patient. Perioperative core temperature management may thus serve as a an ideal example of the paradigm change in anaesthesiology looking 'beyond the drapes' with a focus shift from intraoperative analgesia and hypnosis towards long-term patient outcome and the perspective of 'personalized, perioperative medicine'.

References

1. Lopez M, Sessler DI, Walter K, Emerick T, Ozaki M: Rate and gender dependence of the sweating, vasoconstriction, and shivering thresholds in humans. Anesthesiology. 1994; 80: 780–8.

2. Torossian A: TEMMP Study Group. Survey on intraoperative temperature management in Europe. Eur.J.Anaesthesiol. 2007; 24: 668–75.

3. Smith JJ, Bland SA, Mullett S: Temperature – the forgotten vital sign. Accid.Emerg.Nurs. 2005; 13: 247–50.

4. Sawka MN, Latzka WA, Matott RP, Montain SJ: Hydration effects on temperature regulation. Int.J.Sports.Med. 1998; 19 Suppl 2: S108–10.

5. Lenhardt R, Sessler DI: Estimation of mean body temperature from mean skin and core temperature. Anesthesiology. 2006; 105: 1117–21.

6. Tayefeh F, Plattner O, Sessler DI, Ikeda T, Marder D: Circadian changes in the sweating-to-vasoconstriction interthreshold range. Pflugers.Arch. 1998; 435: 402–6.

7. Frank SM, Raja SN, Bulcao CF, Goldstein DS: Relative contribution of core and cutaneous temperatures to thermal comfort and autonomic responses in humans. J.Appl.Physiol. 1999; 86: 1588–93.

8. van Marken Lichtenbelt W: Brown adipose tissue and the regulation of nonshivering thermogenesis. Curr. Opin.Clin.Nutr.Metab.Care. 2012; 15: 547–52.

9. De Witte J, Sessler DI: Perioperative shivering: physiology and pharmacology. Anesthesiology. 2002; 96: 467–84.

10. Matsukawa T, Kurz A, Sessler DI, Bjorksten AR, Merrifield B, Cheng C: Propofol linearly reduces the vasoconstriction and shivering thresholds. Anesthesiology. 1995; 82: 1169–80.

11. Ikeda T, Kurz A, Sessler DI, et al: The effect of opioids on thermoregulatory responses in humans

and the special antishivering action of meperidine. Ann.N.Y.Acad.Sci. 1997; 813: 792–8.

12. Annadata R, Sessler DI, Tayefeh F, Kurz A, Dechert M: Desflurane slightly increases the sweating threshold but produces marked, nonlinear decreases in the vasoconstriction and shivering thresholds. Anesthesiology. 1995; 83: 1205–11.

13. Xiong J, Kurz A, Sessler DI, et al: Isoflurane produces marked and nonlinear decreases in the vasoconstriction and shivering thresholds. Anesthesiology. 1996; 85: 240–5.

14. Mekjavic IB, Sundberg CJ: Human temperature regulation during narcosis induced by inhalation of 30% nitrous oxide. J.Appl.Physiol. 1992; 73: 2246–54.

15. Kurz A, Sessler DI, Annadata R, Dechert M, Christensen R, Bjorksten AR: Midazolam minimally impairs thermoregulatory control. Anesth.Analg. 1995; 81: 393–8.

16. Cornett PM, Matta JA, Ahern GP: General anesthetics sensitize the capsaicin receptor transient receptor potential V1. Mol.Pharmacol. 2008; 74: 1261–8.

17. Kurz A, Ikeda T, Sessler DI, et al: Meperidine decreases the shivering threshold twice as much as the vasoconstriction threshold. Anesthesiology. 1997; 86: 1046–54.

18. Kurz A, Go JC, Sessler DI, Kaer K, Larson MD, Bjorksten AR: Alfentanil slightly increases the sweating threshold and markedly reduces the vasoconstriction and shivering thresholds. Anesthesiology. 1995; 83: 293–9.

19. Leslie K, Sessler DI: Reduction in the shivering threshold is proportional to spinal block height. Anesthesiology. 1996; 84: 1327–31.

20. Kim JS, Ikeda T, Sessler DI, Turakhia M, Jeffrey R: Epidural anesthesia reduces the gain and maximum intensity of shivering. Anesthesiology. 1998; 88: 851–7.

21. Joris J, Ozaki M, Sessler DI, et al: Epidural anesthesia impairs both central and peripheral thermoregulatory control during general anesthesia. Anesthesiology. 1994; 80: 268–77.

22. Emerick TH, Ozaki M, Sessler DI, Walters K, Schroeder M: Epidural anesthesia increases apparent leg temperature and decreases the shivering threshold. Anesthesiology. 1994; 81: 289–98.

23. Doufas AG, Morioka N, Maghoub AN, Mascha E, Sessler DI: Lower-body warming mimics the normal epidural-induced reduction in the shivering threshold. Anesth.Analg. 2008; 106: 252–6.

24. Arkiliç CF, Akça O, Taguchi A, Sessler DI, Kurz A: Temperature monitoring and management during neuraxial anesthesia: an observational study. Anesth. Analg. 2000; 91: 662–6.

25. Caldwell JE, Heier T, Wright PM, et al: Temperature-dependent pharmacokinetics and pharmacodynamics of vecuronium. Anesthesiology. 2000; 92: 84–93.

26. Leslie K, Sessler DI, Bjorksten AR, Moayeri A: Mild hypothermia alters propofol pharmacokinetics and increases the duration of action of atracurium. Anesth. Analg. 1995; 80: 1007–14.

27. Lenhardt R, Marker E, Goll V, et al: Mild intraoperative hypothermia prolongs postanesthetic recovery. Anesthesiology. 1997; 87: 1318–23.

28. Kurz A, Sessler DI, Narzt E, et al: Postoperative hemodynamic and thermoregulatory consequences of intraoperative core hypothermia. J.Clin.Anesth. 1995; 7: 359–66.

29. Badjatia N, Strongilis E, Prescutti M, et al: Metabolic benefits of surface counter warming during therapeutic temperature modulation. Crit.Care.Med. 2009; 37: 1893–7.

30. Rajagopalan S, Mascha E, Na J, Sessler DI: The effects of mild perioperative hypothermia on blood loss and transfusion requirement. Anesthesiology. 2008; 108: 71–7.

31. Hohn DC, MacKay RD, Halliday B, Hunt TK: Effect of O_2 tension on microbicidal function of leucocytes in wounds and in vitro. Surg.Forum. 1976; 27: 18–20.

32. van Oss CJ, Absolom DR, Moore LL, Park BH, Humbert JR: Effect of temperature on the chemotaxis, phagocytic engulfment, digestion and O_2 consumption of human polymorphonuclear leucocytes. J. Reticuloendothel.Soc. 1980; 27: 561–5.

33. Hunt TK, Pai MP: The effect of varying ambient oxygen tensions on wound metabolism and collagen synthesis. Surg.Gynecol.Obstet. 1972; 135: 561–7.

34. Kurz A, Sessler DI, Lenhardt R: Perioperative normothermia to reduce the incidence of surgical-wound infection and shorten hospitalization. Study of Wound Infection and Temperature Group. N. Engl.J.Med. 1996; 334: 1209–15.

35. Melling AC, Ali B, Scott EM, Leaper DJ. Effects of preoperative warming on the incidence of wound infection after clean surgery: a randomised controlled trial. Lancet. 2001; 358: 876–80.

36. Frank SM, Higgins MS, Breslow MJ, et al: The catecholamine, cortisol, and hemodynamic responses to mild perioperative hypothermia. A randomized clinical trial. Anesthesiology. 1995; 82: 83–93.

37. Frank SM, Fleisher LA, Breslow MJ, et al: Perioperative maintenance of normothermia reduces the incidence of morbid cardiac events. A randomized clinical trial. JAMA. 1997; 277: 1127–34.

38. Alfonsi P: Postanaesthetic shivering. Epidemiology, pathophysiology and approaches to prevention and management. Minerva.Anestesiol. 2003; 69: 438–42.

39. Crossley AW, Mahajan RP: The intensity of postoperative shivering is unrelated to axillary temperature. Anaesthesia. 1994; 49: 205–7.

40. Zwischenberger JB, Kirsh MM, Dechert RE, Arnold DK, Bartlett RH: Suppression of shivering decreases oxygen consumption and improves hemodynamic stability during postoperative rewarming. Ann.Thorac. Surg. 1987; 43: 428–31.

41. Ralley FE, Wynands JE, Ramsay JG, Carli F, MacSullivan R: The effects of shivering on oxygen consumption and carbon dioxide production in patients rewarming from hypothermic cardiopulmonary bypass. Can.J.Anaesth. 1988; 35: 332–7.

42. Pauca AL, Savage RT, Simpson S, Roy RC: Effect of pethidine, fentanyl and morphine on post-operative shivering in man. Acta.Anaesthesiol. Scand. 1984; 28: 138–43.

43. Delaunay L, Bonnet F, Liu N, Beydon L, Catoire P, Sessler DI: Clonidine comparably decreases the thermoregulatory thresholds for vasoconstriction and shivering in humans. Anesthesiology. 1993; 79: 470–4.

44. Panneer M, Murugaiyan P, Rao SV: A comparative study of intravenous dexmedetomidine and intravenous clonidine for postspinal shivering in patients undergoing lower limb orthopedic surgeries. Anesth.Essays.Res. 2017; 11: 151–4.

45. Dal D, Kose A, Honca M, Akinci SB, Basgul E, Aypar U: Efficacy of prophylactic ketamine in preventing postoperative shivering. Br.J.Anaesth. 2005; 95: 189–92.

46. Alfonsi P, Adam F, Passard A, Guignard B, Sessler DI, Chauvin M: Nefopam, a nonsedative benzoxazocine analgesic, selectively reduces the shivering threshold in unanesthetized subjects. Anesthesiology. 2004; 100: 37–43.

47. Wadhwa A, Sengupta P, Durrani J, et al: Magnesium sulphate only slightly reduces the shivering threshold in humans. Br.J.Anaesth. 2005; 94: 756–62.

48. Komatsu R, Sengupta P, Cherynak G, et al: Doxapram only slightly reduces the shivering threshold in healthy volunteers. Anesth.Analg. 2005; 101: 1368–73.

49. Komatsu R, Orhan-Sungur M, In J, et al: Ondansetron does not reduce the shivering threshold in healthy volunteers. Br.J.Anaesth. 2006; 96: 732–7.

50. Asl ME, Isazadefar K, Mohammadian A, Khoshbaten M: Ondansetron and meperidine prevent postoperative shivering after general anesthesia. Middle.East.Anaesthesiol. 2011; 21: 67–70.

51. Mokhtarani M, Mahgoub AN, Morioka N, et al: Buspirone and meperidine synergistically reduce the shivering threshold. Anesth.Analg. 2001; 93: 1233–9.

52. Lin CM, Neeru S, Doufas AG, et al: Dantrolene reduces the threshold and gain for shivering. Anesth.Analg. 2004; 98: 1318–24.

53. Kimberger O, Ali SZ, Markstaller M, et al: Meperidine and skin surface warming additively reduce the shivering threshold: a volunteer study. Crit.Care. 2007; 11: R29.

54. Campbell G, Alderson P, Smith AF, Warttig S: Warming of intravenous and irrigation fluids for preventing inadvertent perioperative hypothermia. Cochrane. Database.Syst.Rev. 2015CD009891.

55. Madrid E, Urrútia G, Roqué i Figuls M, et al: Active body surface warming systems for preventing complications caused by inadvertent perioperative hypothermia in adults. Cochrane.Database.Syst.Rev. 2016; 4: CD009016.

56. Wartzek T, Mühlsteff J, Imhoff M: Temperature measurement. Biomed.Tech.(Berl). 2011; 56: 241–57.

57. Henker RA, Brown SD, Marion DW: Comparison of brain temperature with bladder and rectal temperatures in adults with severe head injury. Neurosurgery. 1998; 42: 1071–5.

58. Rossi S, Zanier ER, Mauri I, Columbo A, Stocchetti N: Brain temperature, body core temperature, and intracranial pressure in acute cerebral damage. J. Neurol.Neurosurg.Psychiatry. 2001; 71: 448–54.

59. Liu SK, Chiang YY, Poon KS, et al: Thoracotomy for lung lesion does not affect the accuracy of esophageal temperature. Acta.Anaesthesiol.Taiwan. 2013; 51: 116–19.

60. Lefrant JY, Muller L, de La Coussaye JE, et al: Temperature measurement in intensive care patients: comparison of urinary bladder, oesophageal, rectal, axillary, and inguinal methods versus pulmonary artery core method. Intens.Care.Med. 2003; 29: 414–18.

61. Mekjavić IB, Rempel ME: Determination of esophageal probe insertion length based on standing and sitting height. J.Appl.Physiol. 1990; 69: 376–9.

62. Makic MB, Lovett K, Azam MF: Placement of an esophageal temperature probe by nurses. AACN Adv. Crit.Care. 2012; 23: 24–31.

63. Wallace CT, Marks WE, Adkins WY, Mahaffey JE: Perforation of the tympanic membrane, a complication of tympanic thermometry during anesthesia. Anesthesiology. 1974; 41: 290–1.

64. Wang M, Singh A, Qureshi H, Leone A, Mascha EJ, Sessler DI: Optimal depth for nasopharyngeal temperature probe positioning. Anesth.Analg. 2016; 122: 1434–8.

65. Sinha PK, Kaushik S, Neema PK: Massive epistaxis after nasopharyngeal temperature probe insertion after cardiac surgery. J.Cardiothorac.Vasc.Anesth. 2004; 18: 123–4.

66. Ciuraru NB, Braunstein R, Sulkes A, Stemmer SM: The influence of mucositis on oral thermometry: when fever may not reflect infection. Clin.Infect.Dis. 2008; 46: 1859–63.

67. Torossian A, Bräuer A, Höcker J, Bein B, Wulf H, Horn EP: Preventing inadvertent perioperative hypothermia. Dtsch.Arztebl.Int. 2015; 112: 166–72.

68. Nierman DM: Core temperature measurement in the intensive care unit. Crit.Care.Med. 1991; 19: 818–23.

235

69. Bräuer A, Martin JD, Schuhmann MU, Braun U, Weyland W: Accuracy of intraoperative urinary bladder temperature monitoring during intra-abdominal operations. Anasthesiol.Intensivmed. Notfallmed.Schmerzther. 2000; 35: 435–9.

70. Greenes DS, Fleisher GR: When body temperature changes, does rectal temperature lag? J.Pediatr. 2004; 144: 824–6.

71. Weingart S, Mayer S, Polderman K: Rectal probe temperature lag during rapid saline induction of hypothermia after resuscitation from cardiac arrest. Resuscitation. 2009; 80: 837–8.

72. Kuremu RT, Hadley GP, Wiersma R: Gastro-intestinal tract perforation in neonates. East.Afr.Med.J. 2003; 80: 452–5.

73. Kimberger O, Cohen D, Illievich U, Lenhardt R: Temporal artery versus bladder thermometry during perioperative and intensive care unit monitoring. Anesth.Analg. 2007; 105: 1042–7.

74. Lefrant JY, Muller L, de La Coussaye JE, et al: Temperature measurement in intensive care patients: comparison of urinary bladder, oesophageal, rectal, axillary, and inguinal methods versus pulmonary artery core method. Intens.Care.Med. 2003; 29: 414–18.

75. Niven DJ, Gaudet JE, Laupland KB, Mrklas KJ, Roberts DJ, Stelfox HT: Accuracy of peripheral thermometers for estimating temperature: a systematic review and meta-analysis. Ann.Intern.Med. 2015; 163: 768–77.

76. Dollberg S, Mincis L, Mimouni FB, Ashbel G, Barak M: Evaluation of a new thermometer for rapid axillary temperature measurement in preterm infants. Am.J.Perinatol. 2003; 20: 201–4.

77. Kimberger O, Thell R, Schuh M, Koch J, Sessler DI, Kurz A: Accuracy and precision of a novel non-invasive core thermometer. Br.J.Anaesth. 2009; 103: 226–31.

78. Vaughan MS, Cork RC, Vaughan RW: Inaccuracy of liquid crystal thermometry to identify core temperature trends in postoperative adults. Anesth.Analg. 1982; 61: 284–7.

79. Chaturvedi D, Vilhekar KY, Chaturvedi P, Bharambe MS: Reliability of perception of fever by touch. Indian.J. Pediatr. 2003; 70: 871–3.

80. Dodd SR, Lancaster GA, Craig JV, Smyth RL, Williamson PR: In a systematic review, infrared ear thermometry for fever diagnosis in children finds poor sensitivity. J Clin.Epidemiol. 2006; 59: 354–7.

81. Moran JL, Peter JV, Solomon PJ, et al: Tympanic temperature measurements: are they reliable in the critically ill? A clinical study of measures of agreement. Crit.Care.Med. 2007; 35: 155–64.

82. Iden T, Horn EP, Bein B, Böhm R, Beese J, Höcker J: Intraoperative temperature monitoring with zero heat flux technology (3 M SpotOn sensor) in comparison

with sublingual and nasopharyngeal temperature: An observational study. Eur.J.Anaesthesiol. 2015; 32: 387–91.

83. Mäkinen MT, Pesonen A, Jousela I, et al: Novel zero-heat-flux deep body temperature measurement in lower extremity vascular and cardiac surgery. J. Cardiothorac.Vasc.Anesth. 2016; 30: 973–8.

84. Dahyot-Fizelier C, Lamarche S, Kerforne T, et al: Accuracy of zero-heat-flux cutaneous temperature in intensive care adults. Crit.Care.Med. 2017

85. Gunga HC, Werner A, Stahn A, et al: The Double Sensor – A non-invasive device to continuously monitor core temperature in humans on earth and in space. Respir.Physiol.Neurobiol. 2009; 169 Suppl 1: S63–8.

86. Kimberger O, Thell R, Schuh M, Koch J, Sessler DI, Kurz A: Accuracy and precision of a novel non-invasive core thermometer. Br.J.Anaesth. 2009; 103: 226–31.

87. Kimberger O, Saager L, Egan C, et al: The accuracy of a disposable noninvasive core thermometer. Can.J.Anaesth. 2013; 60: 1190–6.

88. Mendt S, Maggioni MA, Nordine M, et al: Circadian rhythms in bed rest: monitoring core body temperature via heat-flux approach is superior to skin surface temperature. Chronobiol.Int. 2016; 1–11.

89. Seip R, Ebbini ES: Noninvasive estimation of tissue temperature response to heating fields using diagnostic ultrasound. IEEE.Trans.Biomed.Eng. 1995; 42: 828–39.

90. Winter L, Oberacker E, Paul K, et al: Magnetic resonance thermometry: methodology, pitfalls and practical solutions. Int.J.Hyperthermia. 2016; 32: 63–75.

91. Fernandes AA, Moreira DG, Brito CJ, et al: Validity of inner canthus temperature recorded by infrared thermography as a non-invasive surrogate measure for core temperature at rest, during exercise and recovery. J.Therm.Biol. 2016; 62: 50–5.

92. Pereira CB, Heimann K, Czaplik M, Blazek V, Venema B, Leonhardt S: Thermoregulation in premature infants: a mathematical model. J.Therm.Biol. 2016; 62: 159–69.

93. Grundstein AJ, Duzinski SV, Dolinak D, Null J, Iyer SS: Evaluating infant core temperature response in a hot car using a heat balance model. Forensic.Sci. Med. Pathol. 2015; 11: 13–19.

94. Laxminarayan S, Buller MJ, Tharion WJ, Reifman J: Human core temperature prediction for heat-injury prevention. IEEE.J.Biomed.Health.Inform. 2015; 19: 883–91.

95. Hirshberg A, Sheffer N, Barnea O: Computer simulation of hypothermia during "damage control" laparotomy. World.Surg. 1999; 23: 960–5.

96. Chan LS, Cheung GT, Lauder IJ, Kumana CR, Lauder IJ: Screening for fever by remote-sensing infrared thermographic camera. J.Travel.Med. 2004; 11: 273–9.

97. Bräuer A, English MJ, Sander H, Timmermann A, Braun U, Weyland W: Construction and evaluation of a manikin for perioperative heat exchange. Acta. Anaesthesiol.Scand. 2002; 46: 43–50.

98. Bräuer A, English MJ, Steinmetz N, et al: Comparison of forced-air warming systems with upper body blankets using a copper manikin of the human body. Acta.Anaesthesiol.Scand. 2002; 46: 965–72.

99. Nightingale S, Wynne L, Cassey J: Convection heating in pediatric general surgery – a comparison of warming alternatives in a mannequin study. Paediatr. Anaesth. 2006; 16: 663–8.

100. Buisson P, Bach V, Elabbassi EB, et al: Assessment of the efficiency of warming devices during neonatal surgery. Eur.J.Appl.Physiol. 2004; 92: 694–7.

101. Bussmann O, Nahm W, Konecny E: A model for simulating heat transfer and thermoregulation of premature infants. Biomed.Tech.(Berl). 1998; 43 Suppl: 300–1.

102. Lam TK, Leung DT: More on simplified calculation of body-surface area [letter]. N.Engl.J.Med. 1988; 318 (17): 1130.

103. Ultman JS: Computational model for insensible water loss from the newborn. Pediatrics. 1987; 79: 760–5.

104. Fiala D, Havenith G, Bröde P, Kampmann B, Jendritzky G: UTCI-Fiala multi-node model of human heat transfer and temperature regulation. Int.J.Biometeorol. 2012; 56: 429–41.

105. Yang J, Weng W, Wang F, Song G: Integrating a human thermoregulatory model with a clothing model to predict core and skin temperatures. Appl.Ergon. 2017; 61: 168–77.

106. Havenith G, Fiala D: Thermal indices and thermophysiological modeling for heat stress. Compr. Physiol. 2015; 6: 255–302.

107. Fu M, Weng W, Chen W, Luo N: Review on modeling heat transfer and thermoregulatory responses in the human body. J.Therm.Biol. 2016; 62: 189–200.

108. Sun Z, Honar H, Sessler DI, et al: Intraoperative core temperature patterns, transfusion requirement, and hospital duration in patients warmed with forced air. Anesthesiology. 2015; 122: 276–85.

109. Perl T, Peichl LH, Reyntjens K, Deblaere I, Zaballos JM, Bräuer A: Efficacy of a novel prewarming system in the prevention of perioperative hypothermia. A prospective, randomized, multicenter study. Minerva. Anestesiol. 2014; 80: 436–43.

110. Engorn BM, Kahntroff SL, Frank KM, et al: Perioperative hypothermia in neonatal intensive care unit patients: effectiveness of a thermoregulation intervention and associated risk factors. Paediatr. Anaesth. 2017; 27: 196–204.

111. Wetz AJ, Perl T, Brandes IF, Harden M, Bauer M, Bräuer A: Unexpectedly high incidence of hypothermia before induction of anesthesia in elective surgical patients. J. Clin.Anesth. 2016; 34: 282–9.

112. Sessler DI, McGuire J, Sessler AM: Perioperative thermal insulation. Anesthesiology. 1991; 74: 875–9.

113. Hynson JM, Sessler DI: Intraoperative warming therapies: a comparison of three devices. J.Clin.Anesth. 1992; 4: 194–9.

114. Kimberger O, Held C, Stadelmann K, et al: Resistive polymer versus forced-air warming: comparable heat transfer and core rewarming rates in volunteers. Anesth.Analg. 2008; 107: 1621–6.

115. Brandes IF, Müller C, Perl T, Russo SG, Bauer M, Bräuer A: Efficacy of a novel warming blanket: prospective randomized trial. Anaesthesist. 2013; 62: 137–42.

116. Bernard SA, Smith K, Cameron P, et al: Induction of prehospital therapeutic hypothermia after resuscitation from nonventricular fibrillation cardiac arrest. Crit.Care.Med. 2012; 40: 747–53.

117. Hegazy AF, Lapierre DM, Butler R, Althenayan E: Temperature control in critically ill patients with a novel esophageal cooling device: a case series. BMC. Anesthesiol. 2015; 15: 152.

118. Davis JS, Rodriguez LI, Quintana OD, et al: Use of a warming catheter to achieve normothermia in large burns. J.Burn.Care.Res. 2013; 34: 191–5.

Chapter 16

Effects of Perioperative Management on Kidney Function

Xavier Borrat and Jordi Mercadal

Introduction

Normal kidney function is essential to maintain whole body homeostasis. An acute decline in kidney function, 'acute kidney injury' (AKI), is in and by itself a major cause of perioperative morbidity and mortality. Maintaining preexisting kidney function therefore is a key task of the anaesthesiologist in the perioperative period [1].

Studies on perioperative AKI (including worsening of chronic renal failure) have mainly focused on the postoperative/ICU setting because (1) renal dysfunction does not alter intraoperative haemodynamics or oxygenation (provided a neutral fluid balance is maintained); (2) we lack readily available biomarkers to monitor intraoperative renal function (intraoperative oliguria is a poor marker of AKI, and creatinine value takes hours to rise); (3) medical treatment of AKI is mainly performed in the ICU (managing fluid overload, hyperkalaemia, drug dosing adjustments or renal replacement therapies); (4) patients at risk for AKI are likely to be admitted to the ICU postoperatively.

Despite being 'silent' in the operating room, measures to prevent postoperative AKI must be implemented pre- and intraoperatively and include identifying risk factors related to the type of surgery and the patient (*pre*operative condition), carefully managing fluid balances (both fluid overload and hypovolaemia should be avoided) and carefully considering the indication for nephrotoxic drugs.

Epidemiology and Definition of Acute Kidney Injury

Definition and Incidence

In 2004, the Acute Dialysis Quality Initiative reached a consensus definition of AKI based on the RIFLE criteria (see below) [2]. RIFLE is the acronym of Risk, Injury, Failure, Loss and End-Stage Kidney. It provides a structured classification of AKI severity and recovery. Prior to this consensus, the use of inconsistent definitions

caused the incidence of AKI to widely range from 1% to 31%. The KDIGO (Kidney Disease: Improving Global Outcomes) guidelines define AKI as:

1. An increase in serum creatinine ≥ 0.3 mg/dL within the last 48 h
2. A 1.5 increase in baseline serum creatinine, known or presumed to have occurred within the last seven days
3. Urine output < 0.5 mL/kg/h for six hours.

When this KDIGO criteria were applied in a meta-analysis of 312 studies [3], the pooled incidence of AKI during an episode of hospital care was 21.6% in adults and 33.7% in children. It was highest in critical care patients (31.7%) and in patients who underwent cardiac surgery (24.3%). AKI-associated mortality was 23.9% in adults and 13.8% in children.

AKI is further stratified in three stages (see Table 16.1). Mortality increases with each stage.

Special Considerations in the Perioperative Period

While the diagnosis of postoperative AKI obviously considers urine output as well, it has to be recognized that oliguria in the postoperative period is often secondary to the normal physiological retention of salt and water in response to tissue damage, pain, mild degrees of hypovolaemia, hypotension and positive pressure ventilation [4]. Few prospective studies have

Table 16.1. Stages of AKI.

Stage	Serum Creatinine Increase	Urine Output
1	1.5–1.9 times baseline or ≥ 0.3 mg/dL increase	< 0.5 mL/kg/h for 6-12 h
2	2–2.9 times baseline	< 0.5 mL/kg/h for $\geq$12 h
3	Three times baseline or serum creatinine ≥ 4 mg/dL Initiation of renal replacement therapy	< 0.3 mL/kg/h for $\geq$ 24 h or anuria for $\geq$ 12 hours

examined the contribution of oliguria to postoperative prognosis, in particular the ability of oliguria to predict subsequent creatinine changes. A study of critically ill surgical and medical patients reported that oliguria was not a useful predictor of subsequent increases in creatinine, and that there was no consistent relationship between the duration of oliguria and RIFLE criteria [5]. Another study confirmed that intraoperative oliguria is common but not usually followed by a rise in creatinine, with the authors suggesting that the relationship between oliguria and renal failure should be further investigated [6].

Risk Factors for Perioperative Acute Kidney Injury

In a review of 28 studies involving 10,865 patients that underwent either vascular, cardiac, general or biliary surgery, preexisting chronic renal failure was the most important and consistent risk factor for postoperative AKI [7]. As mentioned above, the incidence of AKI during an episode of hospital care was highest in critical care patients (31.7%) and in patients that underwent cardiac surgery (24.3%). In a single centre prospective study involving 15,102 patients undergoing non-cardiac surgery and without preexisting renal dysfunction (creatinine clearance > 80 mL/min), the incidence of postoperative renal failure was 0.8%, and was associated with the following seven independent preoperative risk factors [6]: age > 59, emergency surgery (as defined by ASA physical status), chronic liver disease, body mass index > 32, peripheral vascular disease, COPD requiring bronchodilator therapy and finally high risk surgery: intrathoracic, intraperitoneal, supra-inguinal vascular and other surgeries with a potential for large fluid shifts such as multilevel spine fusions, intracranial aneurysm clippings, transhiatal oesophagectomy and pelvic exenteration.

Pathophysiology
Renal Autoregulation

While a detailed description of renal physiology is outside the scope of this chapter, some basic concepts should be reviewed. Traditional teaching holds that autoregulation maintains renal blood flow in response to changes in mean arterial pressure within the 50 to 150 mmHg range in normotensive patients by vasodilating and vasoconstricting the afferent arteriole in response to a decrease and an increase of blood

pressure, respectively. In the hypertensive patient, the curve is shifted to the right. The renal perfusion pressure is calculated as the difference between mean arterial pressure and central venous pressure. The perfusion pressure needs to remain above the lower autoregulation limit in order to maintain renal blood flow and hence glomerular filtration rate – once the perfusion pressure drops below the lower autoregulation limit, renal blood flow decreases proportionally with perfusion pressure.

While the above is true in the experimental environment in the isolated kidney, the intact kidney is extensively innervated by the sympathetic nervous system and influenced by systemic and locally released hormones and vasoactive substances. In fact, the response to circulatory failure (low blood pressure) consists of activation of the sympathetic nervous system and the renin axis, which results in afferent arteriolar vasoconstriction that maintains renal perfusion pressure [8]. Lack or exhaustion of this compensatory response (typical in distributive shock due to e.g. sepsis, high risk surgery, anaphylaxis) leads to systemic hypotension with kidney ischaemia despite the high cardiac output. In this context, noradrenaline has been demonstrated not to cause deterioration in kidney function [9], and for now is considered the best intraoperative approach to restore systolic blood pressure to minimize the incidence of AKI if combined with the judicious use of fluid therapy avoiding fluid overload [10].

Classification of Acute Kidney Injury and Limitations in Perioperative Care

Of all AKI cases, one-third are related to previous surgical procedures [4]. The diagnosis of AKI and its aetiology must be performed based on clinical criteria supported by ultrasound studies, biochemistry and urinalysis (urea/creatinine ratio, sodium, fractional sodium and urea excretion). The aetiology can be pre-, intra-, and post-renal (see Table 16.2), a distinction that helps guide treatment and prognosis.

While they rarely are the origin of renal dysfunction (1–2%), post-renal causes can be easily diagnosed and thus have to be excluded first. They are most often marked by *sudden* oliguria or anuria. Intraoperatively, sudden oliguria or anuria has to prompt a search for a kinked Foley catheter. An ultrasound exam may reveal other causes in the perioperative period, e.g. renal vascular occlusion.

After having excluded post-renal causes, pre-renal and intra-renal causes have to be considered. This

239

Table 16.2. Potential causes of perioperative AKI. NSAIDs (Non-steroidal anti-inflammatory drugs), ACEI (Angiotensin converting enzyme inhibitors), ARB (Angiotensin receptor blockers).

Pre-renal

- Hypovolaemia (surgical haemorrhage, gastrointestinal losses)
- Hypotension [sepsis, cardiac failure, drugs (including most anaesthetics), anaphylaxis, cardiopulmonary bypass, vena cava cross-clamping]
- Increased intra-abdominal pressure
- NSAIDs, ACEI, ARB
- Hepatorenal syndrome
- Aortic cross-clamping

Renal

- Inflammatory damage
- Diabetes mellitus, vasculopathy, chronic kidney disease, obesity
- Nephrotoxic drugs (aminoglycosides, vancomycin, colistin, amphotericin B, radiocontrast agent, immunosuppressants)
- Fluid solutions (overuse of hydroxyethyl starch and chloride rich solutions)

Post-renal

- Urinary bladder tumour, retroperitoneal fibrosis, neurogenic bladder, renal calculi, urinary bladder haemorrhage
- Urinary catheter obstruction

distinction is important because most cases of AKI during the perioperative period (70% in the recent EPI-AKI study [11]) are considered to be caused by renal ischaemia secondary to haemodynamic derangements (haemorrhage, perioperative losses, sepsis, low cardiac output). The effect of renal ischaemia goes through two phases. In the first phase, there are no structural changes, and renal function will recover rapidly (pre-renal or functional) after restoring perfusion. In the second phase, persistent hypoperfusion will cause structural renal damage, the deterioration of renal function will be more protracted, and prognosis will be worse.

Recent data suggest that the commonly used biochemical and urinalyses are not very useful in differentiating pre- and intra-renal causes in the context of sepsis and the critically ill surgical patient [12, 13]. In addition, renal hypoperfusion may involve more than just haemodynamic factors [14], and renal hypoperfusion *per se* may not be the leading cause of AKI in the critically ill and high risk surgery patient (defined as a patient with high risk of worsening or developing organ dysfunction postoperatively). There is evidence that fluid overload should be avoided because it might cause and propagate AKI [12, 15, 16], but also that aggressive fluid restriction should be avoided [16b].

Biomarkers of Acute Kidney Injury

In the last years, much research has been devoted to the validation of new biomarkers for AKI to try to better characterize both the clinical syndrome and

its pathophysiological course [17]. They vary in their anatomical and cellular origin, physiological function, time of release after the onset of renal injury and kinetics after their release.

The main objective of a biomarker in this context would be to allow an early diagnosis of AKI, predict evolution and prognosis, and define basic pathophysiological mechanisms. Biomarkers for AKI can be stratified according to the part of the nephron that has been affected and/or the specific markers released by these sites if injured.

The availability of these new markers has led to a new classification of AKI based on the alteration of glomerular filtration (marked by creatinine levels) and the presence of structural damage (marked by elevated biomarkers). The complex clinical syndrome of AKI can thus be stratified in three new classes with prognostic significance:

- **Subclinical AKI**: patients with elevated biomarkers but no elevation of serum creatinine.
- **Functional AKI**: patients with elevated serum creatinine but no elevation of biomarkers.
- **Structural AKI**: patients with both elevated serum creatinine and biomarkers.

A New Acute Kidney Injury Paradigm for Sepsis and its Applicability to the High Risk Surgical Patient

As mentioned above, sepsis is considered to be a cause of (or a major factor contributing to) AKI in the

Table 16.3. Potential biomarkers of AKI according to their mechanism of damage.

Glomerular filtration	Serum Cystatin C
Glomerular permeability	Albuminuria Proteinuria
Tubular stress	Insulin-like growth factor binding protein 7 (IGFBP-7) Tissue inhibitor metalloproteinase 2 (TIMP2)
Tubular damage	Neutrophil gelatinase-associated lipocalin (NGAL) Kidney injury molecule-1 (KIM-1) N-acetyl-β- D-glucosaminidase (NAG) Liver fatty acid-binding protein (L-FAB)
Intra-renal inflammation	Interleukin-18

critically ill patient [11, 18], with absolute or relative hypovolaemia and the concomitant use of vasoconstrictors resulting in ischaemic kidney injury. Even though physiologically plausible, recent experimental and clinical data challenge the vision that both septic and non-septic AKI are caused by ischaemia:

- AKI is not a universal outcome after cardiac arrest. Cardiac arrest is the best model of clinical ischaemia with periods of low or absent renal flow, especially if there is no hypoperfusion after return of spontaneous circulation [12].
- During sepsis, the proportion of cardiac output received by the kidneys does not change, implying that renal blood flow is high in patients with a hyperdynamic circulation. A hyperdynamic circulation is the most frequent form of haemodynamic derangement during sepsis [19].
- AKI during sepsis can develop without any clinical evidence of hypovolaemia and haemodynamic instability [20].
- Pathological findings in kidneys of patients dying from septic shock demonstrate heterogeneous tubular damage with apical vacuolization without extensive necrosis rather than acute tubular necrosis, the pathological correlate of ischaemic renal damage [21].

Based upon clinical data and robust experimental models, the following theory has been developed to explain the aetiology of sepsis induced AKI [22]. During early sepsis, the predominant mechanism of kidney dysfunction is a vasodilation state causing low glomerular filtration pressures and low glomerular filtration rates, despite the hyperdynamic circulation with a high cardiac output and high renal blood flow. In this early phase, treatment with vasoconstrictors can prevent AKI, but sometimes restoring haemodynamics will not be enough to restore kidney function because microcirculatory glomerular and peritubular dysfunction will inflict inflammatory damage. Filtration of the resulting inflammatory mediators will induce endothelial dysfunction that contributes to a sluggish peritubular blood flow that promotes adhesion of activated leucocytes to the endothelium that will infiltrate the kidney interstitium. The resulting inflammation will initially only affect proximal tubular cells because these are the cells first to be exposed to the inflammatory milieu. Next, these proximal tubular cells will secrete paracrine factors that trigger more distal tubular cells to enter into a sort of hibernating state to avoid further damage and possibly to facilitate recovery once the inflammatory insult has ceased.

This theory integrates clinical and experimental data and reinforces the concept that AKI may not be just a haemodynamically mediated phenomenon. While the above focuses on events occurring during septic AKI, inflammation could also play a pivotal role in perioperative (not septic related) AKI but this remains speculative at this time.

Prevention of Acute Kidney Injury

Because of the high mortality and morbidity associated with renal dysfunction, prevention of AKI in different clinical scenarios has been the topic of intense research. Yet while the exact underlying pathophysiological mechanisms remain to be fully elucidated, those factors known to contribute to AKI should be targeted to help minimize its incidence.

Nephrotoxic Drugs

Common sense recommends that nephrotoxic drugs should be avoided whenever possible. These include drugs like NSAIDs and certain classes of antibiotics such as aminoglycosides, glycopeptides or amphotericin (Table 16.2).

Fluid Administration and Haemodynamic Management

There is no consensus about what the optimal haemodynamic goals and interventions have to be to prevent AKI because these will depend on the clinical situation such as anticipated changes during surgery and the comorbidities of the patient. Currently, the only way to manage fluids is through haemodynamic monitoring, titrated to maintain a stable cardiac output and mean arterial pressure (also see Chapter 14). Fluid and vasoactive drug administration must also be titrated to meet the demand and characteristics of the individual patient: it is not the same for an old and frail patient with critical aortic stenosis scheduled to undergo femoral neck fracture surgery and a young healthy man to undergo abdominal surgery for a (peri)appendicular abscess.

There is general agreement that hypovolaemia should be avoided and a minimum renal perfusion pressure should be maintained by titrating fluids and vasoconstrictors [23]. Again, this recommendation is based on studies performed in the context of sepsis. There is growing evidence that suggests that once initial resuscitation has been finished, fluid overload should be avoided because it has been associated with worsening renal function and poor renal recovery. A high central venous pressure was recently found to be the haemodynamic variable most closely associated with AKI during sepsis, which suggests congestion may worsen AKI during septic episodes [24]. But while evidence is accumulating that fluid overload should be avoided because it might cause and propagate AKI [12, 15, 16], there is evidence that aggressive fluid restriction should also be avoided to prevent AKI in patients undergoing abdominal surgery [16b]. According to the previous information, current evidence suggests that the clinician should judiciously administer fluids based on preexisting renal function, individual risk factors, the type of surgery and intraoperatively monitored haemodynamic parameters.

Pharmacological Agents

Dopamine, fenoldopam, atrial natriuretic peptide, insulin-like growth factor-1 and diuretics have no role in the management of AKI [25]. Diuretics, however, may be useful in the management of volume overload.

The Special Case of Contrast Induced Nephropathy

The incidence of contrast induced AKI remains high, despite the introduction of novel iso-osmolar and low-osmolar contrast agents. The most important and effective measure to be taken is obviously to avoid contrast exposure: minimize the number of diagnostic or therapeutic procedures that require the injection of contrast and minimize the amount of contrast dye, especially in patients with preexisting renal dysfunction. Fluid loading with normal saline is the only preventive measure found to have a consistent protective effect. Because the benefits of n-acetylcysteine or a bicarbonate sodium infusion remain unproven, they cannot be recommended as a standard of care.

Recent data indicate that the use of CO_2 as a contrast agent should be considered if iodinated contrast agents are contraindicated, either absolutely (contrast agent allergy) or relatively (preexisting renal dysfunction). In certain procedures such as in TIPS (transvenous intrajugular portosystemic shunt placement) CO_2 may be superior to iodinated contrast agents.

Application of Mathematical Modelling to Predict Acute Kidney Injury

Risk Prediction: Difficulties in Applying Models to Acute Kidney Injury

Digitalization has allowed large amounts of data to be stored and analysed. Electronic Health Records (EHR) and Hospital Information Systems (HIS) contain huge amounts of clinical data that can be used to discover new relationships between clinical data and outcomes. The Acute Dialysis Quality Initiative (ADQI) Group proposed to conduct data mining of the EHR to derive models with predictive ability for AKI [26]. This proposal comes from the fact that AKI is associated with poor short- and long-term outcomes [27] and because there still is no effective therapy to prevent AKI. It is expected that predictive models can help modify clinical care pathways and implement preventive interventions to improve outcome.

For a predictive model to be useful, the ADQI Group recommends that it must be able to predict AKI as far as 48–72 h in advance of the scheduled intervention because that is the time interval that would be needed to take proactive measures.

This 48–72 hour period seems a reasonable tradeoff between model accuracy and the time needed for the care team to implement the necessary measures to prevent its development, such as considering the use of CO_2, discussing avoiding other nephrotoxic drugs, assessing fluid status, and/or optimizing haemodynamics. The primary focus should be on models that try to predict 'moderate/severe' AKI, defined as KDIGO [25] stage 2 or 3, including those with renal replacement therapy.

During model derivation, well established risk factors from literature should be considered, along with novel risk factors identified via machine learning techniques. Models must include general variables with known renal implications (i.e. baseline renal function, medications, hypertension, age, diabetes, etc.). In addition to these factors, a positive fluid balance has been associated with increased mortality in both paediatric and adult patients with AKI.

New data analysis techniques should detect and extract significant and clinically reasonable trends, and extract new variables that will improve the predictive accuracy of the model. The recommended approaches range from neuronal networks, random forests, cluster analysis and principal component analysis, to support vector machines.

Finally, after having detected and selected variables and having developed a predictive model, the AQDI Group proposes that the final predictive algorithm be directly integrated into theatre so that it can be used in real time, e.g. to issue special alerts to try to prevent AKI development.

Conclusions

AKI most often becomes apparent during the postoperative period or in the intensive care unit. Intraoperatively, oliguria is probably the only direct biomarker of renal function, but unfortunately its predictive value for AKI is poor. Avoiding nephrotoxic drugs and maintaining stable haemodynamics should be considered as constituting preventive measures to avoid AKI. Finally, because of its late diagnosis and the limited treatment options, prediction tools for AKI may gain relevance in the near future. New insights and technology offer the exciting possibility to predict the occurrence of AKI well before the surgical procedure is scheduled, so that pro-active measures taken during the perioperative period (before, during and after anaesthesia and surgery) may allow a personalized approach that might alter outcome.

References

1. Bartels K, Karhausen J, Clambey ET, Grenz A, Eltzschig HK: Perioperative organ injury. Anesthesiology. 2013; 119: 1474–89.

2. Bellomo R, Ronco C, Kellum JA, Mehta RL, Palevsky P: Acute renal failure – definition, outcome measures, animal models, fluid therapy and information technology needs: the Second International Consensus Conference of the Acute Dialysis Quality Initiative (ADQI) Group. Crit.Care 2004; 8: R204–12.

3. Susantitaphong P, Cruz DN, Cerda J, Abulfaraj M, Alqahtani F, Koulouridis I, Jaber BL: World incidence of AKI: a meta-analysis. Clin.J.Am.Soc.Nephrol. 2013; 8: 1482–93.

4. Goren O, Matot I: Perioperative acute kidney injury. Br.J.Anaesth. 2015; 115 Suppl 2: ii3–14.

5. Prowle JR, Liu Y-L, Licari E, Bagshaw SM, Egi M, Haase M, Haase-Fielitz A, Kellum JA, Cruz D, Ronco C, Tsutsui K, Uchino S, Bellomo R: Oliguria as predictive biomarker of acute kidney injury in critically ill patients. Crit.Care 2011; 15: R172.

6. Kheterpal S, Tremper KK, Englesbe MJ, O'Reilly M, Shanks AM, Fetterman DM, Rosenberg AL, Swartz RD: Predictors of postoperative acute renal failure after noncardiac surgery in patients with previously normal renal function. Anesthesiology. 2007; 107: 892–902.

7. Novis BK, Roizen MF, Aronson S, Thisted RA: Association of preoperative risk factors with postoperative acute renal failure. Anesth.Analg. 1994; 78: 143–9.

8. Lote CJ: Renal blood flow and glomerular filtration rate. In Lote CJ, *Principles of Renal Physiology*. New York, NY: Springer, 2013: 83–92.

9. Bellomo R, Giantomasso DD: Noradrenaline and the kidney: friends or foes? Crit.Care. 2001; 5: 294–8.

10. Marik PE: Iatrogenic salt water drowning and the hazards of a high central venous pressure. Ann.Intens. Care. 2014; 4: 21.

11. Hoste EAJ, Bagshaw SM, Bellomo R, Cely CM, Colman R, Cruz DN, et al.: Epidemiology of acute kidney injury in critically ill patients: the multinational AKI-EPI study. Intens.Care.Med. 2015; 41: 1411–23.

12. Prowle J, Bagshaw SM, Bellomo R: Renal blood flow, fractional excretion of sodium and acute kidney injury: time for a new paradigm? Curr.Opin.Crit.Care. 2012; 18: 585–92.

13. Schneider AG, Bellomo R: Urinalysis and pre-renal acute kidney injury: time to move on. Crit.Care. 2013; 17: 141.

14. Sharfuddin A, Molitoris B: Pathophysiology of ischemic acute kidney injury. Nat.Rev.Nephrol. 2011; 7: 189–200.

15. Prowle JR, Kirwan CJ, Bellomo R: Fluid management for the prevention and attenuation of acute kidney injury. Nat.Rev.Nephrol. 2014; 10: 37–47.

16a. Prowle JR, Echeverri JE, Ligabo EV, Ronco C, Bellomo R: Fluid balance and acute kidney injury. Nat.Rev. Nephrol. 2009; 6: 107–15.

16b. Myles PS, Bellomo R, Corcoran T, Forbes A, Peyton P, et al: Restrictive versus liberal fluid therapy for major abdominal surgery. N.Engl.J.Med. 201; 378: 2263–74.

17. Ostermann M, Joannidis M: Acute kidney injury 2016: diagnosis and diagnostic workup. Crit.Care 2016; 20: 299.

18. Uchino S, Kellum JA, Bellomo R, Doig GS, Morimatsu H, Morgera S, Schetz M, Tan I, Bouman C, Macedo E, Gibney N, Tolwani A, Ronco C: Acute renal failure in critically ill patients. J.Am.Med.Assoc. 2005; 294: 813–18.

19. Langenberg C, Bellomo R, May C, Wan L, Egi M, Morgera S. Renal blood flow in sepsis. Crit.Care 2005; 9: R363–74.

20. Murugan R, Karajala-Subramanyam V, Lee M, Yende S, Kong L, Carter M, Angus DC, Kellum JA: Genetic and inflammatory markers of sepsis (GenIMS) investigators. Acute kidney injury in non-severe pneumonia is associated with an increased immune response and lower survival. Kidney.Int. 2010; 77: 527–35.

21. Langenberg C, Bagshaw SM, May CN, Bellomo R: The histopathology of septic acute kidney injury: a systematic review. Crit.Care 2008; 12: R38.

22. Gomez H, Ince C, De Backer D, Pickkers P, Payen D, Hotchkiss J, Kellum J: A unified theory of sepsis-induced acute kidney injury. Shock. 2014; 41: 3–11.

23. Joannidis M, Druml W, Forni LG, Groeneveld ABJ, Honore P, Oudemans-van Straaten HM, Ronco C, Schetz MRC, Woittiez AJ: Prevention of acute kidney injury and protection of renal function in the intensive care unit. Expert opinion of the Working Group for Nephrology, ESICM. Intens.Care.Med. 2010; 36: 392–411.

24. Legrand M, Dupuis C, Simon C, Gayat E, Mateo J, Lukaszewicz AC, Payen D: Association between systemic hemodynamics and septic acute kidney injury in critically ill patients: a retrospective observational study. Crit.Care 2013; 17: R278.

25. Group KDIGO (KDIGO) AKIW. KDIGO clinical practice guideline for acute kidney injury. Kidney.Inter. 2012; 2: 1–138.

26. Sutherland SM, Chawla LS, Kane-Gill SL, Hsu RK, Kramer AA, Goldstein SL, Kellum JA, Ronco C, Bagshaw SM: Utilizing electronic health records to predict acute kidney injury risk and outcomes: workgroup statements from the 15(th) ADQI Consensus Conference. Can.J.Kidney.Heal.Dis. 2016; 3: 11.

27. Chertow GM, Burdick E, Honour M, Bonventre J V, Bates DW: Acute kidney injury, mortality, length of stay, and costs in hospitalized patients. J.Am.Soc. Nephrol. 2005; 16: 3365–70.

Effects on Liver Function

Andre M. De Wolf and Jan F. A. Hendrickx

Summary

Liver surgery can be remarkably safe: a zero mortality rate has been achieved with liver resections when patients are properly selected and with meticulous perioperative care [1]. In order to maintain liver function in individual patients undergoing anaesthesia and surgery, the single most important factor is maintaining its perfusion. In order to avoid hypoxic liver injury, preserving sinusoidal blood flow is best done by maintaining an adequate perfusion pressure and avoiding a high central venous pressure. Reducing intraoperative blood loss and maintaining systemic haemodynamics likely play major roles in avoiding hypoxic liver injury. It is still unknown which vasoactive drugs are preferred when haemodynamic instability occurs; Noradrenaline seems to be well tolerated as long as hypovolaemia is avoided. Ischaemic preconditioning and pharmacological preconditioning and postconditioning are promising, but their clinical relevance remains to be determined. Finally there are no good markers of hepatocyte damage that could be used intraoperatively to optimize anaesthetic management.

Introduction

The goal of every anaesthesiologist is not just to anaesthetize the patient but also to protect the patient from potential harm, including that as a result of tissue injury caused by the surgical procedure. One of the key organs that has to be protected is the liver, because a properly functioning liver is required for survival. With minor surgery, there is virtually no chance that the liver can be harmed to any significant degree, and this is true whether the liver is healthy or diseased. In this situation the anaesthetic technique that is chosen plays virtually no role in the overall outcome of the liver, as long as global haemodynamics and oxygenation are maintained. Nevertheless, signs of minor liver injury postoperatively are not uncommon even in healthy patients [2]. The situation becomes more complex when the procedure is more extensive, with more tissue injury due to the surgery, with major abdominal

procedures influencing splanchnic blood flow, when the liver is the subject of the surgical procedure, and when dealing with a diseased liver. Thus factors that play a role are changes in global and regional circulation, liver versus non-liver surgery, and presence or absence of preexisting liver dysfunction as the diseased liver is more susceptible to further injury. Liver trauma or vascular injury during any liver surgery can result in major bleeding requiring temporary interruption of liver blood flow through the Pringle manoeuvre, achieved by placing a vascular clamp on the hepatic pedicle, thereby interrupting arterial and portal venous inflow into the liver. However, it should be of limited duration because the degree of tissue injury is related to the duration of ischaemia [3], and preferably it should be avoided completely unless the risk of major bleeding justifies its use.

There are two main mechanisms to injure the liver perioperatively: reduce its blood flow, or submit it to toxins. Since in general modern anaesthetic agents are not hepatotoxic, we will focus on reduced liver blood flow as the cause of perioperative liver dysfunction. Liver blood flow can be reduced as a result of global haemodynamic instability, or as a result of hepatic pedicle clamping (Pringle manoeuvre). The Pringle manoeuvre, in combination with low CVP, is used to reduce blood loss during parenchymal transection.

It is imperative to first discuss normal liver blood flow at a macro- AND a micro-level. It is also important to recognize why the diseased liver is more vulnerable to a further reduction in blood flow. How exactly the hepatic sinusoidal blood flow in liver disease is abnormal (liver fibrosis, liver cirrhosis) will be presented in order to appreciate that perioperative hepatic injury is more likely to occur in the already diseased liver.

Physiology

Liver Anatomy and Histology

Liver anatomy by itself is not really relevant to this topic. What is important is the histology: rows of hepatocytes are neatly lined up with the capillaries called sinusoids, separated by highly fenestrated endothelial cells; this results in an optimal environment for extensive bidirectional metabolic exchange between sinusoidal blood and hepatocytes. The space between the sinusoids and the hepatocytes is called the space of Disse and it contains loose connective tissue, phagocytic Kupffer cells and hepatic stellate cells (Ito cells). The excessive fluid in the space of Disse is drained into the lymphatic system (Fig. 17.1 and Fig. 17.2) [4, 5].

Liver Function

The function of the liver is complex; the liver is involved in production of most proteins in the blood (except immunoglobulins), including albumin, most coagulation factors and several inhibitors of the coagulation system. The liver plays a key role in carbohydrate metabolism, including storage (glycogen), glucose breakdown and gluconeogenesis. Lipid metabolism as well as cholesterol synthesis is complex. Bilirubin is cleared from the blood and after conjugation secreted into the intestinal tract with the bile. Bile production and secretion into the gut facilitates the digestion of ingested fats. Finally, biotransformation (deactivation but sometimes activation) of drugs, chemicals such as alcohol and endogenous substances occurs in the liver.

Global Liver Blood Flow

The liver receives a dual blood supply: the hepatic artery delivers oxygenated blood to the hepatic sinusoids, while the portal vein delivers partially deoxygenated but nutrient- and hormone-rich blood from the splanchnic organs. Hepatic arterial blood flow represents about 25–30% of total liver blood flow, and portal venous blood flow about 65–70%; each contributes about 50% of the oxygen supply to the liver. A decrease in hepatic oxygenation results in increased oxygen extraction rather than an increase in hepatic arterial blood flow [6]. A decrease in portal vein blood flow leads to dilatation of the hepatic artery, increasing hepatic arterial blood flow, and vice versa: this is the so-called hepatic arterial buffer response that is based on changes in adenosine concentrations [7, 8, 9].

Sinusoidal Blood Flow

Blood from the portal vein and hepatic artery perfuses the liver sinusoids, flowing towards the central vein of each liver lobule, eventually draining into the hepatic

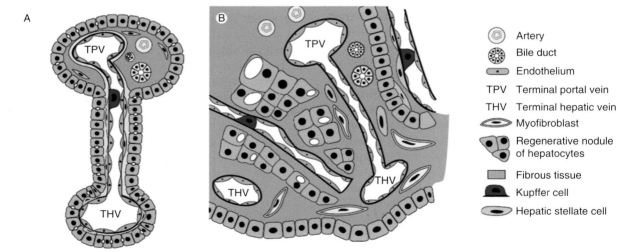

Fig. 17.1 Vascular and architectural alterations in cirrhosis. Hepatic sinusoids receive blood from the portal vein and hepatic artery. (A) Healthy liver: terminal portal tract blood runs through hepatic sinusoids where fenestrated sinusoidal endothelia that rest on loose connective tissue (space of Disse) allow for extensive metabolic exchange with the lobular hepatocytes; sinusoidal blood is collected by terminal hepatic venules that drain into one of the three hepatic veins and finally the inferior vena cava. (B) Cirrhotic liver: activated myofibroblasts that derive from perisinusoidal hepatic stellate cells (Ito cells) and portal or central-vein fibroblasts proliferate and produce excess extracellular matrix. This event leads to fibrous portal-tract expansion, central-vein fibrosis and capillarization of the sinusoids, characterized by loss of endothelial fenestrations, congestion of the space of Disse with extracellular matrix, and separation or encasement of perisinusoidal hepatocyte islands from sinusoidal blood flow by collagenous septa. Blood is directly shunted from terminal portal veins and arteries to central veins, with consequent (intrahepatic) portal hypertension and compromised liver synthetic function [4].

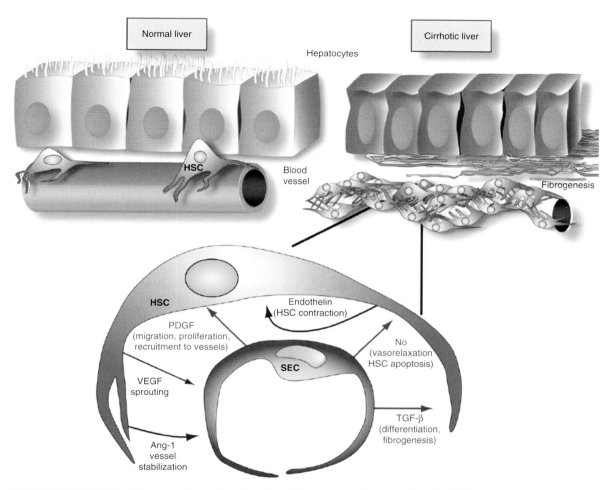

Fig. 17.2 Pathological sinusoidal remodelling in cirrhosis and portal hypertension. Hepatic stellate cells (HSC) align themselves around the sinusoidal lumen in order to induce contraction of the sinusoids. While in normal physiological conditions HSC contractility and coverage of sinusoids is sparse, in cirrhosis, increased numbers of HSC with increased cellular projections wrap more effectively around sinusoids, thereby contributing to a high-resistance, constricted sinusoidal vessel. At the cellular level, a number of growth factor molecules contribute to this process through autocrine and paracrine signalling between HSC and sinusoidal endothelial cells (SEC). A number of these molecules are depicted along with their proposed role in paracrine function. PDGF: platelet-derived growth factor; VEGF: vascular endothelial growth factor; Ang-1: angiopoietin 1; NO: nitric oxide; TGF-β: transforming growth factor beta [5].

veins. In the healthy liver the vascular resistance in the liver sinusoids is low.

Effects of Anaesthesia and Surgery on Liver Blood Flow and Liver Function

Every major anaesthetic technique (general anaesthesia, spinal and epidural anaesthesia) results in a reduction in total liver blood flow. The modern inhaled agents (sevoflurane, desflurane, isoflurane) reduce liver blood flow less than halothane. The reduction in liver blood flow is mainly the result of a reduction in cardiac output and portal venous blood flow; hepatic arterial blood flow usually increases as a result of the hepatic arterial buffer response, but this does not restore liver blood flow to normal levels [10]. In general, hypotension is associated with a reduction in liver blood flow. Halothane reduces total hepatic blood flow more than other agents because it also increases hepatic arterial vascular resistance [11]. Major surgery, but especially upper abdominal surgery, results in a further reduction in liver blood flow [10].

247

Intravenous anaesthetics and opioids probably have less effect on liver blood flow than inhaled anaesthetics, although they have not been studied as well. While thiopental and etomidate seem to decrease total liver blood flow, it is unchanged with ketamine and increased with propofol, likely the result of splanchnic vasodilatation which results in increased portal inflow [12]. Intravenous anaesthetics have little or no adverse effect on liver function when haemodynamics are maintained.

Liver function tests are usually mildly increased after surgery and anaesthesia [13, 14], but anaesthesia with modern potent inhaled anaesthetics without surgery does not result in abnormalities in liver function tests [15, 16, 17].

There are very few studies determining the effect of general anaesthesia on liver blood flow and hepatic function in patients with preexisting liver disease. Overall, current inhaled anaesthetics do not seem to affect liver function in adult surgical patients with chronic liver disease [18].

Xenon has no direct haemodynamic effects and does not seem to influence total liver blood flow. In addition, liver function tests remain unchanged after xenon anaesthesia. It may be the ideal anaesthetic with regard to hepatic perfusion and function although its potential hepatic protective effects remain unstudied [19].

Pathophysiology: Liver Fibrosis and Cirrhosis

Changes in Histology and Sinusoidal Blood Flow

The most typical forms of liver disease are fibrosis and cirrhosis. Fibrosis is an abnormal healing response to liver injury, with activation of Ito cells resulting in their proliferation. The Ito cells transform into active fibroblasts that deposit an excessive amount of fibrin strands in the peri-sinusoidal areas, and into myofibroblasts that can contract and increase the resistance to flow in the sinusoids. There is the formation of fibrous septa, interfering with the metabolic exchange between hepatocytes and sinusoidal blood (Fig. 17.1 and Fig. 17.2).

Cirrhosis is the progression of fibrosis with the creation of regenerative nodules whereby there is distortion of the hepatic vasculature resulting in a further increase in intrahepatic vascular resistance, causing portal hypertension. An abnormal balance between intrahepatic vasoconstrictors and vasodilators contributes to the increased intrahepatic vascular resistance. The space of Disse contains fibrous tissue, and in addition the endothelial fenestrations are lost; as a result the sinusoidal blood drains into the terminal hepatic veins without undergoing adequate metabolic exchange (Fig. 17.1 and Fig. 17.2).

Metabolic Changes

Liver fibrosis but especially liver cirrhosis has significant metabolic consequences; these are the direct result of the inadequate metabolic exchange between sinusoidal blood and hepatocytes. Cirrhosis results in hepatocellular dysfunction, leading to hyperbilirubinaemia, reduced synthesis of albumin and coagulation factors, and reduced clearance of toxins and intestinal vasoactive substances. Pharmacokinetics of drugs that undergo hepatic metabolism is altered. Portosystemic collateral circulation worsens the effects of hepatocellular dysfunction.

Changes in Sinusoid Blood Flow and Liver Blood Flow

Cirrhosis results in reduced sinusoidal perfusion due to the mechanical obstruction of the sinusoids by regenerative nodules and constriction of sinusoids by contraction of surrounding myofibroblasts, resulting in hepatocellular dysfunction and portal hypertension. The portal hypertension is aggravated by the reduced local production of nitric oxide and excessive production of vasoconstrictors, both the result of endothelial dysfunction. An increase in nitric oxide production in the splanchnic circulation, however, leads to an increased intestinal inflow, again worsening portal hypertension. Release of vascular endothelial growth factor in the splanchnic system results in the development of portosystemic shunts (collateral vessels between the portal vein and the azygos system), further contributing to overall hepatic dysfunction (portal blood bypassing the liver). Although poorly studied, it seems that the arterial inflow into the hepatic sinusoids in the cirrhotic liver is reduced.

Changes in Macrohaemodynamics

There is a change in global haemodynamics: hyperdynamic circulation with high cardiac output, low systemic vascular resistance and relatively low systemic blood pressure. The hepatocellular dysfunction and the blood bypassing the liver result in globally increased concentrations of nitric oxide, prostaglandins, oestrogen, bradykinin and vasoactive intestinal peptide. In addition, there is a reduced sensitivity to vasoconstrictors such as noradrenaline, vasopressin and endothelin-1 due to a decreased number of receptors and post-receptor defects. The low splanchnic vascular resistance is a major contributor to the low systemic vascular resistance. Although there is an increase in total blood volume, central blood volume is reduced, resulting in activation of baroreceptors with subsequent activation of compensatory mechanisms that are proportional to the degree of liver disease [20]. These profoundly affect the macrohaemodynamics: there is activation of the sympathetic nervous system, activation of the ADH–arginine–vasopressin pathway, activation of the renin–angiotensin–aldosterone system and increased concentrations of circulating endothelin. These compensatory systems result in further increases in heart rate and cardiac output, reduced renal perfusion (sodium and water retention) and overall a gradual decrease in effective organ perfusion. With progressive liver failure, these compensatory systems become insufficient to maintain effective tissue perfusion, ultimately resulting in multiorgan failure.

Although cirrhosis is typically associated with an increased cardiac output, there is impairment of cardiac function as a result of cirrhotic cardiomyopathy. Cirrhotic cardiomyopathy is characterized by the following triad: systolic and diastolic dysfunction in combination with electrophysiological abnormalities. Pathophysiological mechanisms of cirrhotic cardiomyopathy include downregulation of beta-receptors, abnormal excitation–contraction coupling, circulating myocardial depressant substances and areas of myocardial fibrosis and subendothelial oedema. Cardiac systolic dysfunction may initially not be apparent at rest because it is masked by the low systemic vascular resistance, but it can be provoked by cardiac stress such as placement of TIPS or liver transplantation, or increase in afterload as a result of vasopressin, terlipressin or noradrenaline administration. Left atrial enlargement is frequently seen on echocardiography, with a reduction in E/A ratio across the mitral valve (E wave reflects passive flow through the mitral valve, and A wave is the flow that results from atrial contraction). The change in E/A ratio is a reflection of LV diastolic dysfunction.

Anaesthetic Management in Patients with Liver Cirrhosis

The basic management of general anaesthesia changes little in the presence of cirrhosis. The main concern is the altered pharmacokinetics of anaesthetic agents, and the maintenance of liver blood flow. The use of drugs that are metabolized by the liver needs to be adjusted. For example, rocuronium has an increased duration of action in patients with liver cirrhosis, but this likely has become clinically irrelevant with the availability of sugammadex. Other aspects of anaesthetic management (global haemodynamic goals and management, choice of anaesthetic agents for their ischaemic preconditioning effect) will be discussed later in this chapter.

Perioperative Liver Injury

Hypoxic Liver Injury: Overview

Hypoxic liver injury is also called ischaemic hepatitis, shock liver or hypoxic hepatitis. Hypoxic liver injury is the result of an imbalance between hepatic oxygen supply and demand in the absence of other acute causes of liver damage, resulting in a diffuse hepatic injury. The direct cause is inadequate oxygen delivery to the liver. Most frequently it is caused by severe and prolonged hypotension and low cardiac output, but sometimes severe hypoxaemia or low haemoglobin concentration is the culprit. The Pringle manoeuvre interrupts liver blood flow completely and is obviously a risk factor. Rarely, increased oxygen consumption by the liver, seen with hyperthermia, could contribute to the imbalance. The severity of hypoxic liver injury depends on the duration of the insult. It is manifested by a large (usually > 10-fold) increase in serum transaminase levels which normalizes quickly over several days. During liver injury, intracellular enzymes such as AST and ALT are released into the plasma because of increased hepatocellular permeability. If the hypoxic injury is relatively mild, there will be acute hepatic impairment consisting of synthetic dysfunction (increased bilirubin, INR) and elimination dysfunction (e.g. reduced ICG clearance). Its more severe form is acute hepatic failure, characterized by encephalopathy, coagulation abnormalities, jaundice and intracranial hypertension; this has a high risk of mortality without liver transplantation. On liver biopsy centrilobular necrosis is seen because the area around the central vein is most prone to ischaemic damage. Differential diagnosis includes toxin-or drug-induced hepatitis (e.g. paracetamol) and acute viral hepatitis. It should be distinguished from hepatic infarction, which represents a focal injury to the liver. Treatment and prognosis are determined by the underlying disease. In the intensive care unit, hypoxic liver injury has a 50% mortality rate [21].

Risk Factors for Hypoxic Liver Injury

The diseased liver (liver fibrosis but especially cirrhosis) already has a reduced sinusoidal blood flow with inadequate metabolic exchange between sinusoidal blood and hepatocytes due to fibrosis; this makes the hepatocytes more susceptible to ischaemic injury, including in the perioperative setting. Portosystemic collaterals further reduce sinusoidal blood flow. Variceal bleeding, a common complication of cirrhosis, may result in hypotension, ultimately leading to hypoxic liver injury. Clinical experience has shown that anaesthesia and surgery in patients with cirrhosis carries increased risks, with an increase in perioperative mortality rate proportional to severity of liver cirrhosis, with abdominal and emergency procedures further increasing mortality [22].

Also, chronic hepatic congestion and sepsis increase the liver's susceptibility to hypoxic liver injury [23]. The increased hepatic vein pressure not just reduces hepatic perfusion but also promotes translocation of intestinal bacteria into the portal vein as a result of congested ischaemic bowel, leading to the exposure of the hepatocytes to endotoxins, as is the case with sepsis. Endotoxins cause Kupffer cells to release pro-inflammatory cytokines that result in translocation of neutrophils. Substances released by both Kupffer cells and activated neutrophils activate platelets, causing the formation of microthrombi in the hepatic vessels. The inflammatory process also results in a worsening of the hepatocyte function.

Mechanisms of Ischaemia–Reperfusion Injury

Injury to the liver after ischaemia becomes apparent only after restoration of blood flow. A complete discussion of the mechanisms of ischaemia–reperfusion injury is beyond the scope of this chapter. Briefly, the initial injury is the deprivation of the organ of tissue oxygen. The severity of organ injury depends on the extent of activation of the Kupffer cells, the degree of platelet and leucocyte activation, and the extent of production of inflammatory mediators [24]. Reperfusion of the tissues following a period of ischaemia results in the generation of oxygen-derived radicals or reactive

oxygen species and other mediators; this leads to production of pro-inflammatory mediators and activation of neutrophils, eventually resulting in tissue damage and potentially cell death. Sinusoidal endothelial cells are susceptible to cold ischaemia, leading to increased expression of vWF on their surface, resulting in platelet adhesion to the endothelial cell surface. Activation of Kupffer cells results in the release of reactive oxygen species and cytokines. Thus, hepatic injury occurs as the result of increased hepatic reactive oxygen species production, cellular pH changes, increased inflammatory responses and reduced hepatic microcirculation by sinusoidal vasoconstriction. Hepatic steatosis worsens the outcome of ischaemia–reperfusion because steatotic livers are less tolerant to the ischaemia–reperfusion insult [25]. Techniques that may temper this ischaemia–reperfusion injury will be discussed later.

Other Causes of Perioperative Liver Injury

Drug-related hepatotoxicity is fairly uncommon (except for paracetamol). Other potential causes of acute liver injury include toxins, acute hepatitis and autoimmune hepatitis. Early administration of intravenous N-acetylcysteine in non-paracetamol acute liver failure patients with encephalopathy is associated with an improved outcome [26].

Management of Perioperative Liver Injury

Management is based on the correct diagnosis and identification of the cause of the perioperative liver injury. Obviously if drug toxicity is suspected the causative agent should be discontinued. Supportive therapy should be initiated, but there is little direct intervention. It seems logical to maintain adequate organ perfusion, fluid balance and electrolyte concentrations.

Intraoperative Monitoring of Liver Well-being

Macrohaemodynamic Monitoring

Although there is an unclear relationship between global haemodynamics and liver perfusion, it is generally accepted that low cardiac output and hypotension result in hypoperfusion of the liver. Therefore, monitoring to allow proper maintenance and correction of cardiac output and perfusion pressure may include the use of a central venous catheter, pulmonary artery catheter and arterial catheter, depending on the expected haemodynamic instability and bleeding during the procedure. Also, it remains unclear whether monitoring of global oxygen delivery (DO_2) can improve liver outcome. Finally transoesophageal echocardiography (TEE) helps in the early detection of liver outflow obstruction, allowing swift correction [27]; this does not mean that TEE should be used routinely during liver resection.

Microhaemodynamic Monitoring

Currently there are no microhaemodynamic monitoring tools available for routine clinical use. However, there are a few technologies that have been used experimentally, for example laser Doppler flowmetry, near-infrared spectroscopy, and in vivo fluorescence microscopy [28]. Although some of these are promising, none of these techniques is currently ready for clinical use.

Monitoring of Splanchnic Microcirculation

There may be a relationship between the microcirculation in sublingual and intestinal vascular beds during haemorrhagic shock [29, 30]. Preoperative abnormalities in sublingual microvascular flow seem to predispose to postoperative complications after major abdominal surgery, while global oxygen delivery or cutaneous tissue oxygenation did not correlate with the postoperative complication rate. It is unclear whether this monitoring technique has true value in monitoring liver tissue well-being. Gastric tonometry attempts to estimate gastric mucosal perfusion by determining the mucosal carbon dioxide partial pressure. However, outcome of clinical management based on gastric tonometry was no better than control, and the use of gastric tonometry has waned [31].

Markers of Liver Injury

Traditional Markers of Liver Injury

The most commonly used markers of liver injury include plasma concentrations of bilirubin, albumin, coagulation factors (the last one frequently assessed indirectly by PT and overall coagulation tests) and 'liver enzymes'.

Hyperbillirubinaemia is a common marker of liver injury. Total bilirubin represents both conjugated ('direct') bilirubin and unconjugated ('indirect') bilirubin. Enzymes in the microsomes of hepatocytes convert unconjugated bilirubin into the more water-soluble conjugated bilirubin, allowing excretion in bile. Unconjugated hyperbilirubinaemia is seen in haemolysis or Gilbert syndrome, while conjugated hyperbilirubinaemia suggests cholestasis or hepatocellular dysfunction. Bile acids may be a better marker of hepatic biotransformation and cholestatic dysfunction than bilirubin [32, 33]. However, changes in bilirubin concentrations are not fast enough to detect intraoperative liver dysfunction.

Plasma concentrations of proteins synthesized by the liver do help in the assessment of liver function. However, since albumin has a half-life of about 21 days, it is not suited to detect acute liver dysfunction.

Because the half-life of clotting factors II, VII, IX and X is < 24 h, prothrombin time or INR could be a better marker of acute liver dysfunction. However, this one too may not be very helpful for the intraoperative determination of hepatic well-being because the half-lives of the clotting factors are still too long. Furthermore, coagulation changes can be induced by other factors, such as haemodilution, activation of the coagulation system (release of tissue factor) or activation of the fibrinolytic system. Therefore, changes in INR or in viscoelastic measures of coagulation (such as TEG and ROTEM) still don't reflect acute changes in liver function intraoperatively.

The so-called liver function tests [such as aspartate aminotransferase or AST (not specific for liver damage), and alanine transaminase or ALT] reflect the release of these enzymes from damaged or necrotic hepatocytes. Another enzyme that is released with hepatocyte injury is lactate dehydrogenase, also a non-specific marker of ischaemic damage. However, the intraoperative and early postoperative determination of liver enzymes suffers from the same shortcomings as the ones previously mentioned: they reflect hepatocyte damage but provide no information about the function of the remaining hepatocytes. Thus, mild elevations of liver enzymes are common during and immediately after liver surgery but have little prognostic value.

Hepatic Clearance Tests

There are other tests that have the potential to determine liver function in a hyperacute setting: indocyanine green (ICG) and lactate clearance tests. Although these tests clearly are much more indicative of true liver function than the so-called liver function tests, they are also dependent on liver perfusion. It is well known that anaesthesia and surgery (especially major and upper abdominal surgery) affect total liver blood flow, and this will affect the clearance tests. In addition, the results are much less reliable in the presence of hyperbilirubinaemia (for ICG, due to competition for the same carrier) and severe peripheral hypoperfusion [34]. Furthermore, in the case of lactate, there are variable degrees of lactate production and metabolism during surgery. And then these tests take too long to allow intraoperative management changes. Therefore, the main use of clearance tests is in the determination of liver function preoperatively (before liver resection) [35], and to determine liver function postoperatively after liver resection and transplantation [36]. Even if these tests could be done in a timely manner, it is unclear how intraoperative management would be affected. In conclusion, there are no good intraoperative tests to determine liver function or hepatocyte well-being.

Prevention of Perioperative Liver Injury

Prevention of hepatic injury is based mainly on preservation of liver blood flow. How this should be clinically accomplished is unclear, since we can only determine global haemodynamics, such as blood pressure, central venous pressure or pulmonary artery pressures, and cardiac output. The relationship between these global haemodynamic parameters and liver blood flow is vague. Also, the liver blood flow is complex, with a portal venous component and a hepatic arterial component. Although we have some knowledge about the effect of global haemodynamics on liver blood flow, it is unclear how quickly haemodynamic instability results in ischaemic injury to the liver.

Haemodynamic Monitoring

Intraoperative haemodynamic monitoring is determined by the expected changes in volume status and haemodynamics, and may include direct invasive arterial pressure monitoring, central venous pressure monitoring and pulmonary artery catheterization. TEE is virtually never used during liver surgery except in the intraoperative management of a specific cardiac issue (e.g. asymmetrical septal hypertrophy with left ventricular outflow tract obstruction). These monitors serve as a guide to normalize global haemodynamics. However, they are not really helpful to improve or optimize the hepatic microcirculation. For example, splanchnic blood flow does not necessarily increase with an increase in cardiac output. Nevertheless, most

agree that a decrease in cardiac output and systemic vascular resistance, and an increase in central venous pressure all reduce hepatic blood flow [37, 38, 39]. Because there is no clinical monitoring tool available to guide our interventions to improve microcirculatory blood flow to the liver, we continue to use macro-haemodynamic variables to guide us.

Haemodynamic Management

It is obvious that hypovolaemia should be appropriately corrected to restore cardiac output, perfusion pressure and oxygen delivery to the tissues while avoiding overfilling the patient, since high central venous pressure reduces liver blood flow and increases perioperative blood loss. Cardiac dysfunction as the cause of low cardiac output should be appropriately treated, if necessary with inotropic agents. Hypoxaemia should be managed depending on its cause. Excessively low systemic vascular resistance as the cause of severe hypotension in patients with liver cirrhosis has been treated with infusions of noradrenaline and/or vasopressin (or analogues) without significant detrimental effects on liver function but with improvement in renal function [40, 41, 42]. It is very difficult to determine the effects of vasoactive agents on liver perfusion. First of all, these agents have a complex effect on splanchnic perfusion, and therefore on portal venous blood flow. In addition, they also affect hepatic arterial blood flow and sinusoidal vascular resistance. There is some information regarding this in specific situations and in certain species. For example, in a sepsis model in pigs, adrenaline and noradrenaline increased systemic blood flow but did not improve splanchnic microcirculation because they appeared to divert blood flow away from the splanchnic organs. Phenylephrine, however, increased blood pressure and splanchnic microperfusion without changing blood flow distribution [43]. A meta-analysis comparing noradrenaline with vasopressin in patients with septic shock found no difference in outcome [44]. In patients with shock (any cause), noradrenaline may be safer than dopamine [45, 46]. It is unclear whether these observations stand in humans with liver disease. Thus, the effects of vasoactive agents on splanchnic and liver blood flow are complex, difficult to monitor, differ from species to species and may be affected by the anaesthetic that is used [47]. It may be difficult to draw conclusions regarding tissue oxygenation and perfusion based on systemic oxygen transport parameters.

Preconditioning and Postconditioning

Preconditioning attempts to protect the organ from ischaemia–reperfusion injury. Postconditioning attempts to modulate cell injury and cell death after periods of ischaemia/anoxia by administering drugs after the ischaemic insult has occurred.

Ischaemic preconditioning is achieved by briefly interrupting blood flow to the organ to generate a few minutes of ischaemia, followed by reperfusion. It is still unclear how long the initial ischaemic period should last; 10 min may be better than 5 min [48]. This process induces intracellular responses to ischaemia which render the tissues more resistant to the subsequent ischaemic insult of longer duration [49]. However, a systematic review concluded that currently the routine use of ischaemic preconditioning in liver surgery cannot be supported nor refuted due to the unproven clinical benefit [50]. A variant of this is remote ischaemic preconditioning: transient warm ischaemia–reperfusion of other tissues (e.g. limbs) may have a protective effect on the organ that will be rendered ischaemic.

Pharmacological preconditioning makes use of drugs to reduce the ischaemia–reperfusion injury. Agents that have been studied include potent inhaled anaesthetics (isoflurane, sevoflurane). Sevoflurane has been shown to have ischaemic preconditioning effects on hepatic function [51, 52]. These agents have also been used for pharmacological postconditioning: mitigating the deleterious ischaemia–reperfusion injury by administering these drugs after the insult has occurred. Propofol also has preconditioning effects in patients undergoing partial hepatectomies [53]. Opioid preconditioning via inducible NO synthase expression and early neuronal and delayed inducible NO synthase blockade has been shown to attenuate liver injury [54, 55].

Surgical Interventions to Prevent Perioperative Liver Injury

Surgeons should try to minimize liver injury by resecting as little liver tissue as possible, and by paying meticulous attention to haemostasis. As mentioned in the introduction, the Pringle manoeuvre should be avoided if at all possible. It is obvious that, when indicated, intraoperative liver blood should be measured in the field with magnetic flow probes or with Doppler probes; this would allow early revision of vascular anastomoses when indicated.

A recently recognized issue is the small-for-size syndrome: resection of part of the liver may result in deleterious excessive portal flow, beyond a certain threshold (portal hyperperfusion syndrome), to the remaining liver tissue. There are several surgical techniques available to prevent this complication, such as splenic artery ligation or embolization, splenectomy or the creation of a portocaval shunt [56, 57].

Preoperative selective portal vein embolization has been utilized when liver resection is expected to result in insufficient remnant liver volume, because this intervention stimulates growth of the future remnant liver [58].

Extracorporeal artificial liver support systems could be used to provide support until the liver function has recovered. The most commonly used systems are molecular adsorbents recirculatory systems (MARS), fractionated plasma separation and adsorption (EPSA or Prometheus) and single-pass albumin dialysis (SPAD). These systems contain live hepatocytes, but they all suffer from poor functionality over longer time periods. Modern stem cell technology may allow the development of bioactive systems that can provide support for longer periods of time [59].

Conclusion

There are remarkably few intraoperative adjustments that can be made in order to avoid liver damage during general anaesthesia. This is the case for patients undergoing non-liver surgery, liver surgery or any surgery in the presence of liver disease. In general it is strongly recommended to maintain liver perfusion through maintenance of volume status and cardiac output. If it is absolutely required to reduce or stop liver blood flow during liver resection in order to avoid major blood loss, then the ischaemic time should be as short as possible. Intraoperative markers of hepatocyte well-being are currently not available. Finally the value of ischaemic and pharmacological preconditioning remains to be determined clinically.

References

1. Imamura H, Seyama Y, Kokudo N, Maema A, Sugawara Y, Sano K, Takayama T, Makuuch M: One thousand fifty-six hepatectomies without mortality in 8 years. Arch.Surg. 2003; 138: 1198–206.

2. Pratt DS, Kaplan MM: Evaluation of abnormal liver-enzyme results in asymptomatic patients. N. Engl.J.Med. 2000; 342: 1266–71.

3. Gujral JS, Bucci TJ, Farhood A, et al: Mechanism of cell death during warm hepatic ischemia-reperfusion in rats: apoptosis or necrosis? Hepatology. 2001; 33: 397–405.

4. Schuppan D, Afdhal NH. Liver cirrhosis. Lancet. 2008; 371: 838–51.

5. Thabut D, Shah V: Intrahepatic angiogenesis and sinusoidal remodeling in chronic liver disease: new targets for the treatment of portal hypertension? J. Hepatol. 2010; 53: 976–80.

6. Scholtholt J, Shiraishi T: Effect of generalized hypoxia, hypocapnia and hypercapnia on blood flow in the liver and splanchnic region of the anesthetized dog. Pflugers.Arch. 1970; 318: 185–201.

7. Lautt WW: Mechanism and role of intrinsic regulation of hepatic arterial blood flow: hepatic arterial buffer response. Am.J.Physiol. 1985; 249 (5 Pt 1): G549–56.

8. Lautt WW, Legare DJ, d'Almeida MS: Adenosine as putative regulator of hepatic arterial flow (the buffer response). Am.J.Physiol. 1985; 248 (3 Pt 2): H331–8.

9. Lautt WW: Regulatory processes interacting to maintain hepatic blood flow constancy: vascular compliance, hepatic arterial buffer response, hepatorenal reflex, liver regeneration, escape from vasoconstriction. Hepatol.Res. 2007; 37: 891–903.

10. Gelman S: General anesthesia and hepatic circulation. Can.J.Physiol.Pharmacol. 1987; 65: 1762–79.

11. Gatecel C, Losser MR, Payen D: The postoperative effects of halothane versus isoflurane on hepatic artery and portal vein blood flow in humans. Anesth.Analg. 2003; 96: 740–5.

12. Wouters PF, Van de Velde MA, Marcus MAE, Deruyter HA, Van Aken H: Hemodynamic changes during induction of anesthesia with eltanolone and propofol in dogs. Anesth.Analg. 1995; 81: 125–31.

13. Suttner SW, Schmidt CC, Boldt J, Huttner I, Kumle B, Piper SN: Low-flow desflurane and sevoflurane anesthesia minimally affect hepatic integrity and function in elderly patients. Anesth.Analg. 2000; 91: 206–12.

14. Arslan M, Kurtipek O, Dogan AT, Ünal Y, Kizil Y, Nurlu N, Kamici S, Kavutvu M: Comparison of effects of anaesthesia with desflurane and enflurane on liver function. Singapore.Med.J. 2009; 50: 73–7.

15. Holmes MA, Weiskopf RB, Eger EI II, Johnson BH, Rampil IJ: Hepatocellular integrity in swine after prolonged desflurane (I-653) and isoflurane anesthesia: evaluation of plasma alanine aminotransferase activity. Anesth.Analg. 1990; 71: 249–53.

16. Weiskopf RB, Eger EI II, Ionescu P, Yasuda N, Cahalan MK, Freire B, Peterson N, Lockhart SH, Rampil IJ, Laster M: Desflurane does not produce hepatic or renal injury in human volunteers. Anesth.Analg. 1992; 74: 570–4.

17. Ebert TJ, Messana LD, Ulrich T, Staacke T: Absence of renal and hepatic toxicity after four hours of 1.25 minimal alveolar anesthetic concentration sevoflurane anesthesia in humans. Anesth.Analg. 1998; 86: 662–7.

18. Zaleski L, Abello D, Gold MI: Desflurane versus isoflurane in patients with chronic hepatic and renal disease. Anesth.Analg. 1993; 76: 353–6.

19. Reinelt H, Marx T, Kotzerke J, Topalidis P, Luederwald S, Armbruster S, Schirmer U, Schmidt M: Hepatic function during xenon anesthesia in pigs. Acta. Anaesth.Scand. 2002; 46: 713–16.

20. Møller S, Henriksen JH, Bendtsen F: Extrahepatic complications to cirrhosis and portal hypertension: haemodynamic and homeostatic aspects. World.J. Gastroenterol. 2014; 20: 15499–517.

21. Fuhrmann V, Kneidinger N, Herkner H, et al: Hypoxic hepatitis: underlying conditions and risk factors for mortality in critically ill patients. Intens.Care.Med. 2009; 35: 1397–1405.

22. Wong R, Rappaport W, Witte C, Hunter G, Jaffe P, Hall K, Witzke D: Risk of nonshunt abdominal operation in the patient with cirrhosis. J.Am.Coll.Surg. 1994; 179: 412–16.

23. Ebert EC: Hypoxic liver injury. Mayo.Clin.Proc. 2006; 81: 1232–6.

24. de Rougemont O, Dutkowski P, Clavien PA: Biological modulation of liver ischemia-reperfusion injury. Curr. Opin.Organ.Transplant. 2010; 15: 183–9.

25. Veteläinen R, van Vliet A, Gouma DJ, van Gulik TM: Steatosis as a risk factor in liver surgery. Ann.Surg. 2007; 245: 20–30.

26. Lee WM, Hynan LS, Rossaro L, Fontana RJ, Stravitz RT, Larson AM, Davern TJ 2nd, Murray NG, McCashland T, Reisch JR, Robuck PR: Acute Liver Failure Study Group. Intravenous N-acetylcysteine improves transplant-free survival in early stage non-acetaminophen acute liver failure. Gastroenterology. 2009; 137: 856–64.

27. De Wolf AM, Scott VL, Kang Y, Mandel M, Madariega J: Hepatic venous outflow obstruction during hepatic resection diagnosed by transesophageal echocardiography. Anesthesiology. 1994; 80: 1398–1400.

28. Vollmar B, Menger MD: The hepatic microcirculation: mechanistic contributions and therapeutic targets in liver injury and repair. Physiol.Rev. 2009; 89: 1269–1339.

29. Dubin A, Pozo MO, Ferrara G, et al: Systemic and microcirculatory responses to progressive hemorrhage. Intens.Care.Med. 2009; 35: 556–64.

30. Jhanji S, Lee C, Watson D, et al: Microvascular flow and tissue oxygenation after major abdominal surgery: association with postoperative complications. Intens. Care.Med. 2009; 35: 671–7.

31. The Miami Trauma Clinical Trials Group: Splanchnic hypoperfusion-directed therapies in trauma: a prospective, randomized trial. Am.Surgeon. 2005; 71: 252–60.

32. Vanwijngaerden YM, Wauters J, Langouche L, et al: Critical illness evokes elevated circulating bile acids related to altered hepatic transporter and nuclear receptor expression. Hepatology. 2011; 54: 1741–52.

33. Recknagel P, Gonnert FA, Westermann M, et al: Liver dysfunction and phosphatidylinositol-3-kinase signaling in early sepsis: experimental models in rodent models of peritonitis. PLoS.Med. 2012; 9: e1001338.

34. De Gasperi A, Mazza E, Prosperi M: Indocyanine green kinetics to assess liver function: ready for a clinical dynamic assessment in major liver surgery? World.J. Hepatol. 2016; 8: 355–67.

35. Haegele S, Reiter S, Wanek D, Offensperger F, Pereyra D, Stremitzer S, Fleischmann E, Brostjan C, Gruenberger T, Starlinger P: Perioperative non-invasive indocyanine green-clearance testing to predict postoperative outcome after liver resection. PLoS.One. 2016; 11 (11): e016581.

36. Olmedilla L, Lisbona CJ, Pérez-Peña JM, López-Baena JA, Garutti I, Salcedo M, Sanz J, Tisner M, Asencio JM, Fernández-Quero L, Bañares R: Early measurement of indocyanine green clearance accurately predicts short-term outcomes after liver transplantation. Transplantation. 2016; 100: 613–20.

37. Pannen BH: New insights into the regulation of hepatic blood flow after ischemia and reperfusion. Anesth. Analg. 2002; 94: 1448–57.

38. Brienza N, Ayuse T, O'Donnell CP, et al: Regional control of venous return: liver blood flow. Am.J.Respir. Crit.Care.Med. 1995a; 152: 511–18.

39. Brienza N, Revelly JP, Auyse T, et al: Effects of PEEP on liver arterial and venous blood flows. Am.J.Respir.Crit. Care.Med. 1995b; 152: 504–10.

40. Møller S, Bendtsen F, Henriksen JH: Pathophysiological basis of pharmacotherapy in the hepatorenal syndrome. Scand.J.Gastroenterol. 2005; 40: 491–500.

41. Krag A, Borup T, Møller S, Bendtsen F: Efficacy and safety of terlipressin in cirrhotic patients with variceal bleeding and hepatorenal syndrome. Adv.Ther. 2008; 25: 1105–40.

42. Wong F: Hepatorenal syndrome: current management. Curr.Gastroenterol.Rep. 2008; 10: 22–9.

43. Krejci V, Hiltebrand LB, Sigurdsson GH: Effects of epinephrine, Norepinephrine, and phenylephrine on microcirculatory blood flow in the gastrointestinal tract in sepsis. Crit.Care.Med. 2006; 4: 1456–63.

44. Zhou FH, Song Q: Clinical trials comparing Norepinephrine with vasopressin in patients with septic shock: a meta-analysis. Military.Med.Res. 2014; 1: 6.

45. De Backer D, Biston P, Devriendt J, Madi C, Chrochrad D, Aldecoa C, Brasseur A, Defrance P, Gottignies P, Vincent JL: Comparison of dopamine and Norepinephrine in the treatment of shock. N. Engl.J.Med. 2010; 362: 779–89.

46. De Backer D, Aldecoa C, Njimi H, Vincent JL: Dopamine versus Norepinephrine in the treatment of septic shock: a meta-analysis. Crit.Care.Med. 2012; 40: 725–30.

47. Hasibeder W: Gastrointestinal microcirculation: still a mystery? Br.J.Anaesth. 2010; 105: 393–6.

48. DeOliveira ML, Graf R, Clavien PA: Ischemic preconditioning: promises from the laboratory to patients – sustained or disillusioned? Am.J.Transplant. 2008; 8: 489–91.

49. Morris CF, Tahir M, Arshid S, Castro MS, Fontes W: Reconciling the IPC and two-hit models: dissecting the underlying cellular and molecular mechanisms of two seemingly opposing frameworks. J.Immunol.Res. 2015; 2015: 697193.

50. Chu MJJ, Vather R, Hickey AJR, Phillips ARJ, Bartlett ASJR: Impact of ischemic preconditioning on outcome in clinical liver surgery: a systematic review. BioMed. Res.Intern. 2015; 370451.

51. Bedirli N, Ofluoglu E, Kerem M, Utebey G, Alper M, Yilmazer D, Berdirli A, Ozlu O, Pasaoglu H: Hepatic energy metabolism and the differential protective effects of sevoflurane and isoflurane anesthesia in a rat hepatic ischemia-reperfusion injury model. Anesth. Analg. 2008; 106: 830–7.

52. Beck-Schimmer B, Breitenstein S, Urech S, De Conno E, Wittlinger M, Puhan M, Jochum W, Spahn DR, Graf R, Clavien PA: A randomized controlled trial on pharmacological preconditioning in liver surgery using a volatile anesthetic. Ann.Surg. 2008; 248: 909–18.

53. Laviolle B, Basquin C, Aguillon D, Compagnon P, Morel I, Turmel V, Seguin P, Boudjema K, Bellissant E, Mallédant Y: Effect of an anesthesia with propofol compared with desflurane on free radical production and liver function after partial hepatectomy. Fund. Clin.Pharmacol. 2012; 26: 735–42.

54. Yang LQ, Tao KM, Liu YT, Cheung CW, Irwin MG, Wong GT, Lv H, Song JG, Wu FX, Yu WF: Remifentanil preconditioning reduces hepatic ischemia-reperfusion injury in rats via inducible nitric oxide synthase expression. Anesthesiology. 2001; 114: 1036–47.

55. Lange M, Hamahata A, Traber DL, Nakano Y, Esechie A, Jonkam C, Whorton EB, von Borzyskowski S, Traber LD, Enkhbaatar P: Effects of early neuronal and delayed inducible nitric oxide synthase blockade on cardiovascular, renal, and hepatic function in ovine sepsis. Anesthesiology. 2010; 113: 1376–84.

56. Troisi R, Ricciardi S, Smeets P, Petrovic M, Van Maele G, Colle I, Van Vlierberghe H, de Hemptinne B: Effects

255

of hemi-portocaval shunts for inflow modulation on the outcome of small-for-size grafts in living donor liver transplantation. Am.J.Transplant. 2005; 5: 1397–404.

57. Eshkenazy R, Dreznik Y, Lahat E, Bar Zakai B, Zendel A, Ariche A: Small for size liver remnant following resection: prevention and management. Hepatobil. Surg.Nutr. 2014; 3: 303–12.

58. van Lienden KP, van den Esschert JW, de Graaf W, Bipat S, Lameris JS, van Gulik TM, van Delden OM: Portal vein embolization before liver resection: a systematic review. Cardiovasc.Intervent.Radiol. 2013; 36: 25–34.

59. Sakiyama R, Blau BJ, Miki T: Clinical translation of bioartificial liver support systems with human pluripotent stem cell-derived hepatic cells. World.J. Gastroenterol. 2017; 23: 1974–9.

18

Effects on Fluid Balance

Robert G. Hahn

The anaesthetist has the option to perform fluid therapy by adhering to strict protocols and rules-of-thumb. However, gaining a better understanding of how to guide this therapy adds interest to the anaesthetist's professional life, allows more capable handling of tricky situations, and leads to improved patient outcomes. This author has used, and sometimes developed, methods that aim to give the anaesthetist an opportunity to personalize the art and practice of fluid therapy. This chapter includes tips and suggestions about methods that might be considered.

Fluid Therapy at a Glance

In healthy humans, maintaining the balance between fluid intake and fluid losses is a minor issue. Fluid intake is driven by thirst and hunger (food contains a lot of water) and the kidneys quickly and effectively excrete any fluid overload. Feedback loops then restore the optimal body fluid volumes (Fig. 18.1). However, when our bodies are subjected to extreme environments or physiological strain, it becomes apparent that we only tolerate a deviation of a few percent from our optimal body fluid volumes. For example, during acute exercise, our physiological and mental capacities soon become impaired if fluid losses due to increased evaporation from the airways and sweating are not adequately replaced.

The thirst mechanism becomes gradually impaired with age and often deteriorates further in disease states,

such as serious infection and dementia. Patients coming to hospital may be in such a debilitated state that they cannot eat and drink adequately by themselves. Intravenous (IV) fluid therapy then becomes a way to support the normal intake of fluid; this is referred to as *maintenance fluid therapy*. The minimum fluid requirement in the average man is 1 mL/kg/hour, but a rate of 1.3 mL/kg/hour is frequently used, and a rate of 1.5 mL/kg/hour is recommended in children.

The so-called 4/2/1 rule provides a detailed recommendation for suitable water intake in children. This old rule, which is still practised, suggests 4 ml/kg/hour for infants weighing 3 to 10 kg; 40 ml/kg plus 2 ml/kg/hour for each kg over 10 kg for children ranging from 10 to 20 kg; and 60 ml/h plus 1 ml/kg/hour for each kg over 20 kg in children weighing more than 20 kg.

In adults, the maintenance fluid is given as slow IV drip in the form of a 5% glucose solution. Sodium and potassium, at 1 mmol/kg body weight, should be added. The glucose solution is chosen because it provides a minimum amount of energy (200 kcal/L). Glucose is also the only widely available IV solution that partially hydrates the cells; this hydration is needed if therapy spans over several days, as both evaporation and urinary excretion cause losses of intracellular fluid.

The internal control of the fluid balance becomes grossly impaired during anaesthesia, major surgery and intensive care. The normal feedback loops operate less effectively and are disturbed by stress mechanisms,

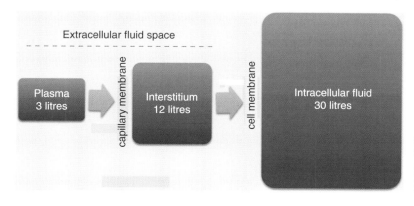

Fig. 18.1 Schematic drawing of the three fluid compartments in the human body. From Hahn RG, Ed. Fluid Therapy in the Perioperative Setting. 2nd ed., Cambridge, 2016.

which usually act to retain fluid. For example, the diuretic response to crystalloid fluid during general anaesthesia and surgery is only about 10% of the response seen in conscious subjects [1]. During surgery, fluid evaporation from the skin and open wounds cannot be replaced by oral intake of fluid. Haemorrhage losses should be substituted with crystalloid electrolyte or colloid fluid until the blood haemoglobin concentration has decreased to the point that the 'transfusion trigger' is reached. This 'trigger' is the haemoglobin concentration where the body is no longer able to compensate for the reduced haemoglobin mass by increasing cardiac output in order to maintain oxygen delivery (in humans, 60–100 g/L). Furthermore, maintenance fluid therapy has to continue as long as patients are unable to eat and drink on their own.

On top of this, a patient might come to surgery in a state of fluid deficit due to vomiting, starvation, ketoacidosis, ileus, or a combination of these factors. Compensation of these losses is called *replacement fluid therapy*. My practice is to provide at least half of this fluid deficit before general anaesthesia for acute surgery is induced, while giving careful consideration to the cardiovascular situation.

The need for high-rate substitution of fluid during surgical procedures necessitates the use of *resuscitation fluids*, such as isotonic or nearly isotonic salt-based crystalloid and colloid solutions. These include buffered Ringer's or Hartmann's solution, hydroxyethyl starch and gelatin.

Urine Analysis

Detection of a fluid deficit in a healthy human is not as easy as one might think. Anamnesis is helpful, but routinely used clinical tests (such as skin-fold thickness) are poor guides. If the problem is purely a lack of water, the serum osmolality is increased (> 300 mOsmol/kg) but this is a fairly late sign [2]. Serum creatinine rises in a severe fluid deficit, but one must then have another sample to compare with. Lack of diuresis is an even later sign of dehydration

(approximately 7% of the body weight) and the anaesthetist should be concerned at a much earlier stage (2–3% of the body weight).

A sensitive and simple method for detection of dehydration is to examine whether the kidneys are set to excrete or retain water. This can be assessed by taking a urine sample and measuring the concentrations of waste products that are excreted at a fairly stable rate. These measurements can include urine specific gravity (summary of solids), osmolality (salt balance), creatinine (from the metabolism of muscle) and urine colour (from the metabolism of erythrocytes).

The ranges of colour, osmolality and creatinine concentrations have been published for subjects aged 17–69 years, and each range paralleled the specific gravity scale [3]. These ranges were assigned a score, where a higher value indicated more severe dehydration (Table 18.1).

The mean of the four scores is termed the *fluid retention index (FRI)*. In sports medicine, urine sampling has been evaluated as a means of detecting a fluid deficit, but only one marker is then commonly employed [4–6]. In hospital care, potential confounders due to diet and disease might affect the result. The use of an aggregate index is therefore recommended to obtain a more robust measure. An index value of ≥ 4.0 corresponds to the degree of renal water conservation that accompanies dehydration amounting to 3% of the body weight (specific gravity ≥ 1.02, creatinine ≥ 12 mmol/L, colour ≥ 4 and osmolality ≥ 600 mOsmol/kg) [3].

In hospital care, a high content of metabolic waste products in the urine is associated with a greater plasma volume expansion in response to crystalloid fluid [7]. For example, a lower cardiac index and greater need for fluid optimization has been reported before abdominal surgery, where the waste products show high values [8]. In hip fracture surgery, a high preoperative FRI has been associated with a greater rise in neutrophil gelatinase-associated lipocalin; a sensitive biomarker of kidney injury (NGAL) [9] and a higher number of

Table 18.1. Scheme for calculating the fluid retention index (FRI), which is the mean of the fluid retention scores for four urinary markers.

Dehydration score	1	2	3	4	5	6
Specific gravity	≤ 1.005	1.010	1.015	1.020	1.025	1.030
Osmolality (mOsmol/kg)	< 250	250–450	450–600	600–800	800–1000	> 1000
Creatinine(mmol/)	< 4	4–7	7–12	12–17	17–25	> 25
Colour (shade)	1	2	3	4	5	6

postoperative complications [10]. In acute geriatric care, an admission FRI of ≥4.0 was associated with higher 30-day mortality [11].

The FRI score *after* surgery can less clearly be attributed to dehydration (indeed, a previous name was the Dehydration Index) because of the overlapping effects of trauma-induced fluid retention. However, in a study of hip fracture patients, the FRI hardly changed at all during surgery [9]. The FRI score also remained unchanged during the course of lengthy (3–4 h) abdominal cancer surgery when hydroxyethyl starch was used as infusion fluid, whereas a minor decrease occurred when Ringer's solution was administered [12]. Therefore, FRI could be a useful index to the fluid status in a fasting patient before surgery while its value during surgery is more uncertain.

BioImpedance

Whole-body bioimpedance (BIA) is a method of estimating the volumes of the body fluid spaces (intra- and extracellular) by analysing a series of weak electrical currents of different frequency that run between the arm and the foot [13]. The method is based on the fact that electric currents have more difficulty passing through large amounts of water than through small amounts. Moreover, the preference for the current to pass through or outside the cells varies with the frequency. The patient must be at complete rest (no movement allowed) during the time when the series of currents are sent through the body. The risk of mechanical and electrical interference must be considered.

The best use of bioimpedance for the anaesthetist would be for detection of pre- and postoperative dehydration [14]. Of course, the purpose is to compensate for any deficit that is detected. This author has found the method to be useful for groups but perhaps not sufficiently accurate for clinical use in individuals.

Blood Volume Changes

The blood volume changes assessed from variations in haemoglobin (Hb) concentration can serve as a practical guide to fluid therapy during and after surgery. The basic idea is to calculate the total amount of Hb in the circulation, which is then corrected for dilution and estimated Hb losses [15]. For example, assume that $Hb_{mass(0)}$ is the amount of Hb in the circulation at time zero (usually about 1 kg), BV_0 is the estimated blood volume at baseline and Hb_0 is the blood Hb concentration, and that the measurements are repeated at a later time (t). Then:

$$Hb_{mass(0)} = BV_0 Hb_0$$
$$BV(t) = (Hb_{mass(0)} - Hb_{loss(0-t)}) / Hb(t) \qquad (1)$$
$$\Delta BV(t) = BV(t) - BV_0$$

Hb_{loss} is obtained as the product of the Hb_0 and the volume of the surgical bleeding if haemorrhage occurs rapidly. When the bleeding is slow, one multiplies the bled volume by the average of Hb_0 and $Hb(t)$.

BV_0 is most conveniently obtained by some anthropometric measure. A simple equation is that BV_0 is 7% of the body weight, while regression equations provide more precise measures. These are typically based on tracer measurements of body fluid volumes performed in a large number of humans, and usually employ the gender, body weight and height of the subject as predictors. Below are examples of these equations for estimation of the blood volume in women and men [16].

$$BV(L, female) = 0.03308 \text{ weight (kg)} + 0.3561 \text{ height}^3 (m) + 0.1833. \qquad (2)$$

$$BV(L, male) = 0.03219 \text{ weight (kg)} + 0.3669 \text{ height}^3 (m) + 0.6041. \qquad (3)$$

These equations are easy to programme into a pocket calculator for use in the clinic. The following are three examples of how they can be applied. The examples may look similar, but the Hb calculations suggest three completely different treatments.

Example 18.1.

A 50-year-old man weighing 70 kg has undergone a 2-hour open abdominal surgery with a slow continuous bleeding estimated at 500 mL. The nurse calls you from the postoperative care unit. The patient does not feel well, his arterial pressure is 100/65 mmHg, and the nurse wants you to prescribe fluid for the evening. The blood chemistry says that the preoperative Hb was 145 g/L and the just obtained postoperative analysis was 110 g/L. What do you prescribe?

Our pocket calculator says that BV_0 should be approximately 5.0 L; therefore, the $Hb_{mass(0)}$ should be $5 \times 145 = 725$ g. The bleeding of 500 mL was slow, and Hb_{loss} should therefore be calculated based on the mean of the pre- and postoperative Hb values. Hb_{loss} is then $0.5 \times (145+110)/2 = 64$ g. Further is $BV(t) = (725 – 64) / 110 = 6.0$ L.

The blood volume of this patient is 1.0 L larger than before the surgery. Hence, the patient should not have any more resuscitation fluid but should only receive a restrictive amount of maintenance fluid. An injection of furosemide would probably improve this patient's general condition, and this is recommended. A bolus infusion to challenge the patient's fluid status in this setting could possibly have precipitated pulmonary oedema.

Example 18.2.

A 75-year-old woman weighing 80 kg and with a previous myocardial infarction has undergone hysterectomy due to a cancer diagnosis. She has received an epidural catheter for postoperative pain relief. A rapid haemorrhage, estimated to be 800 mL, has occurred during surgery. The operation is about to end, and you are faced with the challenge of prescribing fluid for her stay in the postoperative care unit. Her blood chemistry shows a preoperative Hb of 115 g/L and the just taken postoperative value is 105 g/L. What do you prescribe?

Our pocket calculator says that BV_0 should be approximately 5.5 L; therefore, the $Hb_{mass(0)}$ should be $5.6 \times 114 = 638$ g. The bleeding of 800 mL was rapid, which means that Hb_{loss} can be set to $0.8 \times 114 = 91$ g. The $BV(t)$ then becomes $= (638 - 91) / 105 = 5.2$ L.

The change in blood volume, which is given by $\Delta BV(t) = BV(t) - BV_0$, shows that the patient is hypovolaemic by 300 mL. Slight hypervolaemia in this setting would be beneficial, due to the vasodilatation caused by the epidural analgesia and the fact that an internal organ has been removed, which would be expected to cause some exudation and fluid accumulation in the surgical area. An increase in the blood volume by at least 0.5 L is warranted. However, this cannot be achieved without reducing the Hb concentration to below 100 g/L, which was decided as the transfusion trigger for this patient. My choice would be to prescribe 1 unit of erythrocytes, accompanied by the same amount of buffered Ringer's solution, and to reassess her status thereafter with a new Hb analysis. A likely option is that a second unit of erythrocytes would be prescribed later in the evening.

Example 18.3.

A 75-year-old man weighing 60 kg has undergone transurethral resection of the prostate, during which 90 g of prostate tissue has been removed. The blood loss was 800 mL. In the postoperative care unit, the patient complains of nausea, and he vomits. His arterial blood pressure is 90/60 mmHg. The preoperative Hb concentration was 140 g/L and the postoperative is 132 g/L. What do you prescribe?

The BV_0 should be approximately 4.2 L and $Hb_{mass(0)}$ then $4.2 \times 140 = 588$ g. The bleeding of 800 mL occurred rapidly, which means that Hb_{loss} can be set to $0.8 \times 140 = 112$ g. The $BV(t)$ then becomes $(588 - 112) / 132 = 3.6$ L.

The diagnosis is that the patient is hypovolaemic by 0.6 L. Treatment consists of clear fluids – either 500 mL of colloid or 1.5 L of buffered Ringer's solution. I would prefer the colloid if the patient has already received 2 L of crystalloid during the surgery, because adding even more crystalloids would cause gastrointestinal oedema [17, 18]. This patient has no risk of hitting the transfusion trigger (in his case, probably 90 g/L) due to fluid prescription. One can actually estimate how much the Hb concentration would decrease by adding 500 mL of clear fluid to the $BV(t)$ in the equations above. If more Hb is lost by haemorrhage, that amount is subtracted from Hb_{mass}. Transfused erythrocytes are simply added in the same fashion. It is important to note that the usefulness of the subsequent estimates depends on the accuracy of the quantitation of Hb losses and additions.

The Hb method for estimating blood volume changes is a simplified form of volume kinetics that has also been used in many scientific studies. For example, the BV change that is required before a drop in arterial pressure occurs during a transurethral prostatic resection is determined to be −0.5 L with the legs in stirrups but is +0.5 when the legs are lowered [19]. For this reason, it is good practice to give the patient a fluid bolus just before the legs are lowered at the end of a surgery performed in the lithotomy position when blood loss has occurred.

The Hb method has also been applied to show that as much as 60% of administered buffered Ringer's solution is retained in the bloodstream during ongoing surgery [20] as well as to demonstrate that arterial hypotension acts to retain fluid during induction of epidural anaesthesia [21].

The lesson learnt from these blood volume assessments is that Hb should change in proportion to the haemorrhage (i.e. the lost blood volume) if normovolaemia is to be maintained. The patient is hypovolaemic when the haemorrhage, in proportion to the initial blood volume, is greater than the relative drop in Hb. Conversely, a marked drop in Hb level without a proportional blood loss indicates hypervolaemia. Most anaesthetists make this judgement by mentally extrapolating from the patient's laboratory data, but erroneous conclusions can easily be drawn if the simple equations shown above are not entered into a pocket calculator (or an Excel spreadsheet) to obtain more precise estimates.

Electrolyte Shifts

The electrolyte shifts occurring when a fluid bolus is given can be used to analyse a clinical situation and to refine the fluid therapy. The assumptions in these calculations are quite similar to those made for Hb monitoring of the blood volume, except that ions that distribute across the entire ECF volume are used (i.e. interstitial fluid is included).

When an isotonic fluid is infused, the dilution of ions that are present in blood but not in the fluid indicates the size of the ECF volume. For example, an infusion of 1 L isotonic (5%) mannitol without electrolytes can be used to estimate the ECF space based on the accompanying dilution of serum sodium [22]. However, the calculation is not straightforward because some fluid and sodium are excreted during the experimental period. These losses by excretion can, and should, be accounted for.

Assuming that the ECF volume of water at baseline is 20% of the body weight (BW) and serum sodium is S-Na, the following changes would occur in the ECF content of Na and water in response to an infusion:

Total amount of Na before infusion = ECF × S-Na

Total amount of Na after infusion

= ECF × S-Na + infused Na − voided Na

Total amount of water before infusion = ECF

Expected amount of water in ECF after infusion

= ECF + infused volume − voided volume   (4)

Na ions remain outside the cells, while water can either enter or leave the cells. If no flow of water occurs, the S-Na after infusion, S-Na(t), is given by the ratio of the amount of Na in the ECF after the infusion and the expected amount of water in the ECF. Hence:

$$S-Na(t) \text{ at no flow}$$
$$= \frac{ECF \times S\text{-}Na + \text{infused Na} - \text{voided Na}}{ECF + \text{infused volume} - \text{voided volume}} \quad (5)$$

Using this equation, one can predict the change in serum sodium (or any other electrolyte that distributes in the ECF volume) in response to any type of infusion.

Interestingly, by measuring the serum sodium also after the infusion, we can compare the measured and predicted S-Na and thereby calculate the flow of fluid between the ICF and the ECF volumes that occurs in response to the infusion. This can be done by saying that the measured S-Na after this infusion must be the same as for the theoretical S-Na(t) at no flow, but adding the flow of fluid between the ECF and ICF as a new term in the denominator (ΔICF). Hence:

$$\text{Measured S-Na}(t)$$
$$= \frac{ECF \times S\text{-}Na + \text{infused Na} - \text{voided Na}}{ECF + \text{infused volume} - \text{voided volume} + \Delta ICF} \quad (6)$$

By re-arrangement:

$$\Delta ICF = ECF + \left(\text{infused} - \text{voided}\right)\text{volume}$$
$$- \frac{\left(ECF \times S\text{-}Na - \left(\text{added} - \text{voided}\right)Na\right)}{\text{Measured S-Na}\left(t\right)} \quad (7)$$

This fluid shift is difficult to calculate by alternative methods in a living human. This mass balance equation has mostly been used to estimate how fast and how extensively electrolyte-free irrigating fluid (e.g. used during endo-urologic surgery) distributes to the ICF space [23–25]. It has also demonstrated that a rapid infusion of buffered Ringer's solution in volunteers actually recruits fluid from the ICF to the ECF, because the kidneys in healthy humans are not set to excrete as high an amount of sodium as is contained in this crystalloid fluid [26]. This runs counter to the "logical" and "intuitive" assumption that the slight hypo-osmolarity of the Ringer's solution causes this fluid to hydrate the cells.

The equation shown above can also provide an explanation for the development of rebound oedema when plain 15% mannitol is infused. This infusion causes osmotic diuresis whereby sodium ions are lost. As long as the infused fluid does not contain any sodium, the therapy will reduce serum sodium, which will cause water to diffuse into the cells, i.e. increase the ICF volume (causing cellular edema). The magnitude of the oedema can be estimated from the equation. The amount of sodium that should be infused to withdraw the oedema can also be calculated using the same equation.

The implications of the electrolyte equation can be developed even further. Assume that we have a patient with diabetic ketoacidosis whose fluid balance and glucose concentration has to be corrected. We assume that ECF is low and that circulatory shock can develop if we administer too much insulin. When glucose enters the cells, the osmotic forces drive fluid in along with it, causing a positive ΔICF (and thus cause cellular edema). The therapy must therefore be cautious while still being effective.

By combining two electrolytes, we can actually estimate both ECF at baseline and the changes in ECF and ICF that accompany an infusion of fluid (2 equations, 2 unknowns). Fluid therapy in ketoacidosis usually begins with 1 L of isotonic saline; therefore, the most suitable electrolytes to monitor are sodium and chloride. If we create two equations, one with sodium and the other with chloride, they should both indicate the same ΔICF. For this purpose, one may use the same equation as the one derived above for the calculation of ΔICF based on changes in serum sodium. Based on this equivalence, we combine the equations and mathematically re-arrange them to have ECF on one side of the equation:

$$ECF = \frac{S\text{-}Na(t) \times Cl\,(infused - voided) - S\text{-}Cl(t) \times (infused - voided)\,Na}{S\text{-}Na \times S\text{-}Cl(t) - S\text{-}Na(t) \times S\text{-}Cl}$$

$$(8)$$

In the next step, ΔICF is calculated using the equation shown above, and ΔECF is simply the difference between infused volume, urinary excretion and ΔICF.

The following examples illustrate how this 'electrolyte maths' can be applied.

Example 18.4.

A patient weighing 95 kg with ketoacidosis received 1 L of isotonic saline over 30 min. 15 min later, the urinary excretion since the infusion began was 300 mL. The S-Na had increased from 130.2 to 133.0 mmol/L and S-Cl from 98 to 102 mmol/L. Urinary concentrations of sodium and chloride were 50 and 25 mmol/L, respectively. What is your analysis of the fluid balance situation?

This patient is expected to have an ECF volume amounting to 20% of his body weight, which is 19 L. Isotonic saline contains 152 mmol/L of both sodium and chloride. Insertion of the available data into the equation shows that ECF was only 14.4 L, which is consistent with severe dehydration. All of the infused fluid volume ended up in the ECF space and, worse yet, 0.78 L of the infused fluid entered the ICF, which means that the severe extracellular dehydration was somewhat worsened, despite the infusion of saline (1 L given, of which 0.30 L became urine and 0.64 L became ΔICF). Our conclusion should be that the insulin was administered somewhat too quickly and should be slowed down to prevent circulatory shock due to depletion of the ECF volume. Another way to handle the situation would be to intensify the fluid treatment, perhaps by doubling the rate of infusion of the crystalloid electrolyte fluid for 2–3 hours, after which the situation should be re-assessed.

Example 18.5

The next day, the same patient receives another infusion of 1 L of isotonic saline. 15 min after the end of the infusion, 600 mL of urine has been excreted. The S-Na has increased from 140.5 to 142.0 mmol/L and S-Cl from 110 to 113 mmol/L. Urinary concentrations of sodium and chloride are 95 and 77 mmol/L, respectively. What is your analysis of the fluid balance situation?

The ECF is now 16.3 L and the ΔICF response to the infusion +0.15 L. Some extracellular dehydration still remains, but no hydration of the ECF was achieved during this fluid challenge. There is still room for more resuscitation fluid.

To summarize, the above concepts can greatly help the clinician personalize care of the patient. Unfortunately, evaluations of the fluid balance based on changes in Hb and electrolyte concentrations are grossly underused in clinical medicine, even though the data required are often on hand for other purposes: the changes in body fluid volumes that they reflect are often simply not appreciated as such.

Tracers

The anaesthetist has several ways to measure the sizes of specific body fluid volumes and compare the derived values found with what is 'normal'. The traditional method to do this is to use a tracer technique. However, most of these are cumbersome to apply in the clinic; consequently, they are almost exclusively encountered in research.

A problem with these approaches is the difficulty in knowing what the volumes are that the body strives to maintain. In principle, challenging the body with a fluid load and observing the response, or examining what the body desires in some other way, has begun to be a more widely accepted approach to assess the fluid balance. However, challenging the body with a fluid load and observing the response cannot be applied uncritically in disease states that affect the body's fluid balances, such as heart failure, where other considerations must be made.

The way to measure the size of a body fluid volume is to inject a tracer that distributes only in the volume in question. The concentration of the tracer is then measured after equilibration, and the volume calculated according to the following basic equation:

$$\text{Volume of compartment} = \frac{\text{Injected dose of tracer}}{\text{Plasma concentration of tracer}}$$

$$(9)$$

Radio-iodinated albumin is a tracer used to measure the plasma and blood volumes. The first one is obtained if the radioactivity is measured on a spun sample of blood (i.e. the plasma), and the second is obtained if whole blood is used. Alternatively, one can use the haematocrit to transform one measure into the other.

Ten minutes after a bolus injection of this substance, three or four blood samples are taken every 10 minutes to account for the exponential elimination, and the plasma volume is obtained by backward extrapolation of the radiation to time zero. The tracer is eliminated from the blood by capillary leakage. Therefore, radio-iodinated albumin can also be used to quantify the rate of albumin loss from the bloodstream. The time window required for the assessment is as long as 30–40 min, so the plasma volume needs to be in a reasonably steady state during that time to yield a correct estimate of the plasma volume.

Indocyanine green (ICG) is another frequently used tracer for measuring the plasma volume. ICG has a half-life of only 3 min and is eliminated completely during the first passage through the liver [27]. The short elimination time makes ICG more useful than radio-iodinated albumin in the unstable surgical setting. However, the transit time for the tracer from the site of injection to the site of elimination (the liver) must be considered in the backward extrapolation, which should then be made to 1 min and not to zero time (Fig. 18.2) [28]. Due to the complete elimination of ICG in the liver, the ICG disappearance curve can

be used to extrapolate the plasma volume as well as the liver blood flow.

Erythrocytes may be labelled with radioactive tracers, such as chromium and technetium, to calculate red cell mass. Carbon monoxide binds to haemoglobin and can also be used for this purpose. Drawbacks are mainly safety issues, as carbon monoxide is toxic.

Tracers used to measure the size of the extracellular fluid (ECF) volume include bromide and iohexol. The latter is eliminated by glomerular filtration only and is therefore often used to assess the glomerular filtration rate (GFR) in the clinic. Bromide is eliminated slowly from the body, and taking the mean of a few samples taken about an hour after injection of the tracer is sufficient for estimating the ECF volume with reasonable confidence [22]. Iohexol is eliminated faster than bromide (half-life 100 min) and repeated blood sampling and backward extrapolation is then needed to obtain an accurate measure of the ECF volume [22]. Sampling cannot start within 30–40 min after a bolus injection because the iohexol kinetics show a clear distribution phase.

More rarely, the anaesthetist might want to assess the total body water, which can be measured with water isotopes including tritium (radioactive) and deuterium (not radioactive). Distribution of these molecules in the body is slow and requires about three hours for completion. An alternative approach is to use ethanol, but its relatively short half-life requires frequent sampling of blood or exhaled air [29].

Plasma tracers, possibly with the exception of ICG, slightly overestimate the plasma volume. Therefore, the result should be multiplied by the haematocrit factor (also called F-cell ratio), which is 0.91. Different interpretations of the haematocrit factor have been given over the years. The traditional one is that the peripheral haematocrit differs from the haematocrit in the total cardiovascular system [30]. A more recent explanation is that plasma is hidden in the endothelial glycocalyx layer, distorting these calculations. Yet another explanation rests on the fact that albumin easily enters the liver sinusoids, which is not the case for the erythrocytes.

Goal-directed Fluid Therapy

The anaesthetist still has other ways to estimate how much fluid the patient needs. These include quantification of the urinary excretion (the diuresis) and haemodynamic measurements. The urinary excretion

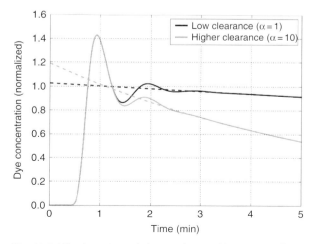

Fig. 18.2 Why the estimated plasma volume will be too small if the backward extrapolation of the concentration–time curve of indocyanine is done to zero time instead of time 1 min, when elimination begins in the liver. The indicated concentration of dye on the y-axis will then be too high [28].

is a poor sign of fluid overload during surgery, due to the generally low clearance of crystalloid fluid in that setting [31]. Hence, hardly any more fluid will become excreted even when the plasma volume is large. By contrast, the urinary excretion is a more sensitive marker of marked hypovolaemia.

The idea underlying goal-directed fluid therapy is to observe the body's physiological response to an infusion of a certain amount of fluid. The infusion is titrated to a specific end-point such as a pre-defined central venous pressure (CVP) or pulmonary artery wedge pressure. However, in recent years, the focus has been on raising the cardiac stroke volume (SV) by successive bolus infusions of a colloid fluid (usually 200–300 mL at a time).

According to Frank–Starling's law of the heart, stretching of the cardiac fibres increases the pumping strength up to a certain level, after which the strength decreases. The goal of goal-directed fluid therapy is then to gradually increase the stretching of the cardiac fibres by these fluid boluses, thereby raising preload until the maximum stroke volume is reached, usually without the use of a vasopressor. As a practical rule, an increase in the SV by more than 10% in response to a fluid bolus indicates that the patient is on the steep part of the Frank–Starling curve. The patient is then said to be 'fluid responsive' and another fluid bolus can be attempted.

Most studies that have evaluated the goal-directed fluid therapy by measuring SV show that the strategy reduces the number of postoperative complications and the length of hospital stay [32–34]. However, this effect might be absent when relatively healthy patients undergo operations that last for only one to two hours. With modern well-designed fluid programmes, a benefit has also been difficult to demonstrate [35]. However, better survival in the sickest patients is more indisputable [36].

Exactly what is being improved by optimizing SV remains elusive. Most scholars believe that the tissue perfusion is better maintained, thereby preventing local tissue acidosis [37]. The SV is reduced by 25–35% due to drug effects when general anaesthesia is induced, and goal-directed fluid therapy by using bolus infusions of a colloid seems to minimize the drop to only 15% when surgery begins [8]. Because the SV is still below baseline in the conscious state, there is probably little reason to perform SV-guided volume optimization in conscious patients.

The area of goal-directed fluid therapy is blurred by the fact that methods other than SV monitoring

can be used to assess whether a patient is fluid responsive. An alternative key approach is to make this conclusion based on a continuous analysis of the arterial pulse wave, either invasively or noninvasively, when the patient is anaesthetized and subjected to controlled ventilation. Unfortunately, some studies cast doubt on how well the commercially available methods correlate [38]. Therefore, the best way of performing goal-directed fluid therapy probably remains to be discovered. This author speculates that a combination of two or three methods might be required.

The CVP is affected by many factors and does not indicate fluid responsiveness. However, the CVP certainly increases when much fluid is infused, and it correlates reasonably well with Hb-indicated changes in blood volume [19]. During volume optimization, the CVP rises when fluid is given to a nonresponder; i.e. when adding more fluid no longer increases the SV.

Goal-directed fluid therapy is a very large area, and the interested reader is recommended to peruse other literature that covers this field in detail [39]. The situation is often that only a few of the anaesthetists in an operation department are able to handle this technique. This author has the opinion that all anaesthetists should be able to manage goal-directed fluid therapy and that the inherent strategy should be applied in the sickest patients, even when they arrive at the hospital during weekends and at night shifts.

Volume Kinetic Analysis

The dehydration status of an individual before surgery can also be studied by a fluid kinetic method. The rationale is the same as for the urine analysis; namely, that the kidneys tend to retain fluid when a preexisting fluid deficit is present. This fluid retention can be detected by less urine being excreted than expected in response to a fluid challenge, but a more precise approach is to include both the urinary excretion and the haemodilution pattern in an aggregate analysis.

In 2012, Zdolsek et al compared the fluid volume kinetics in volunteers in the euvolaemic state, and, on another occasion, after 1.5 L (2% of the body weight) had been removed by diuretic treatment [40]. Dehydration increased the half-life of 5 mL/kg and 10 mL/kg of buffered Ringer's solution from 23 to 76 min. Similar results were found later, when dehydration was indicated by urinary markers [7].

The principle behind volume kinetic analysis is to take repeated blood samples for measurement of the blood haemoglobin (Hb) concentration. The Hb concentration decreases during an infusion of fluid, and it increases again after the infusion due to distribution and excretion of the fluid. The series of Hb concentrations are then converted into the corresponding plasma dilutions by applying the following equation to the data:

Plasma dilution = [(Hb/Hb(t)) − 1]]/(1 − Hct)   (10)

where the absence of an index implies the starting value and (t) the value measured at any later time t. The term (1 - Hct) serves to convert the data from dilution of whole blood to plasma. The series of plasma dilutions are then used as the input variable $(v_c–V_c)/V_c$ and inserted into the mathematical solutions to the following system of differential equations that represent the "volume mass balances" in the two compartments:

$$\frac{dv_c}{dt} = R_o − k_{10}(v_c − V_c) − k_{12}(v_c − V_c) + k_{21}(v_t − V_t)$$ (11)

$$\frac{dv_t}{dt} = k_{12}(v_c − V_c) − k_{21}(v_t − V_t)$$ (12)

The kinetic model is illustrated in Figure 18.3. Fluid is infused at the rate R_o and then expands the central fluid space, V_c. The fluid is assumed to distribute between two body fluid spaces of baseline size V_c and V_t, which roughly correspond to the plasma volume and expandable parts of the interstitial fluid space. The symbols v_c and v_t denote the sum of each baseline volume and the respective excess fluid volume. Distribution from V_c to V_t is governed by a rate constant k_{12} and the return of fluid by another rate constant, k_{21}. Elimination is modelled by the rate constant k_{10}.

Nonlinear regression analysis by computer can be implemented using several types of software, which also solve the differential equations. A stable estimate

of the elimination rate constant k_{10} should be obtained with a series of 12–30 Hb values spread over an appropriate period of time. The half-life of the fluid is then given by $0.693/k_{10}$ (0.693 is the natural logarithm of two). Half-lives longer than about 60 min are consistent with dehydration [40].

The total urinary excretion during the sampling period, if known, can be expected to equal the rate of elimination by the following relationship:

$$k_{10} = \text{urinary excretion / AUC for } (v_c − V_c)$$ (13)

where AUC is the area under the curve. With 'good' data, which are typically due to a well standardized sampling procedure, the model-based k_{10} is usually somewhat higher than the urinary-based k_{10}, which gives room for the estimation of a residual elimination, k_b. This residual term probably represents elimination of infused fluid by lymphatic flow [41].

The sampling period in studies of volume kinetics is usually three to four hours but can be reduced to 90 min if the fluid is given over a short period of time (15–20 min) and the if possibility to fix k_{10} by the urine output is exploited. Because distribution requires 30 min to be completed, the sampling time period in studies of volume kinetics should be at least 90 min for a stable estimate of k_{10} to be obtained.

The fluid volume kinetic method, as described here, is too cumbersome to be used in clinical practice. However, the method is very useful for research, and the insights gained from volume kinetic research are directly applicable to the practice of anaesthesia. One such clinically important concept derived from the study of fluid kinetics is that the distribution of infused crystalloid fluid requires as long as 30 min for completion [31]. This means that the plasma volume expansion during an actual infusion of crystalloid is much greater than is usually believed. Even for 15–20 min after ending an infusion, the plasma volume expansion remains quite good. Thereafter, only 15–20% of the infused volume remains in the bloodstream (Fig. 18.4). However, as long as the fluid is infused, one can count on a plasma volume expansion amounting to approximately 50–60% of the infused volume [20]. This relatively high degree of retention of crystalloid fluid during infusion should be considered when making the choice between infusing a crystalloid versus a colloid fluid.

The transiently greater volume expansion due to the distribution function is important when treating

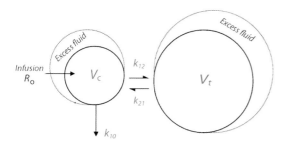

Fig. 18.3 The volume kinetic model. See text for detail.

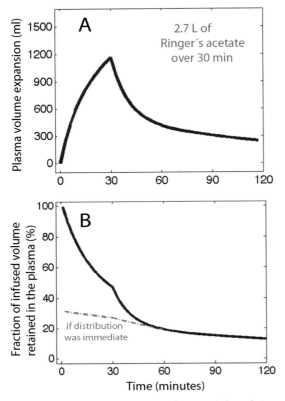

Fig. 18.4 Plasma volume expansion during and after infusion of 2.7 L of Ringer's acetate solution over 30 min in an average normovolaemic adult volunteer weighing 76 kg (A). The fraction of the infused fluid that remains in the blood at any given moment, where the area between the blue and red lines illustrates the impact of distribution on the plasma volume expansion (B).

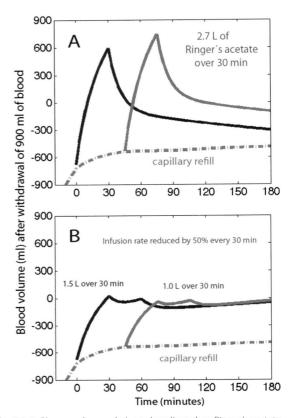

Fig. 18.5 Plasma volume relative to baseline when Ringer's acetate solution is infused over 30 min according to the 3:1 rule, after withdrawal of 900 ml of blood from male volunteers weighing 76 kg (A). To reach normovolaemia, a much smaller amount of Ringer's than suggested by the 3:1 rule should be infused. Titration is necessary to maintain normovolaemia (B). Two situations are shown depending on the delay between the haemorrhage and the onset of the fluid therapy (blue line = 15 min, green line = 60 min). The two differ with regard to the degree of spontaneous capillary refill (red hatched line) that has occurred since the haemorrhage [42].

trauma patients, who may have an injury to a major blood vessel and thereby suffer from 'uncontrolled haemorrhage'. These patients should not be made hypervolaemic at any point in time, because they are at risk of initiating a rebleeding event due to washing away of the immature blood clot that initially arrests the bleeding. Therefore, the commonly recommended substitution of haemorrhage by three times the bled amount with crystalloid fluid is a risky therapy, as it results in hypervolaemia (Fig. 18.5A).

Titration is necessary to prevent episodes of hypervolaemia.

Volume kinetic analysis of hypovolaemic volunteers suggest that 1.5 times the haemorrhage should be infused over 30 min, followed by half that amount over another 30 min, and possibly followed by 30 min when the rate of infusion is 25% of the initial one [42]. The suitable amounts depend to some degree on the delay between the haemorrhage and the onset of the

infusion, because hypovolaemia initiates a spontaneous transfer of fluid from the interstitial fluid space to the plasma ("capillary refill"; Fig. 18.5B).

The plasma volume expansion following crystalloid fluid is even stronger than that indicated above in situations of acute hypotension. When the arterial pressure has dropped to a stable level 20% below baseline, which is very common during induction of anaesthesia, volume kinetic studies show that the intravascular retention of infused fluid is 100% [31]. This effect can be understood from the Starling equation, which holds that the transcapillary flow of fluid is governed by the differences in hydrostatic and colloid osmotic pressures across the capillary wall. Distribution of infused fluid from the plasma to the interstitium becomes retarded, or even arrested, if the hydrostatic pressure

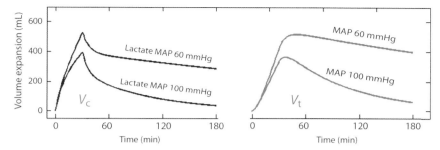

Fig. 18.6 Effect of different levels of mean arterial pressure (MAP) on the distribution of a 30-min infusion of 1 litre of Ringer's lactate between the plasma (V_c) and the interstitial fluid space (V_t). Computer simulation based on volume kinetic data with haemodynamic covariates.

on the luminal side of the capillary wall is suddenly decreased. The pronounced intravascular retention of infused fluid probably lasts until a new Starling equilibrium has been reached; i.e. when the hydrostatic intravascular pressure has been raised sufficiently to match the interstitial fluid pressure. Up to that point in time, crystalloid fluid is likely to be a very effective plasma volume expander.

Hypotension that persists after the normal exchange of fluid between the plasma and interstitial fluid space has been restored by fluid, is characterized by a graded reduction in the urinary excretion so as to result in oliguria. This reduction is powerful and probably explains why the half-life of crystalloid fluid is ten times longer during anaesthesia and surgery than in conscious healthy volunteers [1]. Of course, oliguria during hypotensive states also acts to enhance the fluid retention in the body, which can be estimated by volume kinetics after adding haemodynamic parameters as covariates in the analysis (Fig. 18.6).

Mixed effects modelling of volume kinetic data further shows that rapid infusions of crystalloid fluid (> 30 mL/min) have a natural tendency to cause peripheral oedema, even in healthy volunteers [41]. The reason is probably the loss of elastic properties of the interstitial matrix that occurs when this fluid space is expanded.

Finally, the study of volume kinetics explains why a fixed fluid volume is a more effective plasma volume expander when administered as a slow continuous drip rather than as a bolus. First, fluid volumes up to 5 mL/kg do not seem to expand the interstitial fluid space at all, which is probably due to the resistance to volume expansion that characterizes the interstitial matrix [41]. As the infused fluid then expands only the plasma, the plasma volume expansion per

unit of infused fluid becomes quite strong. Second, a constant-rate infusion represents a zero-order function while both the distribution and the elimination of fluids are exponential functions. The area under the plasma volume–time curve, which is an expression of effect over time, will then be larger for the slow infusion. By the way, the situation is the same for virtually all drugs, as well. Third, and as mentioned above, fluid distributed to peripheral tissues is returned more slowly the faster the fluid is infused, which reduces the volume expanding effect of a fast infusion on the plasma [41].

Ethanol Monitoring of Fluid Absorption

Fluid absorption is a well-known complication of endoscopic procedures, such as transurethral prostatic resection (TURP) and transcervical endometrial resection. Denial of the issue by surgeons is common because fluid absorption is typically believed to be due to lack of surgical skill. Many studies continue to report the incidence of this absorption, and the degree of the problem seems to vary greatly between hospitals. The most common figure is that absorption of 1 L of fluid or more occurs in approximately 5–10% of the transurethral prostatic surgeries performed [43–47]. This volume limit is well founded, as symptoms become statistically more common when > 1 L has been absorbed [45, 46].

Serious consequences of this iatrogenic complication are rare but can be prevented by early detection through perioperative measurements of the absorption. The best evaluated method for this purpose is ethanol monitoring, which is based on using an irrigating fluid that contains 1% ethanol and then measuring the ethanol concentration in the patent's exhaled breath by a hand-held Alcolmeter [48]. Ethanol monitoring can be applied during both regional and general anaesthesia [49]. Thermocatalytic – but not fuel-cell type – breathalyzers may show interference from inhaled anaesthetics. If so, intravenous anaesthesia should be used.

A sample is taken from the patient's breath every ten minutes, but the time interval is reduced to every five minutes once alcohol is detected. The ethanol data are entered into a correlation graph that indicates the amount of absorbed fluid (Fig. 18.7). If electrolyte-free fluid is used, the inflicted degree of hyponatraemia can also be obtained from the same graph.

Uptake of > 3 L of electrolyte-free fluid results in transurethral resection syndrome (TUR syndrome) with a risk of death due to hypovolaemic circulatory collapse and cerebral herniation due to cerebral oedema [50]. With such large-scale absorption, there is a transient hypervolaemic phase when the fluid is absorbed, but this is soon transformed into a

hypovolaemic situation due to osmotic diuresis, concomitant bleeding and intracellular distribution of absorbed fluid [51].

Absorption of isotonic saline, which is used with the bipolar resection technique, will change the scenario of adverse effects in an as yet poorly understood way. Hyponatraemia and brain oedema no longer occur, but fluid absorption is just as common as with monopolar prostate resections [52–54]. Few systematic studies of saline absorption have been performed, but pharmacokinetic data show that the plasma volume expands more in response to isotonic saline than to electrolyte-free irrigating fluids (glycine 1.5%, sorbitol 5%, etc.). Therefore, a higher incidence of pulmonary oedema due to rapid fluid overload is likely. Studies of saline infusions in patients and volunteers demonstrate that saline overload is followed by several symptoms that also are parts of the TUR syndrome, including nausea, swelling of the hands and face, pulmonary congestion, mental blurring and abdominal pain [48, 55, 56].

Adverse effects caused by absorption of isotonic saline are still poorly investigated. The anaesthetist should not accept the widespread belief among urologists that the bipolar resection technique has put an end to problems with adverse effects caused by absorption of irrigating fluid.

In summary, the anaesthetist should be aware that major fluid absorption is a possible event during endoscopic surgery. Precaution by using a monitoring method, of which ethanol is the best evaluated, is recommended.

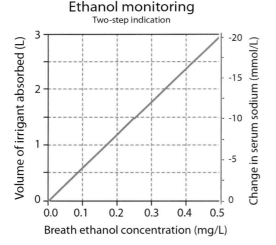

Fig. 18.7 Nomogram for quick reference displaying relationship between the absorbed volume of ethanol containing irrigation fluid absorbed and the breath expired ethanol concentration (calibrated to blood ethanol) and, if the fluid is electrolyte-free, the nomogram can also be used to predict the corresponding decrease in serum sodium. The volume of irrigation fluid absorbed is given by the average absorption time during TURP, which is 20 min in larger cohorts of patients (the absorption time influences the breath ethanol level by means of distribution and elimination of ethanol). The median absolute residual error is 146 ml and is R_2 for the regression 0.80 [48].

References

1. Hahn RG, Lyons G: The half-life of infusion fluids. Eur.J.Anaesthesiol. 2016; 33: 475–82.

2. Cheuvront SN, Ely BR, Kenefick RW, et al: Biological variation and diagnostic accuracy of dehydration assessment markers. Am.J.Clin.Nutr. 2010; 92: 565–73.

3. Hahn RG, Waldréus N: An aggregate urine analysis tool to detect acute dehydration. Int.J.Sport.Nutr.Exerc. Metab. 2013; 23: 303–11.

4. Armstrong LE, Soto JA, Hacker FT, et al: Urinary indices during dehydration, exercise and rehydration. Sport.Nutr.Exerc.Metab. 1998; 8: 345–55.

5. Popowski LA, Oppliger RA, Lambert GP, et al: Blood and urinary measures of hydration status during progressive acute dehydration. Med.Sci.Sports.Exerc. 2001; 33: 747–53.

6. Casa DJ, Armstrong LE, Hillman SK, et al: National athletic trainers' association position statement: Fluid replacement for athletes. J.Athl.Train. 2000; 35: 212–24.

7. Hahn RG, Nyberg Isacson M, Fagerström T, et al: Isotonic saline in elderly men; an open-labelled controlled infusion study of electrolyte balance, urine flow and kidney function. Anaesthesia. 2016; 71: 155–62.

8. Li Y, He R, Ying X, et al: Dehydration, hemodynamics and fluid volume optimization after induction of general anesthesia. Clinics. 2014; 69: 809–16.

9. Hahn RG: Renal injury during hip fracture surgery: an exploratory study. Anaesthesiol.Intensive.Ther. 2015; 47: 284–90.

10. Ylienvaara SI, Elisson O, Berg K, et al:Preoperative urine-specific weight and the incidence of complications after hip fracture surgery. A prospective, observational study. Eur.J.Anaesthesiol. 2014; 31: 85–90.

11. Johnson P, Waldreus N, Hahn RG, et al: Fluid retention index predicts the 30-day mortality in geriatric care. Scand.J.Clin.Lab.Invest. 2015; 75: 444–51.

12. Hahn RG, Li Y, He R: Fluid retention is alleviated by crystalloid but not by colloid fluid after induction of general anesthesia: an open-labeled clinical trial. J. Anesth.Clin.Res. 2016; 7: 1.

13. de Lorenzo A, Andreoli A, Matthie J, Withers P: Predicting body cell mass with bioimpedance by using theoretical methods. J.Appl.Physiol. 1997; 82: 1542–58.

14. Svensén C, Ponzer S, Hahn RG: Volume kinetics of Ringer solution after surgery for hip fracture. Can.J.Anaesth. 1999; 46: 133–41.

15. Hahn RG: A haemoglobin dilution method (HDM) for estimation of blood volume variations during transurethral prostatic surgery. Acta.Anaesthesiol. Scand. 1987; 31: 572–8.

16. Nadler SB, Hidalgo JU, Bloch T: Prediction of blood volume in normal human adults. Surgery. 1962; 51: 224–32.

17. Wuethrich PY, Burkhard FC, Thalmann GN, et al: Restrictive deferred hydration combined with preemptive norepinephrine infusion during radical cystectomy reduces postoperative complications and hospitalization time. Anesthesiology. 2014; 120: 365–77.

18. Li Y, He R, Ying X, et al: Ringer's lactate, but not hydroxyethyl starch, prolongs the food intolerance time after major abdominal surgery; an open-labelled clinical trial. BMC.Anesthesiology. 2015; 15: 72.

19. Hahn RG: Blood volume at the onset of hypotension in TURP performed during epidural anaesthesia. Eur.J.Anaesth. 1993; 10: 219–25.

20. Hahn RG: Volume effect of Ringer's solution in the blood during general anaesthesia. Eur.J.Anaesthesiol. 1998; 15: 427–32.

21. Drobin D, Hahn RG: Time course of increased haemodilution in hypotension induced by extradural anaesthesia. Br.J.Anaesth. 1996; 77: 223–6.

22. Zdolsek J, Lisander B, Hahn RG: Measuring the size of the extracellular space using bromide, iohexol and sodium dilution. Anesth.Analg. 2005; 101: 1770–7.

23. Hahn R, Hjelmqvist H, Rundgren M: Effects of isosmotic and hyperosmotic glycine solutions on the fluid balance in conscious sheep. Prostate. 1989; 15: 71–80.

24. Hahn RG, Stalberg HP, Ekengren J, et al: Effects of 1.5% glycine solution with and without ethanol on the fluid balance in elderly men. Acta.Anaesthesiol.Scand. 1991; 35: 725–30.

25. Hahn RG: Irrigating fluids in endoscopic surgery. Br.J.Urol. 1997; 79: 669–80.

26. Hahn RG, Drobin D: Rapid water and slow sodium excretion of Ringer's solution dehydrates cells. Anesth. Analg. 2003; 97: 1590–4.

27. Menschen S, Busse MW, Zisowsky S, Panning B: Determination of plasma volume and total blood volume using indocyanine green: a short review. J.Med. 1993; 24: 10–27.

28. Polidori D, Rowley C: Optimal back-extrapolation method for estimating plasma volume in humans using the indocyanine green dilution method. Theor.Biol. Med.Model. 2013; 10: 48.

29. Norberg Å, Sandhagen B, Bratteby LE, et al: Do ethanol and deuterium oxide distribute into the same water space in healthy volunteers? Alcohol.Clin.Exp.Res. 2001; 25: 1423–30.

30. Chaplin Jr H, Mollison PL, Vetter H. The body/venous hematocrit ratio: its constancy over a wide hematocrit range. J.Clin.Invest. 1953; 32: 1309–16.

31. Hahn RG. Volume kinetics for infusion fluids. Anesthesiology. 2010; 113: 470–81.

32. Conway DH, Mayall R, Abdul-Latif MS, et al: Randomised controlled trial investigating the influence of intravenous fluid titration using oesophageal Doppler monitoring during bowel surgery. Anaesthesia. 2002; 57: 845–9.

33. Gan TJ, Soppitt A, Maroof M, et al: Goal-directed intraoperative fluid administration reduces length of hospital stay after major surgery. Anesthesiology. 2002; 97: 820–6.

34. Noblett SE, Snowden CP, Shenton BK, et al: Randomized clinical trial assessing the effect of Doppler-optimized fluid management on outcome after elective colorectal resection. Br.J.Surg. 2006; 93: 1069–76.

35. Pearse RM, Harrison DA, MacDonald N, et al: Effect of perioperative cardiac output-guided hemodynamic therapy algorithm on outcomes following major gastrointestinal surgery. A randomized clinical trial and systematic review. JAMA. 2014; 311: 2181–90.

36. Cecconi M, Corredor C, Arulkumaran N, et al: Clinical review: goal-directed therapy – what is the evidence in surgical patients? The effect on different risk groups. Crit.Care. 2013; 17: 209.

37. Mythen MG, Webb AR: Perioperative plasma volume expansion reduces the incidence of gut mucosal hypoperfusion during cardiac surgery. Arch.Surg. 1995; 130: 423–9.

38. Bahlmann H, Hahn RG, Nilsson L: Agreement between Pleth Variability Index and oesophageal Doppler to predict fluid responsiveness. Acta.Anaesthesiol.Scand. 2016; 60: 183–92.

39. Cannesson M, Pearse R, eds. *Perioperative Hemodynamic Monitoring and Goal Directed Therapy*. Cambridge: Cambridge University Press, 2014.

40. Zdolsek J, Li Y, Hahn RG. Detection of dehydration by using volume kinetics. Anesth.Analg. 2012; 115: 814–22.

41. Hahn RG, Drobin D, Zdolsek J: Distribution of crystalloid fluid changes with the rate of infusion: a population-based study. Acta.Anaesthesiol.Scand. 2016; 60: 569–78.

42. Hahn RG: Fluid therapy in uncontrolled hemorrhage – what experimental models have taught us. Acta. Anaesthesiol.Scand. 2013; 57: 16–28.

43. Osborn DE, Rao PN, Greene MJ, et al: Fluid absorption during transurethral resection. Br.Med.J. 1980; 281: 1549–50.

44. Hahn RG, Ekengren J: Patterns of irrigating fluid absorption during transurethral resection of the prostate as indicated by ethanol. J.Urol. 1993; 149: 502–6.

45. Hahn RG, Shemais H, Essén P: Glycine 1.0% versus glycine 1.5% as irrigating fluid during transurethral resection of the prostate. Br.J.Urol. 1997; 79: 394–400.

46. Hahn RG, Sandfeldt L, Nyman CR: Double-blind randomized study of symptoms associated with absorption of glycine 1.5% or mannitol 3% during transurethral resection of the prostate. J.Urol. 1998; 160: 397–401.

47. Yousef AA, Suliman GA, Elashry OM, et al: A randomized comparison between three types of irrigating fluids during transurethral resection in benign prostatic hyperplasia. BMC.Anesthesiology. 2010; 10: 7.

48. Hahn RG: Fluid absorption and the ethanol monitoring method. Acta.Anaesthesiol.Scand. 2015; 59: 1081–93.

49. Stalberg HP, Hahn RG, Jones AW: Ethanol monitoring of transurethral prostatic resection during inhaled anesthesia. Anesth.Analg. 1992; 75: 983–8.

50. Hahn RG: Fluid absorption in endoscopic surgery. Br.J.Anaesth. 2006; 96: 8–20.

51. Hahn RG, Gebäck T. Fluid volume kinetics of dilutional hyponatremia; a shock syndrome revisited. Clinics 2014; 69: 120–7.

52. Hermanns T, Fankhauser CD, Hefermehl LJ, Kranzbühler B, Wong LM, Capol JC, Zimmermann M, Sulser T, Müller A: Prospective evaluation of irrigating fluid absorption during pure transurethral bipolar plasma vaporisation of the prostate using expired-breath ethanol measurements. BJU.Int. 2013; 112: 647–54.

53. Hermanns T, Grossman NC, Wettstein MS, et al: Absorption of irrigating fluid occurs frequently during high power 532 nm laser vaporization of the prostate. J. Urol. 2015; 193: 211–16.

54. Ran L, He W, Zhu Z, et al: Comparison of fluid absorption between transurethral enucleation and transurethral resection for benign prostate hyperplasia. Urol.Int. 2013; 91: 26–30.

55. Wilkes NJ, Woolf R, Mutch M, et al: The effect of balanced versus saline-based hetastarch and crystalloid solutions on acid-base and electrolyte status and gastric mucosal perfusion in elderly surgical patients. Anesth. Analg. 2001; 93: 811–16.

56. Williams EL, Hildebrand KL, McCormick SA, et al: The effect of intravenous lactated Ringer's solution versus 0.9% sodium chloride solution on serum osmolality in human volunteers. Anesth.Analg. 1999; 88: 999–1003.

Chapter 19

Ventilation during General Anaesthesia

Lluís Gallart

Introduction

Even though practices do differ geographically, general anaesthesia often involves some mode of mechanical ventilation different from normal spontaneous ventilation. This chapter will focus on the differences between these conditions, and describe the problems associated with artificial ventilation.

Lung Physiology

The lungs deliver O_2 and remove CO_2, goals that are achieved optimally if ventilation and perfusion are adequately matched. While alveoli are passive 'soft bags' that cannot inflate or deflate themselves, their volumes do range from totally collapsed to fully inflated to overdistended. Alveolar volume is the result of the balance between forces that cause alveolar expansion (thoracic cage, muscle activity, nitrogen) and forces that cause alveolar collapse (elastic recoil of the lung, alveolar surface tension, weight of viscera, hyperoxia).

Lung inflation is achieved by an increase in transpulmonary pressure generated by expansion of the thoracic cage by active contraction of the intercostal muscles (thoracic breathing) and the diaphragm (abdominal breathing). Expiration is most often passive, and ceases when the forces that cause the lung to collapse match the forces that cause it to expand. The lung volume at this equilibrium is the functional residual capacity (FRC).

The relative contribution of thoracic or abdominal breathing during inspiration varies according to body position: thoracic breathing predominates in the upright position, and abdominal breathing in the supine position. These differences reflect the fact that the respiratory system tries to minimize the work of breathing [1]. In the upright position, the abdominal muscles are contracted, and a shortened diaphragm has to make a substantial effort against the abdomen, therefore thoracic breathing prevails. In contrast, in the supine position, the abdominal muscles are relaxed and offer limited resistance to diaphragmatic displacement. In addition, the diaphragm is elongated with actin–myosine alignment optimal to generate maximal force.

During expiration in the supine position in the awake patient, diaphragmatic muscle tone impedes cephalic (non-dependent) displacement of abdominal viscera. This muscle tone is lost during anaesthesia, impairing ventilation/perfusion matching (see below).

Anaesthesia, Mechanical Ventilation and the Respiratory System

During anaesthesia, FRC decreases from an average of 3.5 L in the upright position to 2 L in the supine, anaesthetized subject [2]. This decrease is due to a loss of respiratory muscle tone, mainly in the diaphragm, accompanied by a minor decrease of the thoracic perimeter [3]. The increase in pleural pressure and resulting decrease in aerated lung volume renders the lung parenchyma prone to collapse and leads to airway closure. Airway closure during expiration (dynamic airway collapse) may occur in the healthy awake patient, but worsens with factors such as age, obesity or anaesthesia. These closed airways can reopen during inspiration, but some remain closed and cause alveolar resorption atelectasis, a problem worsened by high inspired O_2 concentrations (FiO_2). Actually, atelectasis is the main problem related to general anaesthesia and mechanical ventilation. It appears in 90% of patients and affects up to 10–20% of the lung during general anaesthesia, regardless of whether spontaneous or mechanical ventilation is used [2]. Ventilation of these atelectatic areas can result in cyclic opening and closing of alveoli, leading to local shear injury called 'atelectrauma' [4, 5]. A second problem is barotrauma or volutrauma, which can be occult in patients apparently ventilated without damage. Atelectrauma and volutrauma lead to biotrauma, i.e. biochemical injury or release of cytokines [6]. We will expand on these elements.

Atelectrauma

Atelectasis during anaesthesia is caused by three mechanisms: absorption of alveolar gas, impairment of surfactant function and compression of lung parenchyma [7].

Absorption of alveolar gas can facilitate alveolar collapse. In the awake subject, alveoli are filled with N_2, O_2, CO_2 and H_2O vapour, and the partial pressure of every gas helps keep the alveoli open. Nitrogen is an inert gas, and thus there is no net uptake from the alveoli across the alveolocapillary membrane. Therefore, N_2 is always present in the alveoli and scaffolds them ('helps keep them open'). Oxygen, however, is consumed: there is a net flow of O_2 into the capillaries that matches O_2 consumption of the patient. Therefore, if the alveolus contains high O_2 partial pressures without other gases to scaffold the alveoli, the net O_2 transfer will cause alveoli to deflate and collapse. This effect is not relevant in the non-dependent (anterior and cephalic) alveolar units with a high ventilation/perfusion (V/Q) ratio, but it is in the dependent (lower and posterior) units with a low V/Q ratio where O_2 uptake from the alveolus exceeds delivery to it. If there is complete airway occlusion after the alveoli have been washed with 100% O_2, lung units behind this obstruction will have all their O_2 removed into the capillary blood and will fully collapse, generating a V/Q unit with absolute shunt.

Surfactant serves to decrease wall tension in the smaller alveoli, preventing them from collapsing. Surfactant function is impaired by inhaled anaesthetics, at least in laboratory studies [7]. In isolated animal lungs, surfactant is released by manoeuvres that increase alveolar size, such as larger tidal volumes or by inflating the lung to total lung capacity [7]. If these effects can be extrapolated to clinical practice, surfactant release could be improved by sighs or recruitment manoeuvres (RM).

Compression of lung tissue is the most important cause of atelectasis. It is caused by an increase of forces compressing the alveoli and a decrease of forces expanding lung units. The main external force is gravity, the effect of which becomes more relevant upon resuming the supine position. Gravity includes the weight of the heart, overweight due to obesity and the weight of abdominal viscera. The weight of abdominal viscera becomes more relevant during anaesthesia, due to the loss of diaphragmatic activity. During spontaneous inspiration, both the anterior and posterior parts of the diaphragm contract, and ventilation will thus be distributed to both the anterior and posterior parts

of the lung. During mechanical ventilation, the diaphragm will act as a passive membrane and inspired gases will choose the path of least resistance, which is towards the non-dependent parts of the lungs – the dependent areas receive less ventilation because the dependent parts of the diaphragm bear the full weight of the abdominal contents. Once the volume and compliance of the dependent alveolar units are reduced, a vicious circle is entered of a lower alveolar radius, requiring higher pressures to open these alveoli with poor ventilation (Laplace's law), causing a further decrease in alveolar volume and compliance, which in turn further worsens ventilation, leading to progressive alveolar collapse.

Atelectrauma is not caused by the atelectasis per se but mainly by the shear stress at the interface of open and closed lung regions [8]. Cyclic opening and closing of alveolar units harms lung parenchyma, mainly because forces acting on lung parenchyma are much higher than the airway pressures. A mathematical model postulated that an airway pressure of 30 cm H_2O results in a pressure of 140 cm H_2O in the interface between open and closed lung units [9].

Volutrauma

Mechanical ventilation with high airway pressures causes lung damage, called barotrauma [10]. Dreyfuss et al proposed using the term 'volutrauma' rather than barotrauma because injury is mainly related to lung deformation by the generated tidal volume (V_T). Both barotrauma and volutrauma act simultaneously. Damaging forces related to pressure are defined as stress, and lung deformation related to volume is called strain [11].

High airway pressures (Paw) can only be harmful if they lead to a high transpulmonary pressure, which is the difference between pressure inside the alveolus (PA) and the pressure outside the alveolus, which is pleural pressure (Ppl). Fig. 19.1 displays two different situations. On the left (A), PA is high (40 cm H_2O) and Ppl low (5 cm H_2O), and the resulting high transpulmonary pressure (35 cm H_2O) will cause tissue deformation and injury. In the example on the right (B), PA is also high (40 cm H_2O) but so is the 'external' pressure Ppl (25 cm H_2O), due to gravity, pleural effusion, compression by a CO_2 pneumoperitoneum, Trendelenburg position or other causes. Transpulmonary pressure thus will be low (15 cm H_2O), so that in this case the high PA will not be harmful. Thus, whenever transpulmonary pressure is high, lung deformation can occur and the lung can be damaged. This happens when high positive pressures are applied but also during spontaneous ventilation with high negative pressure generated during airway occlusion. In both situations, lungs are being damaged [6]. Note that transpulmonary pressure is calculated as PA – Ppl and not as Paw – Ppl. Paw (measured at the mouth) will only match PA (in the alveoli) when there is no airway flow, which, for example, is the case during an end-expiratory pause. This is explained in more detail later.

High V_T (strain) can cause volutrauma when it is combined with high airway pressure (stress). Strain is the ratio of V_T to the functional residual capacity (FRC) [11]. For the same V_T, strain is increased when FRC is low. Because most research on strain has been done in ICU patients with ARDS, these concepts may not exactly apply to the intraoperative setting with low FRC such as obesity or laparoscopy.

Thus, 'high Paw' or 'high V_T' are not synonyms for 'lung trauma'. High Paw can be observed in a trumpet player, but in this setting expiratory muscles create high intrapleural pressures, therefore transpulmonary pressure is low and there is no barotrauma. Also, a high V_T is needed to ventilate a tall basketball player, but this V_T will be easily achieved with a low Paw because his FRC will be larger too.

The harmful threshold for stress is around 27 cm H_2O and the threshold for strain is twice the FRC volume. Stress/strain control is crucial in patients with ARDS with a 'baby lung' [12]. In the operating room, injury related to excessive stress/strain is insignificant in most patients, but should be kept in mind in patients at risk for developing lung injury: those receiving long term ventilation and those likely to experience simultaneous hits on their lungs (see later).

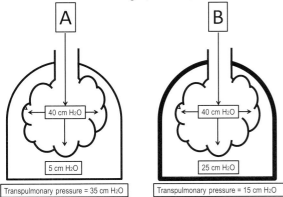

Fig. 19.1 A and B show two lungs receiving the same alveolar pressure (PA) but with different consequences. Patient (B) has lower transpulmonary pressure and lower risk of barotrauma.

Biotrauma

Biotrauma is the biological reaction to mechanical injury [4]. Damage of lung parenchyma causes the release of white cells and pro-inflammatory cytokines – interleukin (IL) IL-1β, IL-6, IL-8, tumour necrosis factor (TNFα) – resulting in lung inflammation.

Biotrauma is obvious when stress/strain is high enough to break lung structure, causing gross, visible anatomical damage. This is mainly caused by repeated recruitment/derecruitment and/or overdistension of the lung [13]. But biotrauma is also measurable with low-intensity damage caused by prolonged mechanical ventilation, fluid overload, hyperoxia, etc., and especially when their effects are combined.

Multiple-hit Theory

Patients submitted to aggressive surgical procedures are at risk of developing postoperative lung injury due to 'multiple-hits' on their lungs in the perioperative phase (Table 19.1) [14]. In the operating room, the lungs may sustain a first injury by sepsis, trauma, infection, or any other harm often related to a surgical problem. These problems are more or less unavoidable. But when we treat the patient in the operating room, we want to avoid second-hits that are under our control yet are also known to cause lung injury: atelectrauma, volutrauma, fluid overload, etc.

Goals of Ventilation during General Anaesthesia

Intraoperatively, mechanical ventilation serves the same goals as physiological ventilation (O_2 delivery and CO_2 removal). Even though mechanical ventilation is innocuous in most surgical patients, we must be cautious in those patients at risk of postoperative pulmonary complications (PPC). We have to identify these patients. Table 19.2 shows a list of risk factors for PPC [14]. Predictive scores such as ARISCAT [15] can

Table 19.1. Postoperative acute lung injury.

First hit	Second hit
Pneumonia	Atelectrauma
Trauma	Volutrauma
Sepsis	Hyperoxia
Shock	Transfusion
Brain injury	Fluid overdose
Pancreatitis	Delayed resuscitation
	Inappropiate antibiotics
	Acid aspiration
	Prolonged surgery

Adapted from Gallart L, Canet J: Best Pract. Res. Clin. Anaesthesiol. 2015; 29: 315–30

Table 19.2. Risk factors for postoperative pulmonary complications[a].

	Level of certainty	Patient-related factors	Procedure-related factors	Preoperative testing
ACP guidelines [19]	Good evidence	Congestive heart failure ASA class ≥ 2 Advanced age COPD Functional dependence	Aortic aneurysm Thoracic Abdominal Upper abdominal Neurosurgery Prolonged surgery Head and neck Emergency Vascular General anaesthesia	Albumin < 30 g/L
	Fair evidence	Weight loss Impaired sensorium Smoking Alcohol use	Transfusion	Chest X-ray BUN > 21 mg/dL
Recently identified risk factors or conflicting results	Insufficient evidence	Respiratory infection in the last month Respiratory symptoms GERD Diabetes mellitus Weight loss BMI ≥ 40 kg/m² Obstructive sleep apnoea Liver disease Sepsis		Positive cough test $SpO_2 < 96\%$ Hb < 10 g/dL

[a] Adapted from Gallart L, Canet J. Post-operative pulmonary complications: Understanding definitions and risk assessment. Best Pract. Res. Clin. Anaesthesiol. 2015; 29 (3): 315–30.
Abbreviations: ACP, American College of Physicians; ASA, American Society of Anesthesiologists; BMI, body mass index; BUN, blood urea nitrogen; COPD, chronic obstructive pulmonary disease; GERD, gastroesophageal reflux disease; Hb, haemoglobin; SpO_2, oxygen saturation measured by pulse oximetry.

also be useful to stratify risk. A common example of patient at risk of PPC would be an 80-year-old patient presenting for a prolonged emergency laparotomy for colon perforation.

Intraoperative Oxygenation

The use of a high FiO_2 during anaesthesia can induce oxygen toxicity and worsen atelectasis. Oxygen toxicity has been demonstrated in animals but the toxic threshold for human adults is unknown. Pulmonary toxicity due to hyperoxia is related to prolonged exposure and high-stretch mechanical ventilation. Hyperoxia can enhance the lung toxicity of drugs such as bleomycin, adriamicin and amiodarone and possibly also other chemotherapy drugs such as cytotoxic antibiotics, alkylating agents, anti-metabolites, alkaloids or biological response modifiers [16]. On the other hand, some have suggested it may be prudent to avoid high O_2 concentrations at the extremes of age, and when

vasoconstriction or ischaemia–reperfusion injury is likely to occur (patients at risk of coronary disease, stroke or postoperative cognitive dysfunction) [17].

To consider what the optimal FiO_2 in the perioperative period might be, we have to consider three different periods: induction, maintenance and emergence.

During induction, a high FiO_2 prior to intubation (i.e. preoxygenation) will increase the time to desaturation during apnoea (e.g. during a dreaded cannot intubate–cannot ventilate scenario). In healthy patients, apnoea time to 90% SpO_2 (oxygen saturation measured by pulse oximetry) was 411 sec after preoxygenation with 100% O_2, but only 200 sec when preoxygenated with 60% O_2 [18]. Thus, routine preoxygenation with a high FiO_2 during induction is likely to improve safety. But the downside is an increase in atelectasis. It is widely accepted that at least 80% O_2 is needed to cause atelectasis, but this is based on research in healthy subjects [18]. In obese, COPD or elderly patients alveolar collapse probably occurs with lower FiO_2. In any case, the use of high FiO_2 is recommended during preoxygenation prior to induction, and atelectasis can be treated after intubation with RM and PEEP.

During maintenance of anaesthesia, an FiO_2 of at least 30% is used routinely to counteract the effect of V/Q mismatching on oxygenation. Hyperoxia ($FiO_2 > 80\%$) to decrease surgical site infection after colorectal surgery has been recommended by Centers for Disease Control (CDC) and World Health Organization (WHO), but this recommendation has generated controversy [19]. A meta-analysis concluded that intraoperative hyperoxia does not increase the risk of atelectasis if PEEP is used [20]. The level of PEEP required is unknown and probably has to be tailored for every patient [21].

During emergence, 100% O_2 is commonly used to avoid diffusion hypoxia (Fink effect) for the first five minutes after discontinuing N_2O or after liberal use of opioids. However, hyperoxia during emergence and after emergence could induce postoperative atelectasis. Although we use RM and PEEP before extubation, these recruitment tools can no longer be used after extubation, a crucial moment because the lung tends to collapse due to pain induced splinting, hypoventilation and decreased muscle activity. This collapse would be impaired by hyperoxia, thus some authorities recommend not to use hyperoxygenation before extubation [22].

Avoid Atelectrauma: Recruitment and Positive End-expiratory Pressure

The pressure needed to recruit alveoli (=critical opening pressure) is much higher than the pressure needed to keep these alveoli open after they have been recruited [23]. This is dictated by Laplace's law: the lower the radius of the alveolus, the higher the pressure needed to open it. Once the alveolus is inflated, the radius increases and the pressure needed to keep the alveolus open decreases. Also, the critical opening pressure is not the same for all alveoli: it is higher in the dependent lung zones (posterior and caudal), it is intermediate in patients with obesity, COPD and/or after prolonged mechanical ventilation, and it is higher still in the presence of pulmonary disorders such as oedema, infection or ARDS.

Lachmann [24] stated: 'open the lung and keep the lung open', which means RM used to open alveoli have to be followed by PEEP to keep them open: both are needed. If RM are not followed by PEEP, alveoli will collapse again. If PEEP is administered without RM,

the pressure will probably be ineffective to open collapsed alveoli.

RM during anaesthesia can be performed by bag squeezing, continuous positive airway pressure (CPAP) or stepwise V_T changes, but probably the best systematized method is the cycling manoeuvre: both inspiratory pressure and PEEP are gradually increasing to 20 cm H_2O (i.e. a total pressure of 20 + 20 cm H_2O) [25]. Once 40 cm H_2O is reached, PEEP is progressively decreased and the optimal PEEP value is determined by looking for the lowest PEEP value that still yields the highest increase in compliance (further explained below).

When might RM be used? Intraoperatively, the use of RM + PEEP could be particularly advantageous (1) after intubation, when atelectasis is common; (2) after any disconnection (especially if combined with airway suctioning), because alveoli have been derecruited; (3) before extubation, to generate the best recruitment conditions for the postoperative period; and (4) when adverse conditions for the lung are present, such as prolonged ventilation, obesity, pneumoperitoneum or relative hypoxaemia (i.e. low SpO_2 despite high FiO_2).

With regard to PEEP, there is no agreement as to the PEEP level that should be used if it is used and as to whether the routine use of intraoperative PEEP affects outcome [21]. While some experts and meta-analysis [26] recommend the routine use of PEEP to reduce PPCs, other studies do not concur this. In the PROVHILO study [27], 12 cm H_2O PEEP with RM did not lower the incidence of PPC after open abdominal surgery compared to ≤ 2 cm H_2O PEEP without RM. One working hypothesis is that patients might benefit from 'individualized PEEP' or 'optimal PEEP' as defined in the classic paper of Suter et al [28]. Gradually increasing PEEP will improve oxygenation by decreasing pulmonary shunt and improving lung compliance. As PEEP is being further increased, oxygenation may still be improving, but at some point, both O_2 delivery and compliance will deteriorate, the former because heart–lung interactions will decrease cardiac output, the latter because high inflation pressure causes alveolar overdistension. 'Best PEEP' therefore is the lowest PEEP that generates optimal O_2 delivery and compliance.

The pressure–volume (P–V) curve explains the above concepts as well as some concepts to be discussed later (Fig. 19.2). The P–V curve is S-shaped, and its slope or steepness ($\Delta P/\Delta V$) defines the compliance. The curve has three segments: an initial only slightly inclined part (collapse zone), a central steep incline (safe zone), and a final part that again has flattened out

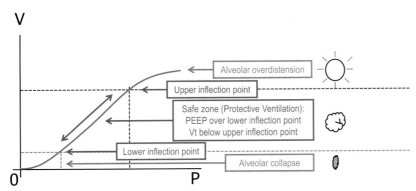

Fig. 19.2 Pressure–volume curve model in patients with mechanical ventilation. The first part of the curve starts from atmospheric pressure. A high pressure is needed to open collapsed alveoli. A lower inflection point indicates the pressure at which alveoli are opened. A second part of the curve shows the ideal zone with best compliance, where high volumes are achieved with low pressures. A third part of the curve, starting at an upper inflexion point, shows the overdistension zone: high pressures scarcely provide changes in volume and risk of barotrauma is increased.

(overdistension zone). These segments are connected by a lower inflection point (between the collapse and the safe zones), and an upper inflection point (between the safe and the overdistension zones). The S-shape is pronounced in patients with ARDS but may be almost imperceptible in healthy subjects.

If the lung is positioned in the collapse zone, compliance (the steepness) is low and a high pressure will be needed to open the collapsed alveoli. Atelectrauma is bound to result from opening and closing alveoli if the lung is being ventilated in this area of the P–V curve. The lower inflection point indicates the airway pressure at which alveoli start to open. In the central safe zone with the steep slope, compliance has increased (improved) because alveoli are open and they are easy to inflate. Thus, low airway pressure increments yield high volume changes. PEEP titrated to this part of the curve is optimal PEEP. The upper inflection point defines the point of (near) maximal lung volume. The absolute volume is high in healthy subjects but low in e.g. ARDS patients ('baby lung' concept) [12]. In this overdistension zone, high pressures will be needed to inflate the already overinflated lungs and volutrauma will ensue.

The alveolar opening pressure is not the same for all alveoli [29, 30]. Some are easily opened at low pressures, others need high pressures, and others still will not open despite recruitment manoeuvres. The S-shape is most consistently observed in patients with ARDS but it is not prominent in healthy subjects, who are less prone to atelectasis and in whom overdistension is observed only with very high V_T. But even though the typical S-shape of the curve is not always present, the concepts of recruitment, safe and overdistension zones apply to all patients.

Optimal PEEP is the level of PEEP that positions the lung above the lower inflection point. Fig. 19.3a shows a theoretical model where the P–V curve would

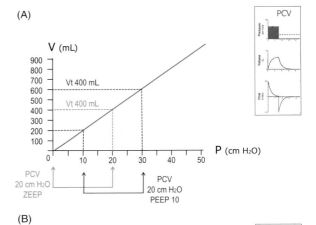

(A)

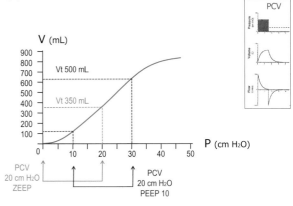

(B)

Fig. 19.3 Pressure–volume curve in patients receiving pressure-controlled ventilation (PCV, see text for details and Fig. 19.6). In a theoretical model with a straight P–V curve (A), Vt delivered with PCV+PEEP or PCV without PEEP (ZEEP) would be the same. With a S-shaped P-V curve (B), the volume delivered with PCV+PEEP will be larger than with PCV+ZEEP. Vt will be the same with different PEEP levels provided these PEEP values are higher than the lower inflection point, which indicates the value of optimal PEEP. See text for details.

be straight. During pressure controlled ventilation (PCV), 20 cm H_2O Paw + 10 cm H_2O PEEP would generate the same V_T as 20 cm H_2O Paw + 0 cm H_2O PEEP

(ZEEP) because these changes occur along a straight line. With an S-shaped P–V curve (Fig. 19.3B), the same pressure difference (i.e. 20 cm H_2O) will generate a different V_T with different PEEP levels. Ventilation with PEEP above the lower inflection point would position the lung on the straight 'safe' line. Ventilation without any PEEP (ZEEP) and thus below the lower inflection point would position the lung on the more horizontal part where compliance is worst, and as a consequence a lower V_T for the same pressure difference will be generated when PEEP is reduced. Thus, the lower inflection point and optimal PEEP can be identified by monitoring the expired V_T while decreasing PEEP during PCV. This procedure is described in Table 19.3.

Avoid Volutrauma: Deliver the Appropriate Tidal Volume (V_T)

Protective lung ventilation is a strategy that includes PEEP, low V_T and RM. Even though widely used during anaesthesia, the benefits on patient outcome remain unclear. Experts and meta-analysis [26, 31] recommend a V_T of 6–8 mL/kg predicted body weight (PBW), with PBW for men = 50 + 0.91(cm of height – 152.4) and PBW for women = 45.5 + 0.91(cm of height – 152.4). An easier alternative is Broca's formula [32]: Ideal body weight = height (cm) – 100.

To avoid volutrauma, we must understand the different components of the airway pressure curve measured at the mouth of the patient and displayed on our anaesthesia workstation. The peak inspiratory pressure (P_{PEAK}) in the pressure–time curve during volume controlled ventilation (Fig. 19.4) is the net result of the sum of three pressures: PEEP, the pressure difference required to expand the lung, and the pressure difference required to overcome the forces opposing airflow. Let us consider all three. Note that the following analysis of airway pressure tracings during volume controlled ventilation requires that the machine generates a constant square flow waveform.

PEEP can be external or internal (also called intrinsic PEEP or auto-PEEP). External PEEP is the PEEP applied by the ventilator (as selected by the clinician). Auto-PEEP is 'hidden': it cannot be derived merely from looking at the pressure wave form on the ventilator but requires additional manoeuvres to be detected. The higher of the two (i.e. PEEP or auto-PEEP) determines the PEEP component that contributes to the P_{PEAK} (see explanation below).

A pressure difference is needed to overcome the static forces of the lung (i.e. in the absence of any gas flow). This is the plateau pressure (P_{PLAT}), measured during the end-inspiratory pause when flow has ceased and the pressure curve has stabilized to a horizontal line. At this time in the ventilatory cycle, pressures have become equal throughout the airway (i.e. from machine tubing to the alveoli) so that P_{PLAT} corresponds to alveolar pressure. This P_{PLAT} is the pressure needed to generate the preset V_T with the current static compliance – 'static' because it is only related to those mechanical characteristics of the respiratory system related to lung inflation without any influence of dynamic elements like flow and resistance.

Finally, a pressure difference is needed to overcome the resistive forces of the lung, i.e. the forces opposing airflow. This dynamic component is determined by the product of inspiratory flow and airway resistance ($\dot{V} \times Raw$) and is reflected in P_{PEAK} (see below). When interpreting P_{PEAK}, it is important to realize that the

Table 19.3. Steps to be taken to determine optimal PEEP (PEEP titration).

- Choose PCV mode (this technique requires a square pressure waveform)
- Perform a RM: use 20 cm H_2O PCV + 20 cm H_2O PEEP
- Decrease PCV to 15 cm H_2O if V_T is high enough
- Progressively decrease PEEP while observing the resulting V_T obtained. Allow sufficient time to let the V_T stabilize after each new PEEP decrement. Once the V_T is stable, take notice of the resulting V_T and proceed with the next PEEP decrement
- Stop when a PEEP decrement results in a lower V_T: this PEEP value lies just below the lower inflection point
- Perform a new RM to re-open the alveoli and set PEEP just above the last PEEP level so it falls above the lower inflection point
- The same procedure could be performed during volume-controlled ventilation (VCV). In this case, a square inspiratory flow is needed and we progressively reduce PEEP (after recruitment), searching for the best compliance. If the ventilator does not display compliance, calculate it by dividing V_T by plateau pressure (measured when it is horizontal, i.e. when flow is absent)
- During PEEP titration, any factor that could alter compliance should be held stable (e.g. neuromuscular blockade, body position, pneumoperitoneum)
- PEEP = Positive end expiratory pressure; PCV = Pressure-controlled ventilation; RM = Recruitment manoeuvre; V_T = Tidal volume; VCV = Volume-controlled ventilation

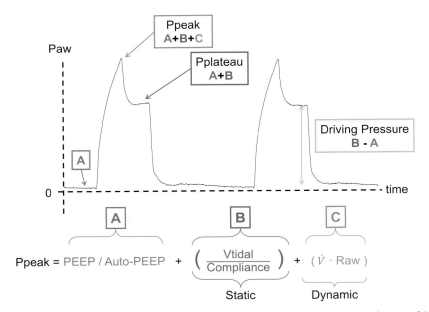

Fig. 19.4 Pressure–time curve displayed in a ventilator. Peak airway pressure (P$_{PEAK}$) is the sum of three components (A+B+C). (A) is the initial pressure at end-expiration. This pressure corresponds to intrinsic or extrinsic PEEP (PEEPi, PEEPe), the highest of both values. PEEPe is displayed by the ventilator but PEEPi is not and has to be measured. (B) is a static component, determined by tidal volume (Vt) and elastance, the reciprocal of compliance. (A+B) is the plateau pressure, which is the same as alveolar pressure during an end-inspiratory plateau during volume controlled ventilation when flow is absent, and indicates the risk of volutrauma. (B – A) is driving pressure, a parameter probably even better than Pplateau as indicative of risk of volutrauma. (C) shows a dynamic component related to inspiratory flow ($\dot{V}$) and airway resistance (Raw). (C) indicates the difference between the pressure generated by the ventilator and the pressure reaching alveoli (Pplateau). If Paw is high with high values of C ($\dot{V}$ or Raw), and the plateau pressure is still normal, there is no increased risk of baro/volutrauma.

monitored 'airway' pressure does not represent the alveolar nor transpulmonary pressure throughout the respiratory cycle. As long as there is inspiratory flow, the measured 'airway pressure' differs from that in the alveoli, and thus a high P$_{PEAK}$ because of increased airway resistance (bronchospasm, tube kinking) or high flow (high respiratory rate) differs from P$_{PLAT}$.

A high P$_{PLAT}$ is the main culprit of volutrauma/barotrauma. But a lung receiving 35 cm H$_2$O P$_{PLAT}$ + 15 cm H$_2$O PEEP (20 cm H$_2$O gradient) will have less stress/strain than a lung receiving 35 cm H$_2$O P$_{PLAT}$ + 5 cm H$_2$O PEEP (30 cm H$_2$O gradient) because the FRC will be higher with 15 cm H$_2$O PEEP. The (P$_{PLAT}$ – PEEP) gradient is the driving pressure (ΔP). In ICU patients with ARDS, Amato et al [33] analysed 3,500 patients from nine randomized trials and demonstrated that ΔP was a better predictor of mortality than P$_{PLAT}$ per se. The notion that driving pressure is associated with better outcomes than P$_{PLAT}$ in the ICU could be applicable to the operating room population, mainly in patients at risk of lung injury (multiple-hit) or in patients ventilated in adverse conditions such as pneumoperitoneum or Trendelenburg, but this requires further study. If we set the V$_T$ while respecting a certain driving pressure

limit, we will generate an adequate V$_T$ that takes the lung characteristics of the individual patient into account [34].

The safe driving pressure limit has not been clearly identified, but 15 cm H$_2$O has been proposed, a value derived from ARDS research [35]. Most surgical patients who need high pressures (obesity, pneumoperitoneum) would probably tolerate them, but a cautious attitude would still be to adhere to certain limits during anaesthesia as well.

The airway pressure waveform morphology itself can also give information about the stress/strain of the lung [36]. During VCV with a square flow pattern, the slope of the airway pressure curve changes if lung compliance changes. Fig. 19.5 simultaneously displays the S shaped P–V curve (at the bottom) and the Paw curve displayed by the ventilator (on top). Part 1 shows the pressure curve that includes the lower inflection point. The initial airway pressure slope is steep and it becomes less steep once collapsed alveoli have been opened and compliance improves. Part 2 shows a straight part of the P–V curve, and the airway pressure is less steep as well as straighter than in part 1 because compliance does not change. Part 3 includes

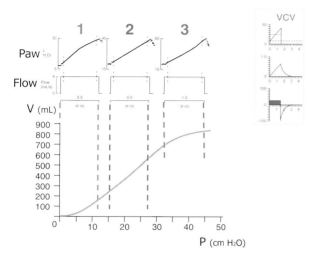

Fig. 19.5 Pressure–time (Paw) curve matched with P–V curve during volume controlled ventilation (VCV). (1) shows a concave down Paw curve denoting an improvement in compliance. (2) shows a straight curve denoting constant compliance. (3) shows a concave up Paw curve denoting an impairment in compliance. A square flow waveform is mandatory. See text for more details.

the upper inflection point. Due to overdistension, compliance is decreased, and the slope of the airway pressure slope increases. In summary, a concave down Paw curve is indicative of recruitment and a concave up Paw curve is indicative of overdistension. Again, a square flow waveform is mandatory to allow data to be interpreted as above.

Auto-PEEP occurs if incomplete expiration is interrupted by the next inspiration [37]. As a result, the V_T delivered during inspiration is not completely exhaled. This volume of non-expired gas remains trapped in the lungs, increasing end-expiratory alveolar pressure. The mechanism of this so-called 'dynamic hyperinflation' can be caused by two factors: increased alveolar time constants (decreased elastic recoil causing increased compliance, or increased airway resistance) and/or insufficient expiratory time.

Auto-PEEP is not detected by the manometer of the ventilator. We can suspect auto-PEEP to be present if the expiratory flow curve does not arrive at zero and/or if the capnogram continues to rise without attaining a horizontal plateau. To measure auto-PEEP, we have to place a clamp between the patient and the Y-piece at the end of expiration and measure the pressure in any point between the clamp and the patient. Some ventilators measure auto-PEEP by occluding the expiratory limb of the breathing system. Another easy method to measure auto-PEEP

[38] is to perform step by step increases of extrinsic PEEP while watching for a rise in the P_{PEAK} (see Fig. 19.4). In normal conditions, an increase in external PEEP will increase P_{PEAK} by the same amount. In patients with auto-PEEP, external PEEP does not increase P_{PEAK} until the extrinsic PEEP exceeds the intrinsic one. The best analogy is that of the waterfall [39]. Expiratory flow can be compared to the flow in a river; auto-PEEP can be compared to a dam in the waterfall; and external PEEP can be compared to the height of the water distal of the dam. As long as the height of the water upstream from the dam is higher than the height of the water downstream, water will continue to flow, regardless of the height of the water downstream of the dam. By analogy, as long as intrinsic PEEP is higher than external PEEP, air can be exhaled. When (and only if) the level of the water downstream of the dam becomes higher than the dam itself, the water upstream of the dam will rise. Again, by analogy, when external PEEP becomes higher than intrinsic PEEP, airway pressure and thus lung inflation will increase, causing P_{PEAK} to rise. A healthy lung is like a river without waterfalls. When there is no waterfall, a minimal dam will increase water height. Similarly, when there is no auto-PEEP, even a minimal external PEEP will increase the P_{PEAK}.

The waterfall model also explains the effect of PEEP during spontaneous breathing in patients with air trapping during a COPD exacerbation. Healthy subjects inspire with a minimal negative pressure (no waterfall) while COPD patients need to generate a negative pressure higher than intrinsic PEEP. External PEEP is the dam that facilitates the inspiratory (upstream) flow. Further details are generated by Rossi et al [38].

Different Mechanical Ventilation Modes: Pressure, Volume and Flow Monitoring

During the inspiratory phase of mechanical ventilation, the morphology of the pressure, flow and tidal volume tracing depends on whether volume or pressure is the variable controlled by the ventilator, i.e. whether volume controlled ventilation (VCV) or pressure controlled ventilation (PCV) is being used, respectively. During VCV, the tidal volume is fixed and the resulting pressure depends on the patient–machine interaction. In contrast, during PCV, pressure is fixed and the resulting volume depends on the patient–machine interaction. Expiration, however, is usually passive and only depends on patient's characteristics, regardless of the ventilator mode.

The next two sections consider the inspiratory phase during VCV and PCV, while a third section considers the expiratory phase. The final section discusses pressure assisted modes of ventilation.

Volume Controlled Ventilation

During volume controlled ventilation (VCV), volume is the controlled variable (Fig. 19.6). VCV ensures a constant V_T regardless of changes in patient compliance and resistance (e.g. due to laparoscopy, Trendelenburg position, neuromuscular blockade, etc.). The resulting Paw curve is determined by patient and equipment factors summarized in Fig. 19.4. The resulting Paw changes can be analysed (Fig. 19.4 and Fig. 19.5) provided a constant square flow waveform or rectangle (■) is present. If flow changes over time, e.g. decreasing (◣) or increasing (◢), the slope of the Paw curve will change accordingly.

The area under the flow curve (flow × time) equals the tidal volume. Whenever time is modified, flow has to be changed in the opposite direction to maintain the same area. Thus, if inspiratory time (Ti) is reduced, the base of the rectangle (time) will be reduced and the ventilator will increase the height of the rectangle (flow) in order to maintain the same area and thus V_T. The increased flow will cause an increase in P_{PEAK} (Fig. 19.4c) but without increasing the risk of barotrauma because P_{PLAT} (V_T/static compliance) will not change. Ti is decreased if the respiratory rate is increased, the inspiratory to expiratory time (I:E) ratio is reduced, or an end-inspiratory pause is applied.

Pressure Controlled Ventilation

During pressure controlled ventilation (PCV), pressure is the variable that the ventilator controls, and the generated pressure is constant (Fig. 19.6). The

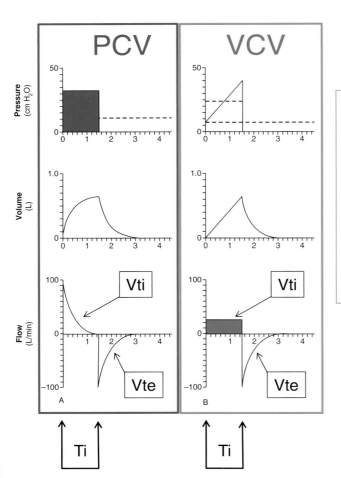

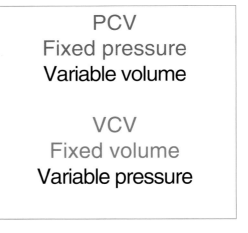

Fig. 19.6 Differences in pressure, volume and flow curves between pressure controlled ventilation (PCV) and volume controlled ventilation (VCV). Vti = inspired tidal volume; Vte = expired tidal volume; Ti = inspiratory time. See text for more details.

resulting flow curve and V_T depend on patient factors (compliance and resistance properties of the lung) and equipment factors (inspiratory flow, Ti, tracheal tube resistance). Opposite to VCV, we now can analyse the flow curve to understand the parameters of the underlying systems, but the pressure curve is fixed.

PCV generates an inspiratory flow curve that more resembles that of physiological inspiration, with an exponential decay pattern towards zero flow in healthy lungs (Fig. 19.6). This flow pattern can be altered by respiratory disorders. When resistance is increased, the inspiratory flow curve is flattened and remains longer above zero. Less frequently, when compliance is reduced without a change in resistance, the decline in the inspiratory flow curve is accelerated and returns quickly to the zero line [40].

Like during VCV, the area under the flow curve is equivalent to V_T. But contrary to VCV, if we change Ti, the ventilator will not modify the flow to guarantee V_T. Thus, if we reduce Ti, the area below the curve will be decreased and V_T will be reduced. The amount of 'lost V_T' is probably minimal in healthy lungs, where 'standard' Ti settings are long enough to deliver an appropriate V_T. But treating the resulting hypercapnia by increasing respiratory rate (RR) will decrease Ti and further decrease V_T. Instead, Ti needs to be prolonged by reducing RR, which will improve V_T and decrease auto-PEEP. Less auto-PEEP will improve lung compliance in an overdistended lung by moving from the upper segment of the S-shaped P–V curve to the central segment, further increasing V_T generated by the same controlled pressure. Close monitoring is needed to prevent and treat hypercapnia during PCV. Watching the shape and area of the flow curve while changing Ti will help to understand these concepts.

PCV can be useful to avoid high Paw that could induce baro/volutrauma because any change in lung and thoracic wall compliance (Trendelenburg position, CO_2 pneumoperitoneum, neuromuscular blockade or other factors) will reduce the delivered V_T. There is no baro/volutrauma because pressure and V_T are limited. The downside is the potential for severe hypoventilation.

During PCV we cannot know whether a high Paw can cause volutrauma because there is no inspiratory zero flow pause (i.e. no P_{PLAT}). We have to switch to VCV with an adequate inspiratory pause, and apply the same V_T that was previously generated by PCV. Then, if P_{PLAT} is low, high pressure is related to airway resistance and there is a low risk of barotrauma. If, however, P_{PLAT} and/or driving pressure is increased, V_T might have to be reduced to avoid volutrauma.

Expiration

Expiratory flow is by definition depicted as a negative flow. The area under this curve is the expired tidal volume (Fig. 19.6). Expiratory flow is passive which means it is only determined by the patient's lung characteristics.

The expiratory flow curve initially drops to a negative peak value, to be followed by a smooth rising exponential curve that progressively returns to zero. The expiratory peak flow is directly proportional to end-inspiratory alveolar pressure, and inversely proportional to the lung time constant (τ, tau) which is the product of compliance × resistance [11]. Peak expiratory flow is increased in patients with low compliance, due to a pathological stiffness of the lung (ARDS, pulmonary fibrosis) or due to transient conditions such as Trendelenburg position or CO_2 pneumoperitoneum. In contrast, peak expiratory flow is decreased in patients with a high compliance (emphysema, with a loss of elastic recoil due to collagen destruction) and/or a high resistance (asthma).

The smooth exponential flow waveform (convex up) is determined by its time constant and thus is affected by compliance and expiratory airway resistance changes. Lung units with a lower resistance and/or low compliance will have a shorter time constant and will require less time to empty [11]. In contrast, lung units with a high compliance and/or a high resistance will have a longer time constant and will need more time to empty.

In a healthy subject, expiratory flow will rapidly rise to zero, but in patients with expiratory airflow obstruction and increased airway resistance, the slope of the expiratory curve becomes more horizontal and may not reach zero value before the start of a new inspiratory cycle, resulting in auto-PEEP (see above). This flow pattern usually coexists with a capnogram that displays a rising slope without reaching a horizontal plateau. Both curves indicate that expiration has not finished and air trapping is likely to be present.

The end-tidal CO_2 ($ETCO_2$) of a capnogram without a horizontal plateau does not reflect real alveolar CO_2 because complete expiration has not been achieved yet. If we want the $ETCO_2$ to better reflect alveolar CO_2, the RR must be briefly reduced, allowing the CO_2 curve to become flat ('true' $ETCO_2$).

Assisted Ventilation Modes: Pressure Support Ventilation or Synchronized Intermittent Mandatory Ventilation

Several ventilation modes can assist the patient's spontaneous breathing efforts to minimize the work of breathing or improve gas exchange [25]. Current ventilators offer assisted or assisted controlled ventilation modes, with different names assigned to them by different manufacturers. The more frequently used modes are pressure support ventilation (PSV) and synchronized intermittent mandatory ventilation (SIMV).

Pressure support ventilation generates a preset pressure after the patient has triggered the ventilator. This mode of ventilation has several advantages: (1) spontaneous muscular activity is maintained; (2) inspiratory negative pressure is preserved, which helps maintain venous return and thus cardiac output; (3) the ventilator's respiratory rate is adapted to the patient's spontaneous breathing rate; (4) stress/strain is reduced; (5) V/Q matching may be improved; (6) opioids can be titrated to respiratory rate; (7) reduced use of muscle relaxants may reduce the incidence of residual curarization and the need for a reversal agent.

The clinician needs to set several parameters [41]. First, the trigger that initiates ventilatory support can be a change in flow or a change in pressure (i.e. flow or pressure triggering). If the ventilator has both types of effort sensors, we will use the one that generates the best response (probably flow triggered). Triggers must be sensitive enough to detect patient effort without demanding an additional inspiratory load or without causing inspiratory dys-synchrony (patient fighting the ventilator). But too sensitive a trigger can cause auto triggering (i.e. the machine starts triggering itself). The breathing system should have no air leaks, no water condensation, and should have rigid, low-compliance tubes to minimize compressible volume and optimize flow and pressure transmission. The management of triggering is probably irrelevant in healthy subjects but it is important in COPD, frail or ICU patients. The second parameter to be set is the degree of positive pressure support. The transpulmonary pressure and consequently V_T is the sum of negative plus positive pressure. The higher the negative pressure effort generated by the patient, the less positive pressure is needed. Third and finally, Ti has to be set. This time can be pre-programmed or can be related to the inspiratory flow, for example, by terminating inspiratory flow once it decreases below e.g. 25% of peak flow.

Synchronized intermittent mandatory ventilation (SIMV) guarantees to deliver a minimum, mandatory ventilation at a low respiratory rate, combined with spontaneous cycles. The mandatory ventilation is automatically adapted to spontaneous ventilation in order to prevent patients from fighting the machine. It is mainly used in ICU patients, but some anaesthesia ventilators offer it too.

Assisted modes of ventilation are not used routinely in anaesthesia, because it is difficult to combine spontaneous ventilation with immobility, mainly during variable pain stimuli. However usage patterns differ widely and the use of other modes may be increasing. If spontaneous ventilation is used, ventilators offer a safety backup if the respiratory drive is suppressed after deepening of anaesthesia. PSV can be particularly useful during emergence from anaesthesia to facilitate the return to spontaneous ventilation and to optimize titration of opioids.

Use of Non-ventilatory Strategies

To avoid postoperative pulmonary complications, the management of mechanical ventilation during anaesthesia includes a series of non-ventilatory strategies as well [14, 42]. These strategies would include moderately restrictive fluid management and/or goal directed fluid therapy to avoid oedema yet also minimize renal insufficiency, avoid the routine use of a nasogastric tube to decrease the risk of pneumonia, minimize transfusion because of its immunosuppressive effects, preoperative dental brushing, appropriate antibiotic use, and possibly the use of inhaled anaesthetics to reduce lung inflammatory response. The relevance of many of these factors is unclear, but they are easy measures which altogether may be beneficial.

Emergence

Most surgical patients were breathing normally before surgery, and this condition has to be regained as soon as possible to avoid postoperative pulmonary complications [43]. Conditions necessary for optimal extubation [43–45] include: (1) absence of postoperative residual curarization (PORC), ensured by using monitoring and administering antagonists if indicated; (2) return of spontaneous respiration, without residual effects of anaesthetics and opioids (short-acting drugs, appropriate titration, and monitoring of consciousness are useful to accomplish this); (3) intact upper airway reflexes to avoid bronchial aspiration; (4) airway patency provided by upper airway muscles [44]; and (5) adequate analgesia to ensure painless breathing, particularly after surgery close to the diaphragm [14]. Regional anaesthesia, mainly epidural, is probably the best choice to attain this objective. In patients with a difficult airway, guidelines for the management of tracheal extubation have to be considered [46]. Slower, more progressive weaning should be considered for patients with acute respiratory disorders (hypoxaemia, fatigue, bronchospasm) and/or after surgical procedures that may impair respiration. Extubation may also have to be delayed in the presence of non-pulmonary problems such as hypothermia, acidosis, sepsis, haemodynamic instability, coma, etc.

Automated Control of Mechanical Ventilation

Automated control of mechanical ventilation has been introduced in intensive care units, mainly to facilitate weaning. This technology is being introduced on anaesthesia machines [47].

Conclusion

In order to properly manage mechanical ventilation and oxygenation during anaesthesia, we must understand the physiology and pathophysiology of the lung, the causes of lung damage, and how to appropriately handle the ventilator settings. The latter involves an understanding of how pressure, flow, volume, resistance, compliance and time are related. Proper understanding of these concepts, integrated with appropriate monitoring, will allow the clinician to personalize oxygenation and ventilation to the individual patient. Future automation of ventilation and oxygenation is looming around the corner.

References

1. Druz WS, Sharp JT: Activity of respiratory muscles in upright and recumbent humans. J.Appl.Physiol.Respir. Environ.Exerc.Physiol. 1981; 51 (6): 1552–61.
2. Hedenstierna G, Edmark L: Effects of anesthesia on the respiratory system. Best.Pract.Res.Clin.Anaesthesiol. 2015; 29 (3): 273–84.
3. Froese AB, Bryan AC: Effects of anesthesia and paralysis on diaphragmatic mechanics in man. Anesthesiology. 1974; 41 (3): 242–55.
4. Tusman G, Bohm SH, Warner DO, Sprung J: Atelectasis and perioperative pulmonary complications in high-risk patients. Curr.Opin.Anaesthesiol. 2012; 25 (1): 1–10.
5. Bersten AD, Kavanagh BP: A metabolic window into acute respiratory distress syndrome: stretch, the "baby" lung, and atelectrauma. Am.J.Respir.Crit.Care.Med. 2011; 183 (9): 1120–2.
6. Slutsky AS, Ranieri VM: Ventilator-induced lung injury. N.Engl.J.Med. 2013; 369 (22): 2126–36.
7. Duggan M, Kavanagh BP: Pulmonary atelectasis: a pathogenic perioperative entity. Anesthesiology. 2005; 102 (4): 838–54.
8. Chiumello D, Carlesso E, Cadringher P, Caironi P, Valenza F, Polli F, et al: Lung stress and strain during mechanical ventilation for acute respiratory distress syndrome. Am.J.Respir.Crit.Care.Med. 2008; 178 (4): 346–55.
9. Mead J, Takishima T, Leith D: Stress distribution in lungs: a model of pulmonary elasticity. J.Appl.Physiol. 1970; 28 (5): 596–608.
10. Gattinoni L, Protti A, Caironi P, Carlesso E: Ventilator-induced lung injury: the anatomical and physiological framework. Crit.Care.Med. 2010; 38 (10 Suppl): S539–48.
11. Hess DR: Respiratory mechanics in mechanically ventilated patients. Respir.Care. 2014; 59 (11): 1773–94.
12. Gattinoni L, Marini JJ, Pesenti A, Quintel M, Mancebo J, Brochard L: The "baby lung" became an adult. Intens. Care. Med. 2016; 42 (5): 663–73.
13. Slutsky AS: Ventilator-induced lung injury: from barotrauma to biotrauma. Respir.Care. 2005; 50 (5): 646–59.
14. Gallart L, Canet J: Post-operative pulmonary complications: understanding definitions and risk assessment. Best.Pract.Res.Clin.Anaesthesiol. 2015; 29 (3): 315–30.
15. Canet J, Gallart L, Gomar C, Paluzie G, Valles J, Castillo J, et al: Prediction of postoperative pulmonary complications in a population-based surgical cohort. Anesthesiology. 2010; 113 (6): 1338–50.
16. Allan N, Siller C, Breen A: Anaesthetic implications of chemotherapy. BJA.Educ. 2011; 12 (2): 52–6.
17. Habre W, Petak F: Perioperative use of oxygen: variabilities across age. Br.J.Anaesth. 2014; 113 Suppl 2: ii26–36.
18. Edmark L, Kostova-Aherdan K, Enlund M, Hedenstierna G: Optimal oxygen concentration during induction of general anesthesia. Anesthesiology. 2003; 98 (1): 28–33.
19. Shankar P, Robson SC, Otterbein LE, Shaefi S: Clinical implications of hyperoxia. Int.Anesthesiol.Clin. 2018; 56 (1): 68–79.
20. Hovaguimian F, Lysakowski C, Elia N, Tramer MR: Effect of intraoperative high inspired oxygen fraction on surgical site infection, postoperative nausea and vomiting, and pulmonary function: systematic review

and meta-analysis of randomized controlled trials. Anesthesiology. 2013; 119 (2): 303–16.

21. Hedenstierna G, Edmark L: Protective ventilation during anesthesia: is it meaningful? Anesthesiology. 2016; 125 (6): 1079–82.

22. Hedenstierna G: Oxygen and anesthesia: what lung do we deliver to the post-operative ward? Acta. Anaesthesiol.Scand. 2012; 56 (6): 675–85.

23. Lachmann B: Open lung in ARDS. Minerva.Anestesiol. 2002; 68 (9): 637–42.

24. Lachmann B: Open up the lung and keep the lung open. Intens.Care.Med. 1992; 18 (6): 319–21.

25. Ball L, Dameri M, Pelosi P: Modes of mechanical ventilation for the operating room. Best.Pract.Res. Clin.Anaesthesiol. 2015; 29 (3): 285–99.

26. Serpa Neto A, Hemmes SN, Barbas CS, Beiderlinden M, Biehl M, Binnekade JM, et al: Protective versus conventional ventilation for surgery: a systematic review and individual patient data meta-analysis. Anesthesiology. 2015; 123 (1): 66–78.

27. Hemmes SN, Gama de Abreu M, Pelosi P, Schultz MJ: High versus low positive end-expiratory pressure during general anaesthesia for open abdominal surgery (PROVHILO trial): a multicentre randomised controlled trial. Lancet. 2014; 384 (9942): 495–503.

28. Suter PM, Fairley B, Isenberg MD: Optimum end-expiratory airway pressure in patients with acute pulmonary failure. N.Engl.J.Med. 1975; 292 (6): 284–9.

29. Rouby JJ, Puybasset L, Cluzel P, Richecoeur J, Lu Q, Grenier P: Regional distribution of gas and tissue in acute respiratory distress syndrome. II. Physiological correlations and definition of an ARDS Severity Score. CT Scan ARDS Study Group. Intens.Care.Med. 2000; 26 (8): 1046–56.

30. Lu Q, Rouby JJ: Measurement of pressure-volume curves in patients on mechanical ventilation: methods and significance. Crit.Care. 2000; 4 (2): 91–100.

31. Schultz MJ, Abreu MG, Pelosi P: Mechanical ventilation strategies for the surgical patient. Curr. Opin.Crit.Care. 2015; 21 (4): 351–7.

32. Rossner S. Paul Pierre Broca (1824–1880). Obes.Rev. 2007; 8 (3): 277.

33. Amato MB, Meade MO, Slutsky AS, Brochard L, Costa EL, Schoenfeld DA, et al: Driving pressure and survival in acute respiratory distress syndrome. N.Engl.J.Med. 2015; 372 (8): 747–55.

34. Loring SH, Malhotra A: Driving pressure and respiratory mechanics in ARDS. N.Engl.J.Med. 2015; 372 (8): 776–7.

35. Bugedo G, Retamal J, Bruhn A: Driving pressure: a marker of severity, a safety limit, or a goal for mechanical ventilation? Crit.Care. 2017; 21 (1): 199.

36. Richard JC, Maggiore SM, Mercat A: Clinical review: bedside assessment of alveolar recruitment. Crit.Care. 2004; 8 (3): 163–9.

37. Brochard L. Intrinsic (or auto-) PEEP during controlled mechanical ventilation. Intens.Care.Med. 2002; 28 (10): 1376–8.

38. Rossi A, Polese G, Brandi G, Conti G: Intrinsic positive end-expiratory pressure (PEEPi). Intens.Care.Med. 1995; 21 (6): 522–36.

39. Tobin MJ, Lodato RF: PEEP, auto-PEEP, and waterfalls. Chest. 1989; 96 (3): 449–51.

40. Blanch PB, Jones M, Layon AJ, Camner N: Pressure-present ventilation. Part 1: Physiologic and mechanical considerations. Chest. 1993; 104 (2): 590–9.

41. Gilstrap D, MacIntyre N: Patient-ventilator interactions. Implications for clinical management. Am.J.Respir.Crit.Care.Med. 2013; 188 (9): 1058–68.

42. Guldner A, Pelosi P, de Abreu MG: Nonventilatory strategies to prevent postoperative pulmonary complications. Curr.Opin.Anaesthesiol. 2013; 26 (2): 141–51.

43. Canet J, Gallart L: Postoperative respiratory failure: pathogenesis, prediction, and prevention. Curr.Opin. Crit.Care. 2014; 20 (1): 56–62.

44. Sasaki N, Meyer MJ, Eikermann M: Postoperative respiratory muscle dysfunction: pathophysiology and preventive strategies. Anesthesiology. 2013; 118 (4): 961–78.

45. Warner DO: Preventing postoperative pulmonary complications: the role of the anesthesiologist. Anesthesiology. 2000; 92 (5): 1467–72.

46. Ogilvie L: Difficult Airway Society guidelines for the management of tracheal extubation. Anaesthesia. 2012; 67 (11): 1277–8.

47. Schadler D, Miestinger G, Becher T, Frerichs I, Weiler N, Hormann C: Automated control of mechanical ventilation during general anaesthesia: study protocol of a bicentric observational study (AVAS). BMJ.Open. 2017; 7 (5): e014742.

Chapter 20

Epilogue: Artificial Intelligence Methods

Sebastián Jaramillo, José F. Valencia and Pedro L. Gambús

Introduction

With the advances in computational technology, artificial intelligence (AI) systems have been growing exponentially and promise to become tools that are able to overcome some of the most difficult issues of medical research and patient care. Current progress in AI systems offers significant advantages in healthcare, with the potential to minimize the gap between data, knowledge and patient care. The purpose of this chapter is to examine how AI methods might affect data analysis in biomedicine and more specifically in anaesthesia. By the time this book has been published, the anaesthesia and critical care literature will be abound with manuscripts that use AI methods. It will therefore become crucial for the clinician to understand what AI is all about. A detailed understanding of AI requires an extensive knowledge of computational science and complex mathematical concepts. This chapter will provide the reader with the main insights needed to understand the basic concepts of the underlying modelling framework used by AI and will briefly review the different AI methods, their applications and limitations.

Basic Concepts

Because AI covers such a wide spectrum, it always needs to be defined in the context of what it is going to be used for. Still, the definition of AI can be reduced to 'a system that mimics human cognition'. This definition might not represent the actual computational basis of AI, but it summarize its current applications in healthcare well. Examples of medical applications of AI include image recognition on chest x-rays or CT Scan, ECG interpretation, surgery assistance, clinical decision making and differential diagnosis support. These are all considered applications derived from human cognition. However,

AI techniques also carry out tasks that cannot be performed by 'human cognition', such as *big data* processing, pattern recognition and other types of data analyses.

To better understand the concept of AI, it is necessary to know how AI works: a system consisting of an *input*, a *black-box*, and a certain *output* (Figure 20.1). The *input* involves any type of information relevant to what the AI is going to be used for (e.g. images, patient data or drug concentration). The *black-box* refers to the underlying AI model, which consists of statistical procedures and computational algorithms that process the information input(s) and link them to the output. AI has used two major approaches, the *rule-based approach*, and the *machine learning (ML) approach* and mainly differs in the underlying *black-box* structure.

Rule-based AI

Rule-based AI is basically an extensive computational algorithm, built from several 'knowledge-based rules' (Figure 20.2). In this approach, the *black-box* is characterized by many inference rules formulated *a priori*, which specify the 'direction' towards an output given the input conditions. In other words, rule-based AI models are constructed by many 'IF–THEN' rules which link the inputs to the outputs. The main difference with other AI approaches is that 'rule-based' AI models do not

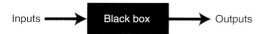

Fig. 20.1 Basic structure of an AI system: *inputs, black-box* (i.e. AI model) and *outputs*.

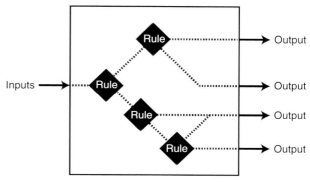

Fig. 20.2 Structure of a rule-based AI system. The information inputs are processed by several static 'rules' which define the pathway to a certain output.

learn from data because the outputs are the direct result from applying the static rules defined by the developer. Therefore, no data are required to develop the model.

This approach was the first AI system to be developed. Examples of this type of AI system are differential diagnosis support systems. In such systems, the inputs are defined by the patient characteristics, symptoms and other clinical data, which are processed by algorithms (e.g. 'is the patient male?' or 'does the patient have anaemia?') to lead to a conclusion (output), such as a disease or condition.

Machine Learning AI

Frequently mixed up with the AI concept, machine learning (ML) models refer to any type of AI model that is able to learn associations from data. In contrast to the rule-based models, ML models are designed to develop their own 'rules' based on the data provided to the system.

ML models are subdivided according to the learning method they employ: *supervised learning, unsupervised learning* and *reinforced learning*. Additionally, ML models can be grouped according to the similarity of the algorithms they use for the specific task they are being used for.

Supervised Learning

In supervised learning, the objective of the ML model is to predict a known output (Figure 20.3). The term 'supervised' means that the output or target is defined *a priori*, and therefore the training process of the model aims to get the most accurate output.

Supervised learning is a two-step process. The first step is the training process, in which the system is 'fed' labelled data (a dataset which contains the outputs). In this step of the process, the system evaluates possible associations between the inputs and the outputs, and then derives a model that links them better. Next, the model is exposed to unlabelled data (dataset not containing outputs), and the estimated outputs ('predicted data') are evaluated to test the accuracy of the model. Supervised learning algorithms and models are classified into two groups:

- *Regression models*: Regression models are quite similar to classic regression approaches. In this type of model, the target is to obtain the most accurate prediction of a predefined output. An example of this type of ML are the risk models such as the Framingham Risk Score and the guide for antithrombotic therapy in atrial fibrillation, in which the output is well defined (e.g. mortality due to cardiovascular disease), and used in the derivation of the model. Other types of regression models include regression trees, ensemble methods and many other types of models, all of them designed to predict or estimate an outcome.

- *Classification models*: With these types of models, the target is to obtain a precise classification or identification of an output. Similar to the regression models, the classification models are also trained with a specific classification output. However, in contrast to regression models, classification models aim to recognize patterns in data inputs to link them to predefined output. Examples of this type of model are the automated EKG interpretation systems and image recognition in chest x-rays, in which the recognition of certain patterns (e.g. ST abnormalities) is linked to a predefined set of diagnoses (e.g. myocardial infarction).

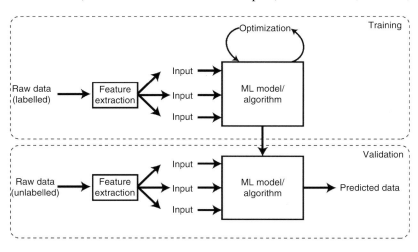

Fig. 20.3 Representation of the development process of a machine learning model using supervised learning. Data are usually split into a *training* and a *validation* dataset. After the extraction of features from raw data, the ML system processes the input/output pairs in order to find the most accurate model. Afterwards, the model is validated by using data without outputs in it (unlabelled data), and the model is evaluated.

Fig. 20.4 Unsupervised learning in ML systems are mainly used to search for patterns or clusters in raw data. As no output is predefined, the ML model is defined by the most relevant patterns observed.

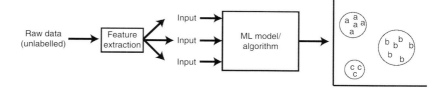

Both types of models, and especially *classification models*, usually need preprocessing of the raw data before they can be properly examined by the model. This process, commonly known as *feature extraction*, is mostly used in image recognition, where the image is processed into a large set of pixels or vectors, and each one of them is handed to the model as a unique input. However, more complex types of ML models, such as neural networks, are designed to also extract features from raw data.

Learning Process

Perhaps the most misunderstood concept is how ML systems actually 'learn' from data. The most basic concept to understand this, and differentiate ML approaches from classical inference statistics, is that ML systems use an optimization algorithm to find the minimum ('simplest') mathematical function that links data to an input. For example, the classic linear regression is determined by the following structure:

$$y = a_0 + a_1 x$$

where *y* is the defined continuous output, a_0 is the intercept of the regression line, and a_1 is the slope of the line.

The most basic concept of the learning process is that the ML system is integrated with a cost function and an *optimization method*. The *cost function* is the overall accuracy estimator of the model, which may vary depending on the ML model used. In the case of the ML linear regression model, the *cost function* is given by the sum of squared errors. Another part of the optimization function is the optimization method. The most frequently used method is the *gradient descendent* method. In simple words, the *gradient descendent* method uses several evaluations of the data (i.e. iterations) to find the model that minimizes the *cost function most*. The goal of adding a *cost function* and the *optimization method* into the ML system is to ensure that (in the case of ML linear regression) the system will continue to update the a_0 and a_1 values until it finds the model that best fits the data. Because both techniques (*cost functions* and *optimization*

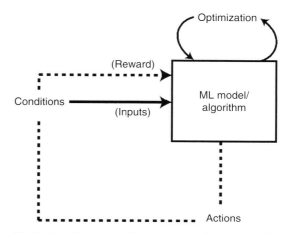

Fig. 20.5 Basic structure of a reinforcement learning-based ML system. The learning process is fundamentally based on the *rewards* obtained from the exploration and exploitation of 'actions' that modify the conditions of the environment.

method) are integrated into the ML system, the system will automatically 'learn' from data and, therefore, no intervention will be required to obtain the most accurate model.

Unsupervised Learning

Unlike supervised learning, the output or target in unsupervised learning is not defined and, therefore, the ML system is 'free' to seek patterns, clusters or groups in data (Figure 20.4). Although this ML approach is not widely known, it is highly relevant in *big data* analysis and *data mining*, where it performs complex tasks such as pattern recognition, clustering and dimensionality reduction. In medical research, unsupervised learning is mostly used to derive information from massive datasets, for instance in genomics or public health-related research.

Reinforcement Learning

Reinforcement learning, infrequently applied in medical care or research, is a ML system that uses continuous learning from data to update the model (Figure 20.5). It resembles supervised learning in that the reinforcement learning uses an optimization method to ensure the accuracy of the model improves. However, in contrast to supervised learning, this type of ML system is in a continuous state of *training* and *validation* because it is constantly exposed to unlabelled new data, and no correct input/output pairs need to be presented. In addition, the learning process of reinforcement learning uses a different optimization method, based on *reward*. The concept of *reward* is complex, and involves finding a balance between data exploration and exploitation.

The main goal of this type of learning is to find the correct 'action' to be taken given a condition or input. However, as no certainty of an 'entirely correct action' is provided, the system is designed to both: (1) search for other new 'actions' that may provide it with *reward* (exploration) and (2) search for 'actions' that the system already knows will provide it with certain *reward* (exploitation).

This type of learning is used mainly in scenarios where dynamic learning is required. Applications in medical care and research are relatively new, and involve data-driven decision support systems and personalized medical decisions systems.

Neural Networks and Deep Learning

Neural networks and *deep learning* are relatively new approaches in machine learning science, yet these are promising tools which have already been proven to be effective in a large variety of contexts, including medical care and research.

The underlying basis of *neural networks* and *deep learning* approaches is distantly based on the structure and physiological functioning of the central nervous system. As neuroscience theories have pointed out, knowledge and learning are processes which may

result from complex interactions between multiple layers of neural systems, including neural systems of perception, processing and storage.

Pretending to simulate the neural system, *neural networks* and *deep learning* approaches are based on a fundamental 'nerve cell-like' entity known as the *perceptron* (Figure 20.6). The perceptron is a machine learning algorithm structure used to classify data into binary outputs. The basic structure of the *perceptron* is composed of multiple information inputs, a *weighing* function for every input, a *weighted sum function* and, finally, a *step function*. Similar to supervised learning, the perceptron uses an optimization method based on several iterations of data, which are used to update the model by modifying the *weights* of each information input. The concept of input *weight* refers directly to the relevance the model gives each input: inputs with a higher *weight* are recognized by the model to be best estimators of the output. The sum of all the input *weights* is then processed by a *step function*, which may be activated if the *sum of weights* is greater than a certain threshold. At the very end of the process, the binary response of the *step function* (activation or no activation) determines the classification of the data.

With a more complex structure and functioning, *neural networks* are fundamentally multiple *perceptrons* combined into a single network (Figure 20.7). However, the configuration of each perceptron is changed from its original structure; in neural networks the *step function* of each perceptron is sigmoid-shaped allowing it to benefit from the interaction between multiple *perceptrons*. The overall structure of the artificial network is composed of three main layers of *perceptrons*. The first layer (*input layer*) receives the information input and processes the information by

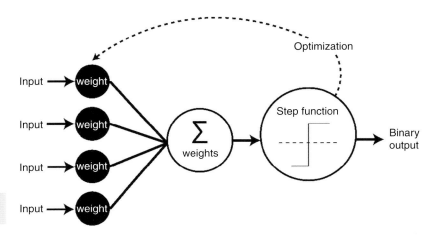

Fig. 20.6 Representation of the *perceptron*. Information input is modified by each *weight*. The sum of all weights determines the activation of the *step function*. The binary functioning of the *step function* (activation/no-activation) is responsible for the binary response of the perceptron.

applying the weights of each input. At the second level, a *hidden layer* of *perceptrons* receives the processed information coming from the *input layer*, and modifies the weight of each information input. Finally, the double-processed information coming from the *hidden layer* is received by the *output layer*. The *perceptrons* of the output layer process the incoming information and provide the final output (binary). The amount of classifications provided by a neural network depends on the number of the *perceptrons* in the output layer.

Optimization methods in *neural networks* may also differ from the original functioning of the *perceptron*. In neural networks, several optimization methods have been proposed and even combined, including methods that modify the step function threshold of *perceptrons* and the information received by them. Many of these optimization methods result in the isolation of a number of *perceptrons*. One of the main optimization methods used in neural networks is *back propagation*. This algorithm optimizes the learning process of the neural networks by calculating the relative contribution of each individual perceptron to the overall error of the model. This method modifies the weights several times on each layer of the *neural network*, starting from the input layers. The importance of this algorithm is that it promotes the 'specialization' of the hidden layer *perceptrons* in recognizing or analysing certain characteristics or features of the input.

One special type of neural network is called the *recurrent neural network*. This type of neural network is the preferred one to analyse time-series data, since it analyses data in a dynamic and temporal way by using an internal 'memory' to process sequences of data inputs. By using this approach, the neural network uses incoming inputs and previously processed inputs to generate an output, making it possible to treat time-dependable tasks such as speech recognition or time-series prediction.

Finally, the deep learning approach refers essentially to an even more complex neural network, which contains multiple *hidden layers* that process the information. This type of AI structure has been recognized as the most sophisticated AI framework and has produced some results superior to human capacities. With the ability to be implemented along with other machine learning systems, the *deep learning* structure has several possible applications. In fact, most of the AI implementations in healthcare are based on the deep learning approach. Some applications include image recognition systems for skin diseases and for diabetic retinopathy. For other proposed medical applications, the technique still has to be improved.

Potentials and Limitations

Given its versatility, AI technology could be applied in many medical contexts, and it has already proven to be effective in performing complex tasks unable to be performed by other methods and even by human experts. One of the most promising applications of AI is related to the exploration of physiological pathways, genomics and proteomics, where it could accelerate target identification for pharmacological interventions and, therefore, improve medical care.

Nevertheless, AI systems still have several limitations. Maybe the most relevant limitations of complex AI systems are directly related to its *black-box* nature. As the complexity of the AI systems grows, the *black-box* gets more and more uninterpretable in terms of underlying physiology, pharmacology, anatomy, pathophysiology, etc. The lack of 'explainability' of these systems is producing distrust because it is felt

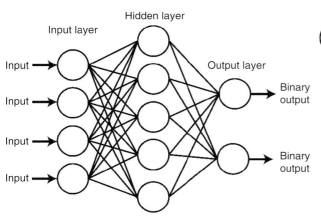

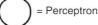 = Perceptron

Fig. 20.7 Schematic representation of a *neural network* with two binary outputs. Each circle represents a unique *perceptron* connected with other *perceptrons* from contiguous layers. Each line symbolizes the information pathway, which is modified in terms of weight in each *perceptron* layer.

289

intuitively by humans that there is not enough control on how the data are being analysed, and whether the derived conclusions are actually sufficiently 'accurate'. Additionally, as AI systems become more complex, over-parameterization and over-fitting become more difficult to control, posing statistical concern.

Another relevant limitation is that complex AI systems require massive datasets in order to derive accurate models. Consequently, more computational resources are required, and computing time can become excessively long for some tasks.

Conclusions

The goal of this chapter was to introduce the basic concepts of different artificial intelligence approaches (that are rapidly becoming alternatives to the classic modelling methods), to briefly describe the different methods that have been and are being developed, and to discuss some of their applications and limitations.

Further Reading

1. Amato F, Lopez A, Peña-Mendez EM, Vaňharan Hampl A, Havel S: Artificial neural networks in medical diagnosis. J.Appl.Biomed. 2013; 11: 47–58.

2. Hinton G: Deep learning—a technology with the potential to transform health care. JAMA. 2018; 320: 1101–2.

3. Deo RC: Machine learning in medicine. Circulation. 2015; 132: 1920–30.

4. Chen JH, Asch SM: Machine learning and prediction in medicine – beyond the peak of inflated expectations. N.Engl.J.Med. 2017; 376: 2507–9.

5. Doi K: Computer-aided diagnosis in medical imaging: historical review, current status and future potential. Comput.Med.Imaging.Graph. 2007; 31: 198–211.

6. Obermeyer Z, Emanuel EJ: Predicting the future – Big data, machine learning, and clinical medicine. N. Engl.J.Med. 2016; 375: 1216–19.

7. Beam AL, Kohane IS: Big data and machine learning in health care. JAMA. 2018; 319: 1317–18.

8. Shen D, Wu G, Suk HI: Deep learning in medical image analysis. Annu.Rev.Biomed.Eng. 2017; 19: 221–48.

9. Stead WW: Clinical implications and challenges of artificial intelligence and deep learning. JAMA. 2018; 320: 1107–8.

10. Zhang Z, Beck MW, Winkler DA, et al: Opening the black box of neural networks: methods for interpreting neural network models in clinical applications. Ann. Transl.Med. 2018; 6: 216.

Index